GERIATRIC MENTAL HEALTH

GERIATRIC MENTAL HEALTH

Edited by

Joel Peter Abrahams, Ph.D.

Senior Psychologist
Geropsychiatric Treatment Unit
Consultant for Gerontology Development
Brentwood Division
West Los Angeles VA Medical Center

Adjunct Assistant Professor
Department of Psychiatry and Biobehavioral Sciences
University of California
Los Angeles, California

Valerie Crooks, D.S.W.

Associate Chief for Evaluation and Training
Geriatric Research, Education and Clinical Center
Wadsworth Division
West Los Angeles VA Medical Center

Adjunct Assistant Professor
Department of Medicine
University of California
Los Angeles, California

G&S

Grune & Stratton, Inc.

(Harcourt Brace Jovanovich, Publishers)

Orlando San Diego New York
London Toronto Montreal Sydney Tokyo

Library of Congress Cataloging in Publication Data
Main entry under title:

Geriatric mental health.

Bibliography.
Includes index.
1. Geriatric psychiatry. 2. Aged—Mental health services. I. Abrahams, Joel Peter. II. Crooks, Valerie. [DNLM: 1. Mental disorders—In old age. 2. Mental health services—In old age. 3. Psychotherapy—In old age. WT 150 G3685]
RC451.4.A5G465 1984 618.97′689 84-699
ISBN 0-8089-1657-2

Grune & Stratton, Inc.
Orlando, FL 32887

Distributed in the United Kingdom by
Grune & Stratton, Ltd.
24/28 Oval Road, London NW 1

Library of Congress Catalog Number 84-699
International Standard Book Number 0-8089-1657-2
Printed in the United States of America

84 85 86 87 10 9 8 7 6 5 4 3 2 1

CONTENTS

IV. SPECIAL ISSUES

V. SOCIAL POLICY, ETHICS, AND PLANNING

ACKNOWLEDGMENTS

A volume such as this owes its existence to many people. The project began as the result of a national conference on geriatric mental health held at the West Los Angeles VA Medical Center. The program was sponsored jointly by the Geriatric Research, Education and Clinical Center, Wadsworth Division, and the Geropsychiatry Program, Brentwood Division of the Medical Center. Our special thanks and gratitude are extended to the Office of Geriatrics and Extended Care and to the Office of Academic Affairs of the Veterans Administration, whose generous funding made the conference possible.

We wish to express our sincerest appreciation to Dr. Milton Greenblatt, Director of the Neuropsychiatric Institute of UCLA, whose kindness and encouragement made possible the translation and expansion of the conference into this volume.

Without the generous assistance of the GRECC staff and support of the following medical center administrators, our endeavor would have been nearly impossible: our thanks go to Doctors T. Makinodan, T. Yoshikawa, H.E. Gordon, S.Y. Tsai, M. Straker, F. Redlich, and C. Frederick. Special thanks also to Jerry Sproul, who typed the manuscript.

FOREWORD

It is an accepted concept in post-industrial societies that individual survival into the post-reproductive and economically post-productive years will increase. This human triumph is cause for celebration. Many of the implications of this change are only now being assessed, however. Aging is associated with an increasing frequency of disabling diseases which also increases the need for support services. For society as a whole, these must be provided by a proportionately declining work force. The ability of humans to anticipate the future makes the specter of increasing disability before death distressing to both the aged and their potential caretakers. It is imperative that these disabilities and dependencies be reduced as much as possible.

There are two traditional approaches to this challenge: (1) to expand those medical, psychiatric, social, and economic programs in which we are already competent, and (2) to explore new ways to prevent and alleviate the problems with intent to improve well-being and contain costs. Both approaches must be pursued.

Psychiatric and intellectual changes, which are common in the aged, are major contributors to disability and dependency. Organic mental disorders, depression, less dramatic mental health problems, treatment of these disorders, and societal responses are all subjects of major concern.

The prevalence of the dementias has long been known, but its quantitative significance must be appreciated. Table 1 indicates frequency of nursing home residence by three cohorts of the aged, and reported frequency of some degree of intellectual impairment in this group. As the data indicate, such patients make up not only the majority of nursing home residents, but also an increasingly significant component of their surviving age cohort.

Table 2 presents comparable data from three other widely dispersed societies, attesting to the universality of the problem. If this is to be the outcome of increasing survival into the ninth decade, it is clear that all lines of investigation must be pursued. Individuals with pseudodementia of depression and reversible dementia must be identified and treated, methods of prevention and cure must be developed, and when all of these fail, adequate and humane care must be made available. There is evidence that

Table 1.
*Age-Specific Incidence of Dementia in Nursing Home Residents**

Age	Population in Nursing Homes (%)		NH Patients with Dementia (%)		Tot. Pop. in NH with Dementia (%)	
	Men	Women	Men	Women	Men	Women
65–74	1.13	1.28	48	48	0.54	0.61
75–84	4.08	7.05	62	63	2.53	4.44
85+	18.04	27.44	68	70	12.27	19.21

*Extrapolated from the National Nursing Home Survey 1973–1974 and census data, Department of Commerce Series P–25, No. 519, April, 1974.

dementia is associated with an extremely high death rate that can be reduced by appropriate, often simple, treatment. The circumstances in which such treatment may or may not be justified has given rise to extensive and unresolved ethical discussion. It is encouraging that there is an accelerating response to these problems.

The potential for depression in senescence is great. It may be the result of social and economic losses, the personal impact of significant physical changes, particularly the presence of early dementia or certain age-related physiological changes, such as changes in biogenic amine metabolism, that may place elders at risk for depression. Given all of the possible causes, it is surprising that depression is not more universal. That it is not inevitable in old age is a tribute to the strength and resiliency of the human spirit.

Although many psychiatrists and psychologists have been pioneers in psychogeriatrics, most have focused on younger individuals in whom it was assumed that overall prognosis was better. In this they have been no different from physicians. But social needs are changing, and there is evidence that professional interest and resources will be increased and redirected

Table 2.
*Cumulative Risk of Chronic Brain Syndrome**

Age	Japan	England	Denmark
60–69	2.3	2.3†	0
70–79	5.9	3.9	1.9
80+	19.8	22.0	13.2

*Adapted from Kay, D.W.K. Epidemiological aspects of organic brain disease in the aged. In C.M. Gaitz (Ed.), *Aging and the brain.* New York: Plenum, 1972.
†65–69

toward the mental health needs of the elderly. It is true that advanced age will make duration of results less impressive, but at the same time relief of symptoms, as opposed to cure, becomes more important. The potential for symptomatic relief is good, and success will certainly be appreciated by patient and family. Researchers and clinicians have been turning their attention to problems of anxiety, adjustment reactions, substance abuse, and benign memory loss, as well as to dementias and depression. Continued examination of these entities will improve diagnosis and service delivery.

The development of adequate treatment resources will be a major challenge. The best available methods have not been established, and there is an increasing public reluctance to support mental health and social programs, particularly those without demonstrated effectiveness and economy. The general public concept is that institutionalization is undesirable, and community alternative are both better and cheaper. These alternatives include home care, a variety of home services, residential housing and congregate housing of several types, and respite care. What seems to be emerging is that patients need to be carefully matched to available resources. In some instances, home care may be best. In others, insitutional care may not only be better, but also cheaper. Studies of the accuracy and effectiveness of placement are under way, and should have a tremendous impact upon policy.

Since this book was encouraged by the Veterans Administration, it is appropriate to comment on VA programs and resources. The VA has long recognized that, from the present time until well into the early years of the twenty-first century, there will be a heavy burden of aged World War II and Korean War veterans requiring care. The VA has attempted to plan a program that will provide to veterans the necessary continuity of care with respect to both time and level of need. Thus, the program includes acute hospital care, long-term intermediate care wards, VA nursing homes, community nursing homes, domiciliaries, hospital-based home care, residential-care homes, and a full range of outpatient facilities. The extent of need has been uncertain, depending as it does on veterans' alternate resources, proximity to a VA facility, status of Medicare, and so on. Like all public facilities, the extent of VA resources will depend upon executive and legislative philosophy and budget priorities, plus the ability of VA staffs to reduce time required to achieve favorable results.

It is with these goals and expectations that *Geriatric Mental Health* is presented.

Ralph Goldman, M.D.
Associate Chief of Staff, Education
West Los Angeles VA Medical Center
Wadsworth Division
Los Angeles, California

PREFACE

The continuing dramatic increase in the number of persons over 65 years of age in this country and elsewhere and the demand to meet their ever-growing and special mental health needs have been well publicized in both the scientific and popular press. As a result of this demand, mental health clinicians are treating greater numbers of older clients and more mental health professionals are conducting geriatric research and specializing in clinical gerontology. Research knowledge and clinical expertise have expanded greatly and this growth in knowledge and services has created a need to communicate emerging techniques, information, and concerns. *Geriatric Mental Health* was conceived to meet this need.

All contributors to this volume are not only recognized experts in geriatric mental health but are also scientist-practitioners. The scientist-practitioner model posits that the mental health professional is best able to provide expert services when techniques of diagnosis and treatment are firmly grounded on empirical and theoretical foundations of the discipline. Each client is not only an individual in need of the best possible care, but also represents an opportunity to expand professional knowledge and understanding. Our contributors are researchers *and* clinicians schooled and practiced in both.

Geriatric Mental Health is designed for clinicians working with elderly patients. Our aim is to provide a guide for the conduct of various aspects of geriatric mental health practice. The esoteric nature of the research has been kept to a minimum to emphasize the applied nature of works presented. Since no volume of this nature can be exhaustive, we decided to focus on those issues of geriatric mental health that we felt would be most useful to our readers.

Part I provides a brief review of experimental psychological research on aging as applied to the diagnosis, treatment, and understanding of the clinical problems of aging. The remainder of the book is divided into four major sections.

In Part II the two most pressing mental health problems of aging are discussed: depression and the dementias. These chapters provide evaluative guidelines and most recent developments in the diagnosis of depression and major dementing illnesses. In addition, current trends in treatment of geriatric depression and special issues in the long-term care of dementia patients are presented in detail.

Part III focuses on three important techniques of psychotherapeutic intervention that have only recently been applied to the functional psychiatric problems of the elderly: family therapy, brief psychotherapy, and behavioral therapies. These are finding increasing acceptance as effective treatment modalities in geriatric mental health. Descriptions of these techniques, as well as ways in which they differ from similar interventions with younger age groups, are discussed.

Part IV presents an examination of four special issues that continually cause problems for patients and practitioners alike. The trials and tribulations of memory, its benign changes, and its more malignant deterioration are examined. The vagaries of geriatric sexuality and recent developments in understanding alcohol abuse and treatment are also presented. The section closes with an examination of the special issues of mental health care of minority elders.

The final section of our book, Part V, centers on issues of social policy, ethics, and planning in delivery of geriatric mental health services. Models of mental health care and the role of the clinical psychologist in community service delivery are examined. The book concludes with discussions of ethics and social policy issues of concern to clinicians working with elders.

CONTRIBUTORS

JOEL PETER ABRAHAMS, PH.D. Senior Psychologist, Geropsychiatry Treatment Unit, Consultant for Gerontology Development, Brentwood Division, West Los Angeles, VA Medical Center; Adjunct Assistant Professor, Department of Psychiatry and Biobehavioral Sciences, Center for Health Sciences, University of California, Los Angeles, California

ROBERT BARNES, M.D. Psychiatrist, Geriatric Research, Education and Clinical Center, Seattle/American Lake VA Medical Center; Assistant Professor, Department of Psychiatry and Behavioral Sciences, University of Washington, Seattle, Washington

JAMES E. BIRREN, PH.D. Director, Andrus Gerontology Center; Professor, Department of Psychology, University of Southern California, Los Angeles, California

CHRISTINE CASSEL, M.D. Assistant Professor, Department of Geriatrics; Acting Chief, Geriatric Inpatient Unit, Mt. Sinai Hospital, New York, New York

ALEX COMFORT, M.D., D.SC. Consultant in Geriatrics, West Los Angeles VA Medical Center, Los Angeles, California; Adjunct Professor, Department of Psychiatry and Biobehavioral Sciences, University of California, Los Angeles, California

THOMAS CROOK, Ph.D. Research Psychologist, Center for the Mental Health of the Aging, National Institute of Mental Health, Rockville, Maryland

VALERIE CROOKS, D.S.W. Associate Chief for Evaluation and Training, Geriatric Research, Education and Clinical Center, Wadsworth Division, West Los Angeles VA Medical Center; Adjunct Assistant Professor, Department of Medicine, University of California, Los Angeles, California

MONY DE LEON, ED.D. Research Associate, Geriatric Study and Treatment Program, Department of Psychiatry, New York University Medical Center, New York, New York

CARL EISDORFER, PH.D., M.D. President, Montefiore Hospital and Medical Center; Professor, Department of Psychiatry, Albert Einstein School of Medicine, Bronx, New York

STEVEN H. FERRIS, PH.D. Executive Director, Geriatric Study and Treatment Program, Department of Psychiatry, New York University Medical Center, New York, New York

RALPH GOLDMAN, M.D. Associate Chief of Staff, Education, Wadsworth Division, West Los Angeles VA Medical Center; Adjunct Professor, Department of Medicine, University of California, Los Angeles, California

JEROME M. GRUNES, M.D. Senior Attending Psychiatrist, Michael Reese Hospital; Assistant Professor of Clinical Psychiatry, Department of Psychiatry, Northwestern University Medical School, Chicago, Illinois

JOHN J. HERR, PH.D. Clinical Psychologist in Private Practice, Campbell, California; Lecturer, Department of Psychiatry, Stanford University, Palo Alto, California

RICHARD A. HUSSIAN, PH.D. Senior Psychologist, Department of Psychology, Terrell State Hospital, Terrell, Texas

ROBERT KASTENBAUM, PH.D. Director, Adult Development and Aging Program, Arizona State University, Tempe, Arizona

PETER R. LEBRAY, PH.D. Clinical Psychologist in Private Practice, Portland, Oregon

LEONARD W. POON, PH.D. Director, Performance and Aging Laboratory, Geriatric Research, Education and Clinical Center, VA Outpatient Clinic; Department of Psychiatry, Massachusetts General Hospital, Harvard Medical School, Boston, Massachusetts

MURRAY RASKIND, M.D. Director, Geriatric Research, Education and Clinical Center Seattle/American Lake VA Medical Center; Associate Professor, Department of Psychiatry and Behavioral Sciences, University of Washington, Seattle, Washington

BARRY REISBERG, M.D. Geriatric Study and Treatment Program, Department of Psychiatry, New York University Medical Center, New York, New York

BARBARA SOLOMON, D.S.W. Professor, School of Social Work, University of Southern California, Los Angeles, California

DENNIS S. STERN, PH.D. Clinical Psychologist, Brentwood Division, West Los Angeles VA Medical Center, Los Angeles, California

JOHN H. WEAKLAND, M.F.C.C. Research Associate and Associate Director, Brief Therapy Center, Mental Research Institute, Palo Alto, California

JUDY M. ZARIT, PH.D. Coordinator of Geriatric Services, Didi Hirsch Community Mental Health Center, Culver City, California; Leonard Davis School of Gerontology, Andrus Gerontology Center, University of Southern California, Los Angeles, California

STEVEN H. ZARIT, PH.D. Associate Professor of Gerontology and Psychology, Leonard Davis School of Gerontology, Andrus Gerontology Center, University of Southern California, Los Angeles, California

GERIATRIC MENTAL HEALTH

PART I

Experimental Psychology and Mental Health

1

CONTRIBUTIONS OF THE EXPERIMENTAL PSYCHOLOGY OF AGING TO GERIATRIC MENTAL HEALTH

James E. Birren
Joel Peter Abrahams

From time to time, national scientific meetings and prestigious scholarly journals question the relevance of laboratory experimental research to issues concerning applied or clinical practice. The fields of psychology and psychological research on aging have a distinguished history translating experimental investigations to applied sectors of gerontology. Such a successful interfacing was published in the *American Psychologist* by Birren (1974), and Schonfield (1974). Such endeavors continue to be an important professional activity. They are, however, usually in response to the direct or implied criticism of experimental investigators by clinicians who perceive a great chasm between basic laboratory research and the needs of clinical practice. The impetus for this chapter is quite different.

The underlying assumption of this chapter is that both clinical research and applied clinical gerontology philosophically and empirically depend on the general knowledge base provided by experimental research on the psychology of aging. The special issues of assessment, diagnosis, and treatment of mental health problems of the aging require the geroclinician to subscribe

GERIATRIC MENTAL HEALTH
ISBN 0-8089-1657-2

to the scientist–practitioner model, which holds that the best mental health care is provided when the techniques and skills of assessment and treatment are firmly grounded in the empirical and theoretical foundations of the discipline. The geriatric scientist–practitioner must not only be competent in the necessary clinical skills and well versed in the psychopathology literature, but must also be thoroughly grounded in normative aging literature.

The experimental psychology of aging has contributed much to the empirical data base, which geroclinicians can translate into practical guidelines for more effective assessment, diagnosis, and treatment. The effective communication of this ever-increasing data base is necessary in order for practitioners to accrue the benefits of research, but it is often impeded by two natural barriers. The first barrier is the exponential growth in the number of publications and the difficulty of efficiently and professionally coping with this knowledge explosion. In a recent review of the psychology of aging, one of the authors located some 6000 articles published during the past 5 years alone. The psychology of aging was once a rather sleepy field, but the explosion of data has created a need for annual reviews in several areas of geropsychology, clinical aging. among them. A recent survey by Hoyer, Raskind, and Abrahams (1984) reported that from 1963 to 1982 the number of research papers on human psychological aging increased from an average of 14.3 per year to 32.9 per year in the *Journal of Gerontology* alone.

The second barrier to effective communication is the impaction of scientific information by discipline; that is, psychiatrists tend to read only psychiatric literature and social workers tend to read only social work literature. This tendency is partially the result of the need of professionals to maintain current knowledge in their particular fields as effectively as possible. It is hoped that this chapter in a multidisciplinary book will ease these barriers to effective communication.

PHILOSOPHICAL ISSUES

Researchers and clinicians alike often use metaphoric speech when discussing theoretical and philosophical concepts on aging. In some instances these metaphors are contradictory; the implicit metaphor of aging is decompensation, which is often in direct opposition to the growth and maturity described for various aspects of psychological and social functioning. Metaphorical aging needs to be delineated into three separate although often co-existing processes. Three metaphors—*senescing, eldering,* and *geronting*—are required in order to adequately describe the processes of aging.

Senescing reflects those biological processes of aging that render us more vulnerable to degradation with the passage of time. The inability to repair and remediate biologically, i.e., the probability of dying, is a function of senescent qualities. Senescence refers to such biological changes as reduced enzyme induction in the liver and decreased cardiorespiratory reserve (Finch & Hayflick, 1977), reduced information-processing efficiency of the brain (Hoyer & Plude, 1980), and decreased efficiency of stress responses (Timiras, 1972). Senescing relates to those functional changes that reflect the deteriorating aspects of aging.

Eldering is another process of aging that is independent from but related to senescing. It is the process of moving into age-appropriate roles. All societies have age-grading and an age-status system (Morgan, 1982). Concurrently with senescing, as one ages, there are changes in social and familial roles, newlyweds become parents, parents become empty-nesters and/or grandparents, and the employed become retired. American society has less well-defined age-related roles than other societies, which often creates behavioral uncertainty. The role ambiguity of eldering often becomes a source of personal and interpersonal problems.

Both senescing and eldering place certain adaptational demands on the aging individual, as social, biological, and psychological changes place a behavioral or cognitive load upon the individual (Birren, 1963). This process of coping with the interaction of senescing and eldering is called *geronting*. The verb form is being used deliberately to imply direction in force. Social structure, with its institutions and sanctions, influences eldering. Our species heritage and individual genetic inheritance define the physical and psychological limits of change and coping. Affected by these interacting forces is the geronting individual—the adapting, strategizing, competent, coping older adult. When the person with a defect in hearing or ambulation so constructs the environment to obviate the full impact of that defect, it is an aspect of geronting.

Theorists and clinicians have written of the necessity of mastering various developmental tasks as a prerequisite to psychosocial adjustment throughout the life span. Butler (1963) and Peck (1956) have discussed the developmental tasks of aging, but it is Erickson (1959, 1963) who is best known for extending psychosocial development into old age. The final stage of Erickson's epigenetic theory is Ego Integrity versus Ego Despair. The successful completion of such developmental tasks as life review and coming to terms with physical decline and one's own mortality are thought necessary to adjustment in old age. These biological, social, and psychological tasks are senescing, eldering, and geronting.

SENSORY DEFICITS, COMMUNICATION, AND CLINICAL ISSUES

Clinical practitioners working with older clients, unlike those working with young to early middle-aged patients, often are presented with simultaneous physical and emotional conditions. Cardiovascular disorders, arthritis, and respiratory diseases represent adjustment challenges to even the most emotionally healthy senior and are often a major theme in geriatric psychotherapy, but sensory deficits, especially vision and audition, may be the most potent and insidious of the physical changes. Some reduction in the acuity of both the visual system (Fozard, Wolf, Bell et al., 1977) and the auditory system (Corso, 1977) occurs in virtually all persons. The decline in sensory functioning begins as early as 35 years for vision and 45 years for hearing, and these changes have potentially significant implications for communication effectiveness, social interaction, and adjustment. The impact of visual and auditory deficits on the psychological functioning and adjustment of elders can be seriously underestimated.

The presence of multiple visual problems in older clients may make optimal eyeglass prescriptions difficult. An older client wearing glasses is not an assurance of optimally corrected vision. Changes in accommodation, refraction, color vision, glare sensitivity, and astigmatism may occur in various combinations, and the influence of visual problems on psychological and neuropsychological assessment can be profound. The glare from fluorescent lights may often obviate the benefits of reading glasses and for example, play havoc with the Picture Arrangement or Picture Completion subtests of the Wechsler Adult Intelligence Scale (WAIS), or with the ability of the elder to develop good quality percepts on the Rorschach.

Perhaps because of the subtle nature of age-related changes in audition, hearing deficits are more often associated with symptoms of psychopathology and abnormal responses to psychological testing than visual deficits. Perhaps the single most common hearing deficit afflicting persons over 65 years of age is presbycusis; it is estimated that 13 percent or more of all older adults suffer from it sufficiently to warrant intervention (Watson & Tolan, 1967). This condition is one in which there is a selective hearing loss for frequencies in the 1000–4000 Hz range. The threshold for perceiving and understanding sounds in this range increases, i.e., the sounds must be louder. Unfortunately, much of the range of the human speaking voice falls within this frequency spread.

Older adults with such auditory disabilities are often extremely sensitive about their decreased capacity for effective communication and social interaction. Denial and covering-up of hearing deficits are common and compound the psychosocial problem. Although deafness alone apparently is not sufficient to foster development of paranoia, pre-existing paranoid tendencies may be exacerbated by a hearing problem. Eisdorfer (1960) has reported that age-related hearing deficits are associated with paranoid responses on Rorschach inkblots. Suspiciousness, oversensitivity, and hostility can be reinforced as a consequence of missed and/or misheard words. Fortunately, many of these symptoms disappear once the auditory deficit is diagnosed or denial is breached.

Other emotional disturbances also have been observed to be related to hearing loss, especially previously unidentified hearing loss. Depression and social withdrawal predominate, but hypochondriasis, anxiety, and compulsive states are also common (Knapp, 1948). As hearing impairment increases, its consequences can be observed on a variety of psychosocial dimensions; the extent and quality of social interactions begin to diminish, ability to maintain control in social situations decreases, and forms of maladaptive behavior manifest themselves (Hyams, 1969).

The conduct of psychotherapy and interviewing are also affected by the need to be aware of the influences of sensory deficits, especially hearing difficulties. Information processing not only slows with aging but is degraded disproportionately by overload situations (Birren, Woods, & Williams, 1980), such as stressful or crosstalk interactions. Group therapy is a primary example, in which even mild auditory deficits add to the possibility that confusion and misunderstanding will result from the often-spirited process. For this reason it is important for the therapist to exert somewhat more control in a group of geriatric patients than would be necessary in a younger group. In an interview, a misunderstood question can produce an apparently inappropriate answer on the part of a hearing-impaired senior. The senior may also ask the interviewer to repeat the question, suggesting to the unsuspecting professional that the older patient is overly distractable or has a significant memory problem. This situation could rapidly lead the clinician to false conclusions about the cognitive functioning of the patient, especially if the elder is unaware of or denies the hearing impairment.

It is vital that professionals delivering geriatric mental health services be aware of the significant impact of sensory deficits on the psychological and psychosocial functioning of their clients. Such awareness can greatly reduce possible clinical misadventures. The development and course of adjustment problems can be influenced by the presence, detection, and remediation of sensory impairments. Assessment, diagnosis, and treatment are all influenced by the effectiveness of interpersonal communication. Learning how to better communicate with hearing-impaired older patients, such as by simply lowering the tonal frequence of one's voice, can improve the quality of care dramatically.

INTELLECTUAL AGING

Do intellectual abilities become less robust as a consequence of aging or senescing or are the assumed declines in intellectual functioning mythical and actually the product of age stereotypes, experimenter expectancies, or methodological artifacts? No other area of psychological aging research has been the focus of an extensive, continued professional argument as has the investigation of various parameters of intelligence. During the past 20 years reports on aging and intelligence have accounted for more than 40 percent of all human psychological research published in the *Journal of Gerontology* (Abrahams, Hoyer, Elias et al., 1975; Hoyer, Raskind, & Abrahams, 1983). Investigators have interpreted and reinterpreted data from their own studies and the studies of others, using a multitude of methodological, theoretical, and philosophical perspectives. A thorough understanding of the nature of intellectual aging is vital for accurate neuropsychological assessment of geriatric patients. Normal aging provides the data base against which pathological changes are measured. Several complex and highly interacting variables are involved in normal intellectual aging. Baltes and K.W. Schaie and their colleagues (Baltes, Nesselroade, K.W. Schaie et al., 1972; Baltes & K.W. Schaie, 1974; K.W. Schaie, 1977, have debated with Botwinick (1973; 1977) the interpretation of the limiting effects of cohort on cross-sectional research. The Riegels (Riegel & Riegel, 1972; Riegel, Riegel, & Meyer, 1967) and Jarvik and Falek (1963) have discussed the effects of selective dropout of nonsurvivors in longitudinal research. Abrahams (1976 a,b), Birren (Birren, Butler, Greenhouse et al., 1963), and Siegler (Siegler, Nowlin, Blumenthal et al., 1980) have reported on the methodological and empirical concerns of subject health status. These variables influence the outcome of research and interpretation of the results. At least until the early 70s, chronological age accounts for less of the variance between age groups in intellectual functioning than subject variables, such as health, socio-economic status, education, and generational cohort. Later in this chapter, we will discuss how the above modifying factors contribute to our understanding of normal aging and individual differences as well as to effective clinical practice.

There are, nevertheless, some very definite conclusions that can be made from the vast empirical literature on intellectual aging. There are often small, but measurable, age-related declines in certain intellectual abilities, many of which may not be seen prior to age 50–60 years. Such functions as vocabulary, general information, and comprehension show remarkable stability even to 70 years and beyond. However, those intellectual abilities involving the speed of response of nonverbal, perceptual–manipulative functions show a pattern of earlier and more rapid decline. Thus, the performance subtests on the Wechsler Adult Intelligence Scale—Revised Form (WAIS-R), for example, show greater susceptibility to aging than verbal subtests. The relative rigor of verbal function is highlighted by the observation that decline in WAIS verbal subtests, especially vocabulary, is a significant marker of altered health status and a predictor of nonsurvival (Eisdorfer & Wilkie, 1973; Jarvik, Eisdorfer, & Blum, 1973).

The relative sensitivity of speeded, non-verbal skills to the effects of normal aging has resulted in the so-called classic aging pattern. This pattern is one of an age difference of one standard deviation or more on the WAIS

Performance subtests and little or no age difference on the verbal subtests. Even when *young*, *young-old* (60–69 years), and *old-old* (70–89 years) age groups were matched for full scale WAIS scores, this classic pattern is observed (Harwood & Naylor, 1971). This pattern cannot be attributed to the timed nature of the performance tasks and the slowed speed of behavior with age. Two studies (Doppelt & Wallace, 1955; Klodin, 1975) eliminated the timing component of the WAIS Performance subtests. They reported a reduction in the magnitude of the age differences but not a negation of the classic pattern. Thus, a speeded component added to tasks of non-verbal, perceptual–manipulative abilities serves to magnify more basic aging changes inherent in intellectual abilities being measured. Because of these factors, the differences between verbal and performance scores on the WAIS/WAIS-R are expected to be greater normatively for older adults than for people in younger age groups. Differences of about one standard deviation, in addition, generally are without diagnostic significance in older age groups.

General adult norms for chronic diffuse deficits cannot be used to assess organic mental disorders in the elderly (Gallagher, Thompson, & Levy, 1980; J.P. Schaie & K.W. Schaie, 1977), nor are signs of neuropathologically-impaired intellect in older adults simply exaggerations of normal aging. The characteristics of such clinical conditions as Senile Dementia of the Alzheimer's Type and its differentiation from pseudodementia of depression must be evaluated against normative aging patterns of disease-related cognitive decline (see Chapter 4).

LEARNING AND MEMORY

The clinical assessment of memory has become a major component of geriatric mental health procedures for several reasons. First, memory deficits play the cardinal role in the age-associated dementias, especially Alzheimer's disease. Second, older clients often come to the attention of clinicians for the first time because of objective or subjective impairment of memory. Third, changes in memory functioning over short periods of time have been observed to be diagnostically relevant. For example, the often-seen memory impairment in pseudodementia of depression responds to the therapeutic effects of antidepressant medications and psychotherapy.

The exact nature of the parameters of age-associated memory changes has yet to be delineated fully (Hartley, Harker, & Walsh, 1980). However, there is no doubt that decrements in memory are normally occurring developments of aging, and the same may be said of verbal and nonverbal learning. A major problem for the geroclinician is the development of age-appropriate normative data against which clinical evaluations can be made.

The different features of memory (e.g., short term, long term, encoding, storage, and retrieval), are affected differently by the processes of aging (K.W. Schaie & J.P. Schaie, 1977).

The translations of relevant experimental research on gerontological learning and memory to clinical practice are different for the tasks of assessment, memory enhancement treatment, and psychotherapy. Poon (see Chapter 9) and Ferris, Reisberg, deLeon, and Crook (see Chapter 4) discuss at length the first two tasks. The impact of learning and memory on geriatric psychotherapy will be focused on here.

Kral (1978) has proposed the term *benign senescent forgetfulness* to describe memory dysfunction characterized by a person's inability to recall minor features of an experience (e.g., a name, date, or place) while still being able to recall the experience itself; the same features may be recalled on one occasion but not on another; faces are familiar but the names have been forgotten temporarily. Persons with this ubiquitous form of memory dysfunction are aware of the problem and often apologize for it and attempt to compensate.

Benign senescent forgetfulness does not appear to be predictive of future development of the devastating amnestic syndrome of dementia; rather, it describes the real-world impairment of memory that is one of the hallmarks of normal aging. Anxiety and depression can exacerbate benign forgetfulness to the extent that the now-worsened memory deficits can be misdiagnosed as dementia (Jarvik, 1980; Miller, 1975).

Psychotherapy is, among other features, a cognitive endeavor. The therapeutic process requires relatively intact intellectual and cognitive functioning. True dementing illness is an unbreakable barrier to psychotherapy, but benign forgetfulness is not. The results of experimental research on geriatric learning and memory provide the clinician with guidelines for improving the effectiveness of individual and group therapy in the presence of normal age-related declines in abilities.

Whether one employs behavioral, cognitive-behavioral, psycho-educational, or psychodynamic techniques, psychotherapy is a learning and problem-solving situation relying heavily on memory. The processes of behavior change, self-understanding, mood-monitoring, or insight, are the result of solving problems, manipulating and integrating new information, or perceiving old information in new ways. Geroclinicians must be prepared to proceed more slowly and in a more concrete fashion with their clients than might be the case with younger patients. They may find that structuring therapy sessions and intervening more actively in the therapeutic processes also greatly facilitates progress.

The following procedures have been observed to maximize performance of older adults on learning, problem solving, and memory tasks: (1) slow, preferably self, pacing; (2) use of concrete, relevant material; (3) repeated exposure to the learning material; (4) narrow focus; (5) structured procedures;

(6) multiple feedback opportunities (Rabbitt, 1977; Giamba & Arenberg, 1980). Such principles have contributed to the success of two recently-developed models of geriatric psychotherapy.

Gallagher and Thompson (1982) and Gallagher, Thompson, Baffa et al. (1981), have reported on the effectiveness of psycho-educational group therapy in treating depressed older patients. Special modifications of cognitive behavior therapy (Beck, Rush, Shaw, et al., 1979) have also been reported to be quite effective in treating geriatric depression (Emery, 1981). These interventions are certainly not the only effective geriatric psychotherapeutic treatments; adaptations of these techniques need to be developed for application to other geropsychiatric disorders, such as anxiety and paranoia. However, the psycho-educational approach in particular, offers an exciting model for development of further cognitively oriented psychotherapeutic interventions, and it also presents an excellent example of benefits to the geroclinician of sound translations of experimental aging research.

More traditional insight-oriented psychotherapy also benefits from clinical application of laboratory research findings. Older clients traditionally have not been considered good candidates for psychotherapy in general and dynamic therapy in particular. Much of the objection has stemmed from the assumed rigidity of elders and a resulting resistance to insight and change. Rigidity can more properly be conceptualized as cautiousness, which can be defined as a general disinclination to respond quickly or to readily alter a behavioral set because of the perceived risk associated with being wrong or the potential cost of giving up familiar, well-established habits for unfamiliar ones. This characteristic of cautiousness can be observed most clearly in unstructured, ambiguous, and stressful situations, which increase the behavioral load on older adults more than on younger ones (Birren, 1965).

Barriers erected by cautiousness can be overcome by the geroclinician, whose structure and active intervention can provide role guidelines for patient and therapist. The behavioral expectancies of this otherwise ambiguous and alien situation become more concrete and less threatening, and may be extended beneficially to the patient's mental health education. Teaching clients about depression, anxiety, medication, and other topics relevant to treatment is well-received by older patients in both group and individual psychotherapy.

Geroclinicians should encourage their patients to take notes during therapy sessions and to maintain a log between sessions. This technique has two definite advantages: First, the burden on memory is eased, and by noting during a session those associations, feelings, and statements of importance, clients have a readily available reference; review and between-session work is facilitated by the notebook entries; reliance on even a benignly forgetful memory is minimized and psychological energy is focused on the therapy material; (2) maintaining a log provides a bridge between therapy sessions and between the sessions and the daily life of the client. Therapy sessions become less isolated, and the therapeutic experience gains both continuity and generalization.

Translations from experimental research on gerontological learning and memory have provided the above techniques, which can facilitate geriatric psychotherapy by providing additional information that older adults often require before behavioral changes are seen and thereby helping to overcome resistance that results from over-cautiousness. The techniques provide an environment in which learning takes place more optimally, and provide simple methods of reducing effects of benign forgetfulness on the psychotherapeutic endeavor. One of the authors of this chapter has been employing these methods successfully for the past seven years.

INDIVIDUAL DIFFERENCES AND NORMATIVE AGING

Individual differences and the establishment of age-appropriate norms for psychological functioning are two of the most difficult problems confronting the geroclinician. These problems are endemic to all of geropsychology and impact significantly on clinical assessment; these issues bring to center stage the need for geroclinicians to function within the scientist–practitioner model. Not only must the skill of clinical practice be mastered, but so must understanding of the psychology of adult development and aging.

Like researchers, geroclinicians must be aware of variables that affect the results of psychological aging research. Age differences derived from cross-sectional data must not be misinterpreted as age changes. The latter are derived from longitudinal designs (K.W. Schaie, 1977). Whether the dependent variable is intellectual functioning, personality characteristics, or symptoms of psychopathology, the results of research on subjects of different ages tested on a single occasion could be based on differences inherent in the cohorts and not just in the processes of aging. In contributing to the results of psychological aging research, cohort variables and subject variables such as education (Birren & Morrison, 1961), health status (Abrahams, 1976a; Spieth, 1964, 1965), or changes in health (Siegler, Nowlin, & Blumenthal, 1980) have been shown to be more important than chronological age or aging. These and other variables influence the adult development of psychological functioning over the later years of life.

Interindividual differences and intraindividual variability across a wide range of psychological measures have been reported to increase markedly with age (Baltes & Willis, 1977). This means that (1) there are greater differences in levels of performance on psychological variables among older adults than among younger adults, a variability that seems to increase further in the very old; (2) a given older adult will demonstrate greater variability of performance than will a younger adult on the same psychological measure, e.g., a group of seniors will have greater differences between each other on a reaction time test than will a group of younger subjects. In addition, the trial-to-trial variability in reaction times will be comparatively greater for the older subjects. Elders are more heterogeneous psychologically than middle-aged or young adults. Much of the between- and within-group differences in psychological functioning is a result of cohort variables and such powerful subject variables as sex, health, and education. This greater heterogeneity of older adults makes the task of establishing age norms and, thus, age-appropriate diagnostic markers difficult (Krauss, 1980).

The slowing of behavior and information processing in the central nervous system is perhaps the most pervasive and generalizing age-related phenomenon (Birren, Woods, & Williams, 1980). Psychological aging research on psychomotor performance, intelligence, learning, memory, and information processing all have indicated the slowing of speed and timing of behavior as a cardinal causative variable. Hicks and Birren (1970) have speculated thoughtfully on the possible neuropathological mechanisms involved in behavioral slowing, but despite the great amount of published research in the area, no age norms have been developed for either speed of central processing or speed of behavior.

Central slowing is currently being studied by neuropsychologists and psychophysiologists as a likely component of observed age- and disease-related alterations in sensory-evoked potentials. The electrocortical responses to meaningful auditory and visual stimuli may prove to be an important marker in the differential diagnosis of pseudodementia of depression and primary degenerative dementia of the Alzheimer's Type. Age-appropriate norms for evoked potential latencies, however, must be established before between-group differences can be meaningfully translated.

Normative aging research has produced results that would have been considered pathological in younger age groups, but were not associated with frankly impaired functioning. For example, Busse and Obrist (1970) reported that the presence of focal slow wave electrocortical activity was not associated with either cognitive or behavioral pathology or with the future development of diffuse slowing. In younger persons, focal slowing on the electroencephalographic record is a definite neuropathological finding and is related to impaired functioning.

Another example of difficulty arising from the attempt to apply normative adult data to senescent populations is readily apparent on the Halstead–Reitan Neuropsychological Test Battery. This battery is the most widely used method of assessing brain damage in the United States. Using the standardized adult scoring and the Impairment Index as the cut-off point for establishing a diagnosis, the majority of normal older adults would be incorrectly classified as brain damaged. Davies (1968) has reported on this problem as it relates particularly to the Reitan Trailmaking Test of the battery. Also, one of the present authors (JPA) has observed the extreme difficulty that unimpaired elders have performing on the Tactile Performance Task of the same battery.

The difficulty of extending normative adult data to the later years of life is also apparent in the assessment of personality and affective status. Self-rating depression scales such as those developed by Zung (1965, 1967) and by Beck (Beck, Ward, Mendelson et al., 1961) overestimate depression in older adults. Elders normally endorse more somatic items on these scales than younger patients, which contributes more to the depression scores of elders than the affective items. Additionally, the somatic items apparently have different meanings to different age groups and are unrelated to psychological distress among the elderly (Gallagher, McGarvey, Zelinsky et al., 1978). The differential meaning of the somatic items is a clear cohort effect.

The use of the Minnesota Multiphasic Personality Inventory (MMPI) presents similar difficulties for the geroclinician. The adult norms for the 10 clinical scales do not provide an accurate, reliable description of personality characteristics and symptoms of psychopathology for older adults. Cohort factors are thought to influence perceptions and attitudes of mental health and deviant behavior. This will affect the likelihood of older age groups endorsing various items (K.W. Schaie & J.P. Schaie, 1977). Scale scores and profile types will then take on different meanings for older patients. Given the popularity of the MMPI, clinicians will no doubt continue to assess older patients with this instrument, but young adult norms cannot be perceived as appropriate for them. Interpretations of the MMPI test results must proceed with great caution.

This discussion of the problems of individual differences and normative aging is not meant to discourage clinicians working with older patients. Rather, it is presented as a caveat: geriatric mental health assessment and treatment require modifications of procedures in order to be reliable and effective. Older adult norms are available for only a limited number of standardized psychological and neuropsychological instruments. In the absence of appropriate normative data and alternative evaluation procedures, clinicians must exercise restraint when interpreting the results of psychological assessment of older patients.

SUMMARY

Aging is not a unitary process. The developmental, time-related changes in psychological functioning are the result of a complex interaction of biologic, personal, and environmental variables imposing their force on the individual. Aging is not the unraveling, or dedifferentiation, of earlier behavioral development. Age-related change patterns are not ordered, or sequential. No monolithic supertheory can provide an adequate system for explaining the manifestations of psychological aging.

Experimental psychological research and normative studies have contributed greatly to our knowledge of the processes of aging. This knowledge can, in turn, be translated into practical clinical tools. Principles have been derived from laboratory results and expanded to mental health practice. Thus, our knowledge of adult learning can be applied to novel situations such as psychotherapy. Our understanding of normative aging provides firmer ground on which to make clinical judgments from psychological evaluations. The techniques and principles of geriatric mental health practice must be established on the data base of the developmental psychology of aging.

REFERENCES

Abrahams, J.P. Health status as a variable in aging research. *Experimental Aging Research,* 1976a, *2,* 63–71.

Abrahams, J.P. Psychological correlates of cardiovascular disease. In M.F. Elias, B.E. Eleftheriou, & P.K. Elias (Eds.), *Special review of experimental aging research: progress in biology.* Bar Harbor, ME: EAR, Inc., 1976b.

Abrahams, J.P., Hoyer, W.J., Elias, M.F., & Bradigan, B. Gerontological research in psychology published in Journal of Gerontology, 1963–1974: Perspectives and progress. *Journal of Gerontology,* 1975, *30,* 668–673.

Baltes, P.B., Nesselroade, K., Schaie, K.W. and Labouvie, E.W. On the dilemma of regression effects in examining ability-level-related differentials in ontogenetic patterns of intelligence. *Developmental Psychology,* 1972, *6,* 78–84.

Baltes, P.B., & Willis, S.L. Towards psychological theories of aging and development. In J.E. Birren & K.W. Schaie (Eds.), *Handbook of the psychology of aging.* New York: Van Nostrand Reinhold, 1977.

Baltes, P.B. and Schaie, K.W. Aging and I.Q.: The myth of the twilight years. *Psychology Today,* 1974, *7,* 35–40.

Beck, A.T., Rush, J., Shaw, B., & Emery, G. *Cognitive therapy of depression.* New York: Guilford, 1979.

Beck, A.T., Ward, C.H., Mendelson, M., Mock, J.E., & Erbaugh, J. An inventory for measuring depression. *Archives of General Psychiatry,* 1961, *4,* 561–571.

Birren, J.E. *The psychology of aging.* Englewood Cliffs, N.J.: Prentice Hall, 1965.

Birren, J.E. Translations in gerontology—from lab to life: Psychophysiology and speed of response. *American Psychologist,* 1974, *29,* 808–815.

Birren, J.E., Butler, R.N., Greenhouse, S.W., et al. (Eds.) *Human aging: a biological and behavioral study.* Washington, D.C.: U.S. Government Printing Office, 1963.

Birren, J.E., & Morrison, D.F. Analysis of the WAIS subtests in relation to age and education. *Journal of Gerontology,* 1961, *16,* 363–369.

Birren, J.E., Woods, A.M., & Williams, M.V. Behavioral slowing with age: Causes, organization, and consequences. In L.W. Poon (Ed.), *Aging in the 1980's.* Washington, D.C.: American Psychological Association, 1980.

Botwinick, J. *Aging and behavior*. New York: Springer, 1973.

Botwinick, J. Intellectual abilities. In J.E. Birren & K.W. Schaie (Eds.), *Handbook of the psychology of aging*. New York: Van Nostrand Reinhold, 1977.

Busse, E.W., & Obrist, W.D. Significance of focal electro-encephalographic changes in the elderly. In E. Palmore (Ed.), *Normal aging*. Durham, N.C.: Duke University Press, 1970.

Butler, R.N. The life review: An interpretation of reminiscence in the aged. *Psychiatry,* 1963, *26,* 65–76.

Corso, J.F. Auditory perception and communication. In J.E. Birren & K.W. Schaie (Eds.), *Handbook of the psychology of aging*. New York: Van Nostrand Reinhold, 1977.

Davies, H.D.M. The influence of age on Trail Making Test performance. *Journal of Clinical Psychology,* 1968, *24,* 96–98.

Doppelt, J.E., & Wallace, W.L. Standardization of the Wechsler Adult Intelligence Scale for older persons. *Journal of Abnormal and Social Psychology,* 1955, *51,* 312–330.

Eisdorfer, C. Rorschach rigidity and sensory decrement in a senescent population. *Journal of Gerontology,* 1960, *15,* 188–190.

Eisdorfer, C., & Wilkie, F. Intellectual changes with advancing age. In L.F. Jarvik, C. Eisdorfer, & J.E. Blum (Eds.), *Intellectual functioning in adults*. New York: Springer, 1973.

Erikson, E.H. Identity and the life cycle. *Psychological issues*. New York: International Universities Press, 1959.

Erikson, E.H. *Childhood and society* (2nd ed.). New York: W.W. Norton, 1963.

Emery, G. Cognitive therapy with the elderly. In G. Emery, S. Hollon, and R. Bedrosian (Eds.), *New directions in cognitive therapy*. New York: Guilford, 1981.

Finch, C.E., & Hayflick, L. (Eds.), *Handbook of the biology of aging*. New York: Van Nostrand Reinhold, 1977.

Fozard, J.L., Wolf, E., Bell, B., et al. Visual perception and communication. In J.E. Birren & K.W. Schaie (Eds.), *Handbook of the psychology of aging*. New York: Van Nostrand Reinhold, 1977.

Gallagher, D., McGarvey, W., Zelinsky, E.M., & Thompson, L.W. Age and factor structure of the Zung Depression Scale. Paper presented at 31st annual meeting of Gerontological Society, 1978.

Gallagher, D., & Thompson, L.W. Treatment of major depressive disorders in older adult outpatients with brief psychotherapies. *Psychology: Theory, Research, and Practice,* 1982, *19,* 482–490.

Gallagher, D., Thompson, L.W., Baffa, G., et al. (Eds.), *Depression in the elderly: A biobehavioral treatment manual*. Los Angeles: University of Southern California Press, 1981.

Gallagher, D., Thompson, L.W., & Levy, S.M. Clinical psychological assessment of older adults. In L.W. Poon (Ed.), *Aging in the 1980's*. Washington, D.C.: American Psychological Association, 1980.

Giamba, L.M., & Arenberg, D. Problem solving, concept learning, and aging. In L.W. Poon (Ed.), *Aging in the 1980's*. Washington, D.C.: American Psychological Association, 1980.

Hartley, J.T., Harker, J.O., & Walsh, D.A. Contemporary issues and new directions in adult development of learning and memory. In L.W. Poon (Ed.), *Aging in the 1980's*. Washington, D.C.: American Psychological Association, 1980.

Harwood, E., & Naylor, G.F.K. Changes in the constitution of the WAIS intelligence patterns with advancing age. *Australian Journal of Psychology*, 1971, *23*, 297–303.

Hicks, L.H., & Birren, J.E. Aging, brain damage, and psychomotor slowing. *Psychological Bulletin*, 1970, *74*, 377–396.

Hoyer, W.J., & Plude, D.J. Attentional and perceptual processes in the study of cognitive aging. In L.W. Poon (Ed.), *Aging in the 1980's*. Washington, D.C.: American Psychological Association, 1980.

Hoyer, W.J., Raskind, C.L., & Abrahams, J.P. Research practices in the psychology of aging: a survey of research published in the Journal of Gerontology, 1975–1982. Journal of Gerontology, 1984, in press.

Hyams, D.E. Psychological factors in rehabilitation of the elderly. *Gerontologia Clinica*, 1969, *11*, 129–136.

Jarvik, L.F. Diagnosis of dementia in the elderly: a 1980 perspective. In C. Eisdorfer (Ed.), *Annual review of gerontology and geriatrics* (Vol. 1). New York: Springer, 1980.

Jarvik, L.F., Eisdorfer, C., & Blum, J.E. *Intellectual functioning in adults*. New York: Springer, 1973.

Jarvik, L.F., & Falek, A. Intellectual stability and survival in the aged. *Journal of Gerontology*, 1963, *18*, 173–176.

Klodin, V.M. *Verbal facilitation of perceptual–integrative performance in relation to age*. Doctoral dissertation, Washington University, St. Louis, 1975.

Knapp, P.H. Emotional aspects of hearing loss. *Psychosomatic Medicine*, 1948, *10*, 203–222.

Kral, V.A. Benign senescent forgetfulness. In R. Katzman, R.D. Terry, & K.L. Bick (Eds.), *Alzheimer's disease: Senile dementia and related disorders* (Aging, vol. 7). New York: Raven Press, 1978.

Krauss, I.K. Between- and within-group comparisons in aging research. In L.W. Poon (Ed.), *Aging in the 1980's*. Washington, D.C.: American Psychological Association, 1980.

Miller, W. Psychological deficit in depression. *Psychological Bulletin*, 1975, *82*, 238–260.

Morgan, L.A. Social roles in later life: Some recent research trends. In C. Eisdorfer (Ed.), *Annual review of gerontology and geriatrics* (Vol. 3). New York: Springer, 1982.

Peck, R. Psychological developments in the second half of life. In J.E. Anderson (Ed.), *Psychological aspects of aging*. Washington, D.C.: American Psychological Association, 1956.

Rabbitt, P. Changes in problem solving ability in old age. In J.E. Birren & K.W. Schaie (Eds.), *Handbook of the psychology of aging*. New York: Van Nostrand Reinhold, 1977.

Riegel, K.F. and Riegel, R.M. Development, drop, and death. *Developmental Psychology*, 1972, *6*, 306–319.

Riegel, K.F., Riegel, R.M., and Meyer, M. A study of the dropout rate in longitudinal research on aging and the prediction of death. *Journal of Personality and Social Psychology,* 1967, *5,* 342–348.

Schaie, J.P., & Schaie, K.W. Psychological evaluation of the cognitively impaired elderly. In C. Eisdorfer & R.O. Freidel (Eds.), *Cognitive and emotional disturbance in the elderly.* Chicago: Yearbook Medical Publishers, 1977.

Schaie, K.W. Quasi-experimental research designs in the psychology of aging. In J.E. Birren & K.W. Schaie (Eds.), *Handbook of the psychology of aging.* New York: Van Nostrand Reinhold, 1977.

Schaie, K.W., & Schaie, J.P. Clinical assessment and aging. In J.E. Birren & K.W. Schaie (Eds.), *Handbook of the psychology of aging.* New York: Van Nostrand Reinhold, 1977.

Schonfield, D. Translations in gerontology—from lab to life: Utilizing information. *American Psychologist,* 1974, *29,* 796–801.

Seigler, I.C., Nowlin, J.B., & Blumenthal, J.A. Health and behavior: Methodological considerations for adult development and aging. In L.W. Poon (Ed.), *Aging in the 1980's.* Washington, D.C.: American Psychological Association, 1980.

Spieth, W. Cardiovascular health status, age, and psychological performance. *Journal of Gerontology,* 1964, *19,* 277–284.

Spieth, W. Slowless of task performance and cardiovascular disease. In A.T. Welford & J.E. Birren (Eds.), *Behavior, aging, and the nervous system.* Springfield, Ill: Charles C. Thomas, 1965.

Timiras, P.S. *Developmental physiology and aging.* New York: Macmillan, 1972.

Watson, L.E., & Tolan, T. *Hearing tests and hearing instruments.* New York: Hafner, 1967.

Zung, W.W.K. A self-rating depression scale. *Archives of General Psychiatry,* 1965, *12,* 63–70.

Zung, W.W.K. Depression in the normal aged. *Psychosomatics,* 1967, *8,* 287–291.

PART II

Depression and Dementia

2

DEPRESSION IN LATER LIFE: THEORY AND ASSESSMENT

Steven H. Zarit
Judy M. Zarit

This chapter and the next will highlight three issues. Prevalence of depression in later life and assessment procedures will be discussed in this chapter, while Chapter 3 will focus on promising treatments. For each issue, the question of whether or not age makes a difference will be considered. For example, does the incidence of depression increase with age? Are there certain procedures that are different when treating an older person? Because of their importance in determining assessment and treatment procedures, models and theories of depression also will be presented.

PREVALENCE OF DEPRESSION

Estimates of the prevalence of depression among people over age 65 are high, although the exact figures depend on the method of gathering information and determining cases. The numbers of depressed vary depending on whether prevalence has been based on diagnosis at admission to mental hospital or clinic, psychiatric evaluation of a non-patient, community sample, or self-report of symptoms by a community sample. Each method has certain advantages and drawbacks which affect estimates. In estimating the relationship between age and depression, it is important also

GERIATRIC MENTAL HEALTH
ISBN 0-8089-1657-2

to consider whether current problems have developed for the first time in later life or are part of a recurrent or chronic pattern.

With respect to prevalence at admission to mental hospitals or psychiatric units, affective disorder has been consistently reported as the most frequent problem among older patients. Estimates of depressive disorders range between 21 and 54 percent of new admissions (Peak, 1973; Redick & Taube, 1980; Vickers, 1976). Using a comprehensive screening a Roth (1955) found that over half of all geriatric admissions to an inpatient psychiatric unit were classified as affective disorders (including manic-depression), and 66 percent of these cases were first admissions.

The total number of older patients admitted with the diagnosis of depression is somewhat lower than those at earlier ages. The peak time for severe depressions appears to be between the ages of 45 and 55 (Gurland, 1976). There may be, however, selection factors which keep the numbers of elderly patients lower. First, some reluctance about admitting older patients to psychiatric facilities appears to exist, probably because of pessimism about their recovery. In general, there has been a shift away from using psychiatric facilities and toward using nursing homes for elders with serious psychiatric disturbances, although the latter typically offer little in the way of assessment or treatment for these problems (Kahn, 1975; Kramer, Taube, & Redick, 1973). Another factor is a tendency to underdiagnose depression in the elderly. In a major cross-national study, it was found that American psychiatrists made fewer diagnoses of depression than British psychiatrists, being more likely to label depressive symptoms as organic brain syndrome (Copeland, Kelleher, Kellett et al., 1974). Finally, depressed older persons may not be referred for treatment as often as younger individuals. There may be some tendency for physicians and mental health professionals to view a certain amount of depression as normal due to the multiple losses many elderly people experience, and therefore not to identify these persons as needing mental health treatment (Gurland, 1973).

The criteria for diagnosis also constitute an important problem for those community studies of nonpatient populations. In perhaps the most comprehensive study to date, Gurland and his associates (1980) used multiple indicators derived from structured interviews to determine cases of depression for a sample of New York City residents over age 65. Their findings indicate that 13 percent of the sample had clinically significant symptoms of depression and another 9 percent met most of the criteria for diagnosis, including the presence of 6 or more symptoms of depression. Depression was higher among women than men between the ages of 65 and 80, but the prevalence of depression among men over 80 was considerably higher and greater than for women. These findings are consistent with other community surveys (Blazer & Williams, 1980; Kay, Beamish, & Roth, 1964; Weissman & Myers, 1978).

When community surveys focus on depressive symptoms rather than diagnosis, the rates are higher for elders than for younger persons (Gurland, 1976). The prevalence of depressive symptoms is especially high among those elderly persons with chronic health problems (Cheah & Beard, 1980; Dovenmuehle & Verwoerdt, 1962). Self-reports have the advantage of assessing directly the concerns of older persons rather than placing diagnostic constructs on symptoms. But they both over- and under-report depressive symptoms. Most self-report inventories include physical complaints, such as insomnia, fatigue, and poor appetite. These symptoms are typical of younger depressed populations, but may reflect health status (Dessonville, Gallagher, Thompson et al., 1982) or even normal changes in an older population. On the other hand, it has been observed that elders sometimes under-report affective symptoms of depression (Salzman & Shader, 1979).

Overall, despite the problems with the various criteria used for estimating prevalence, findings are consistent in indicating that depression in old age is a substantial problem. Rates may or may not be higher than for younger age groups, but it remains that there are large numbers of older persons with depressive complaints who might benefit from treatment.

CONCEPTS AND THEORIES OF DEPRESSION

An implicit problem in the epidemiological studies is that counting of cases is made difficult by the lack of agreement on what constitutes depression. More than being just an academic issue, our concepts of depression influence choices concerning assessment and treatment. For instance, thirty years ago the prevalent view of late-life depression was that it was a manifestation of senile changes, and expectations about the benefits of treatment were minimal (Roth, 1955). Contemporary theories differ significantly in their implications. One who holds that biological factors have primacy in late life depressions is likely to emphasize biological assessments and somatic therapies, while another who adheres to one of the psychosocial theories of depression is more likely to recommend psychotherapy. Since definitive findings about the nature and treatment of depression remain to be discovered, it is important to be aware of the relative strengths and weaknesses of current theories and to draw what is useful from each.

Definitions

Through the years, the terminology used to describe depression has been confusing and imprecise. Recent diagnostic advances, which have been incorporated into the Diagnostic and Statistical Manual of the American Psychiatric Association (DSM III, 1980), represent major improvements in the reliability of diagnostic categories. Because explicit and operational definitions for various diagnoses are given, disagreements between clinicians have been reduced and reliability is at acceptable levels (Spitzer, Endicott, & Robins, 1975, 1978).

The primary distinction in the DSM III is severity: disorders are either "major affective disorders" or "minor depressions." Within the category of major affective disorders there is a further division into "bipolar disorders" and "major depression." Bipolar disorders involve distinct mood shifts, especially involving periods of mania, depression, and apparently normal mood. In contrast, mania is not part of the history of major depressions. A major depression is determined by the presence of a notable dysphoric mood of at least one week's duration and other symptoms typical of severe depression, such as poor appetite, weight loss, sleep difficulty, loss of energy, loss of interest and pleasure in other activities, and thoughts of death or suicide.

Less severe but chronic conditions are classified as cyclothymic (involving mood swings to mild mania), or dysthymic (recurrent and chronic depression). A mild depression following recent life changes is classified as an "adjustment disorder with depressive features."

More detailed subdivisions of the category major depressive disorder are proposed by Spitzer, et al., (1978). In particular, they attempt to provide more precise definitions of such terms as "neurotic depression," "psychotic depression," and "endogenous depression." Each of these terms historically has combined several features, and Spitzer et al. recommend identifying important dimensions separately. For instance, "psychotic depression" has been used to reflect three concepts: (1) "psychotic" symptoms, namely delusions, hallucinations, or stupor; (2) the lack of precipitating events; and (3) severe degree of incapacitation. Spitzer et al. (1978) instead reserve the term "psychotic" only to indicate the presence of psychotic symptoms. "Endogenous" has referred both to history (the apparent absence of precipitating events) and type of symptoms (prominence of vegetative symptoms such as sleep disturbance, loss of appetite, and fatigue), but Spitzer et al. propose its use only where vegetative symptoms are involved. In place of "neurotic depression," they recommend the term "intermittent depressive disorder," to indicate those persons who have been bothered by depressed mood for at least two years. There is usually no clear onset and the person complains of a depressed mood most of the time. By using terminology to reflect the presence or absence of one pattern of symptoms rather than clusters of symptoms, reliability of diagnosis should improve.

Depression: Threshold versus Continuum

The definitions of depression imply that it is a construct, with subtypes that have defined boundaries between each other and from normal variations in mood. To become depressed, one must cross some threshold that distinguishes normal from pathological mood. The question can be raised, however, whether this type of categorizing is premature or even appropriate. An alternative model is that a continuum of fluctuations in mood exists, ranging from normal to severely depressed, with differences a matter of degree, not kind. The boundaries between depressed and normal are not, in fact, all that clear. Although the DSM III improves reliability of diagnosis, the distinction between someone who falls within the boundaries of a category and another who is just outside of them is probably quantitative, rather than qualitative.

Because the word depression refers both to a construct and a set of behaviors, there is a certain degree of ambiguity in its use and, in fact, both meanings are often implied (Lewinsohn, Biglan, & Zeiss, 1976). There are, however, rather different implications for assessment and treatment depending on which view one holds. For instance, if a depressive disorder can best be described as a construct or an illness, then it makes sense to concentrate on identifying boundaries between categories. On the other hand, a continuum model of depression suggests the importance of assessing individual differences.

Both the threshold and continuum models of depression have some degree of empirical support and have practical applications. Diagnosis partly involves determining that someone falls sufficiently outside the realm of normal functioning, so that treatment is appropriate. Therefore, it is important to establish some operational criteria for distinguishing transitory mood fluctuations, such as occasional sadness, from clinically significant episodes of depression. These thresholds determine the boundaries of who is to be assessed, treated, and studied in research. Another use of diagnostic categories is that persons having different clusters of symptoms might have quite different responses to treatment. The most notable example is the bipolar disorders, which generally respond well to lithium carbonate (Prange, 1975), even among the aged (Foster, Gershell, & Goldfarb, 1977).

Other diagnostic constructs are not as consistently useful for planning treatment and they inadvertently minimize potentially important individual differences. Patients with psychotic and endogenous features are more likely to respond to somatic therapies such as antidepressant medications, or electroconvulsive therapy (Klerman, 1971; Prange, 1975), but there are many individuals who do not have optimal responses. Individual differences between persons receiving the same diagnosis may also be substantial. Observing people who meet the criteria of major depressive disorder, Lewinsohn and Lee (1981) describe marked individual variation in behaviors that demonstrate a relationship to depression, which includes social skills and current activities. Despite being diagnostically the same, these persons differ substantially from one another in ways that might be crucial to treatment and subsequent outcome. Clinical experience has indicated another dimension of difference within the category of major depressive disorder. Some individuals, while currently depressed, have long-standing characterological disorders and respond quite differently to treatment than those with more adequate premorbid adjustment. These differences will be discussed further in Chapter 3.

Biological Theories

Speculation about biological components of depression have been present since ancient times. Hippocrates' belief that depression resulted from an imbalance of body fluids in which the person had too much "black bile" dominated European medical thinking until the nineteenth century. Treatment was designed to correct this excess through bleeding, purging, and sweating. Good food, exercise, and regular sleep and bowel movements were also recommended (Diethelm, 1975).

Recent discoveries in two areas have given impetus to biological models of depression. The first area concerns the effects of drugs and other somatic therapies on depression. The second involves basic research in the central nervous and endocrine systems.

Many drugs clearly affect mood. One of the most dramatic examples is Reserpine, which was used widely in the past as an antihypertensive and causes depression in about 20 percent of those taking the drug (Lipton, 1976). The serendipitous discovery that lithium salts mitigate mood swings in bipolar disorders has prompted a search for substances that would have a comparable effect on other depressions (Baldessarini, 1975). Current therapies, including tricyclic medications and electroconvulsive therapy, appear to shorten depressive episodes for many people (Morris & Beck, 1974).

Considerable research has focused on the potential role of neurotransmitters, chemicals which facilitate the transfer of electrical impulses from one brain neuron to another, in mediating depressive disorders. Two groups of chemicals, the catecholamines and the indoleamines, have received special attention. It has been hypothesized variously that excesses or deficits of some of these chemicals, including dopamine, norepinephrine and serotonin, or the balance between neurotransmitters that have antagonistic effects, such as norepinephrine and serotonin, are critical in depression (Baldessarini, 1975; Blazer, 1982; Lipton, 1976; Prange, 1975). Changes in the endocrine system, which mediates stress, also may contribute to depression (Blazer, 1982). Since the levels of neurotransmitters and the body's response to stress both are altered in critical ways with aging (Finch, 1977; Lipton, 1976), the result could be a heightened vulnerability to depression. Genetic factors also have been studied and, while some promising results have been obtained, they appear more relevant to depressions with onset before age 50 (Mendlewicz, 1976).

The implication of biological models is a medical approach to depression.

The advantages of quick-acting drugs and of other somatic therapies should be obvious. But it is important to recognize that current procedures are not consistently effective and, moreover, that some older persons cannot tolerate antidepressant drugs either because of side effects (Gerner, Estabrook, Steuer et al., 1980) or because they have health problems for which the tricyclic medications are contraindicated. From another perspective, biochemical changes may be the result rather than the primary cause, of stresses or personal habits. If that is the case, then treatment might be more effective if it identifies some of those psychosocial risk factors. One comparison of psychotherapy and medications found that therapy had better initial and long-term results (Rush, Beck, Kovacs et al., 1977).

Akiskal and McKinney (1973) have articulated a multidimensional model of depression. Noting the findings that link depression to many different factors, including genetic, biochemical vulnerability, early childhood losses, recent losses, stresses, and personal habits, they propose that there may be several pathways to depression. The amount contributed by each predisposing factor may vary from case to case. In one individual, biological dimensions may be more important, while in another, recent stress plays a larger role. Their model takes into account the interaction between behaviors and stress on one hand and biochemical responses on the other. The notion of multiple pathways to depression also is consistent with the considerable individual differences in symptoms and other behaviors among depressed persons.

Psychoanalytic Theories and the Role of Early Experience

Psychoanalytic approaches to depression have emphasized the primacy of early experience in creating a vulnerability to depression. Freud (1950) notes the resemblance of depression to mourning and speculates that the patient's ambivalent feelings toward the lost object are internalized in a kind of narcissistic identification. Self-torment and self-blame are manifestations of hostility toward the lost person that are turned inward. Other writers have emphasized the relation of depression to the loss of external gratification in someone with excessive dependencies or demands to be loved (Bibring, 1953; Cath, 1966; Fenichel, 1945).

These approaches view the role of recent events as triggering long-standing intrapsychic conflicts, with the source of the depression being personality patterns that were laid down in early life. Actual losses in childhood may heighten this vulnerability. Traumatic separations between mother and child at critical points in development, especially between 9 months and 3 years, can result in a depressive reaction by the child that is characterized by low levels of activity and poor eating (Bowlby, 1973). While the relation between early losses and adult depression has not been supported consistently in empirical studies, the majority of findings point in that direction (Heinicke, 1973). It has not been determined, however, if early losses also have a role in depressions in later life.

The importance of early childhood influences in treatment of adult depression remains controversial. Newer therapy approaches, notably Beck's cognitive treatment of depression (Beck, Rush, Shaw, & Emery, 1979) incorporate the focus of dynamic theories on intrapsychic processes without going back to childhood sources of current problems.

Recent Losses and Learned Helplessness

Life changes usually are implicated in the onset of depression. The amount of life change experienced by a depressed person before the onset of the disorder has been found to be greater and more undesirable, than that experienced by other people, including normal community residents, other psychiatric patients, and medically ill hospital patients (Paykel, 1974). Although no single category of life change consistently predicts depression, depressed people have experienced more losses of others from their lives (Paykel, 1974). Even in cases of endogenous depression, life changes play a role. As noted earlier, the concept of endogenous depression originally denoted the absence of precipitating events, but studies following these patients over time found that distressing life events were eventually reported. What characterizes these patients is that they are initially so lethargic, slow, and unmotivated that interviewers cannot obtain information about life changes. Only as the depression lifts are changes identified (Goodwin & Bunney, 1973; Leff, Roatch, & Bunney, 1970).

Because of the potential for experiencing losses in later life, theorists have emphasized their importance. Taking an Eriksonian approach, Butler (1977; Butler & Lewis, 1982) proposed that the major psychological conflict for older persons is grief versus restitution. According to Butler, adaptation depends on coming to terms with the losses that have occurred and drawing on the resources one has left, rather than grieving perpetually. Erikson's (1963) own concept of aging as a conflict between integrity and despair implicitly refers to loss. Adaptation depends on accepting the mistakes and limitations of the past, as well as the fact that one cannot go back and start over.

There have only been limited studies of the relation of life changes to depression in later life. One problem is that life change inventories sample events more typical of earlier periods of the life cycle, and may not provide an accurate picture of the changes experienced by older people (Chiriboga & Cutler, 1980). Depressed elders generally report that significant life changes preceded depressive episodes (Post, 1962, 1972). Compared to patients with paranoid disorders, depressed persons report more frequent life changes (Kay, Cooper, Garside et al., 1976). Among the various life changes, illness may be more prominent a factor in late-life depressions (Kay, Roth, & Hopkins, 1955; Rubenstein, Zaidi, & Kahn, 1976).

Seligman (1975) has articulated the theory of "learned helplessness," that links losses and depression. Studies have found that when animals are repeatedly exposed to shocks and other noxious stimuli from which they cannot escape, they become inactive, withdrawn, and do not attempt to escape, even when it is possible. By analogy, Seligman proposes that people who are experiencing changes over which they perceive they have no control, learn to view themselves as helpless and therefore no longer take active steps to change their circumstances.

Behavioral and Cognitive Theories

Recent approaches to depression have emphasized identifying and modifying those events which are associated most strongly with depression. In the case of behavioral approaches, primary consideration is given to overt actions that result in increased or decreased feelings of dysphoria (Lewinsohn, Biglan, & Zeiss, 1976). Cognitive approaches, in contrast, use overt behaviors to uncover thoughts that are associated with depressive feelings (Beck, 1976). Despite these differences, there has been considerable convergence of therapy techniques. These approaches will be discussed together.

A behavioral theory of depression has been developed and elaborated by Peter Lewinsohn and his associates (Lewinsohn, Biglan, & Zeiss, 1976; Lewinsohn, Munoz, Youngren et al., 1978). They propose that depression is the result of the person's engaging in few activities that are either reinforced by others or are intrinsically reinforcing. The lack of positive reinforcement leads to a reduction in the output of behavior, and, concurrently, dysphoric mood. Through a series of studies, Lewinsohn and his associates (1976) have demonstrated the relationship between depression and certain behaviors. Depressed persons have been found to engage in few activities that they perceive as pleasant and to improve when they increase these activities. Conversely, they experience high numbers of current life events that they perceive as aversive and report decreased depression when the number of these events decreases. Another dimension emerging from direct observation of depressed patients is that many lack the social skills to elicit positive responses from others. Social skill deficits in depression also have been emphasized by Klerman and his colleagues (Klerman, Rounsaville, Chevron et al., 1979).

The cognitive theory of depression emphasizes the importance of the patient's thoughts in determining both activity and mood (Beck, 1967, 1976). Beck describes what he calls the *cognitive triad* of thoughts that are typical of depressed patients. These thoughts are a negative view of oneself, current experiences, and the future. An important aspect of the theory, which has been supported by clinical examples as well as experimental studies, is that these thoughts represent distortions of reality. For instance, Loeb, Beck, and Diggory (1971) administered a card-sort task to depressed and non-depressed persons, and although performance did not differ between the two groups, the depressed subjects rated their performance as worse than the others. Recently there has been some question about whether depressed persons' evaluations of themselves might be more realistic than those with normal mood, especially for social behaviors (Lewinsohn, Mischel, Chaplin et al., 1980). Whether they are realistic or not, depressed persons consistently have more negative thoughts.

Another major aspect of the cognitive theory is that thoughts determined depressed mood. This can be illustrated by the way depressed patients often react to neutral events. Burns (1980) describes one patient who, as therapy progressed, revealed that she had been initially quite upset at the beginning of treatment. When the therapist started the session late, she interpreted that as indicating that he really was not interested in her and cared more about his other patients. When he saw her early, she interpreted that as evidence that she must be in terrible shape and required extra time. When he saw her on time, she thought to herself that he was just running an assembly line. The patient's thoughts about the situation, in this example, caused her to feel more upset. Experimental evidence tentatively supports the proposition that thoughts can affect mood (Velten, 1968; Baffa, 1981).

Neither cognitive nor behavioral theory discusses etiology or risk factors in detail. Beck (1976; Beck, Rush, Shaw et al., 1979) suggests that recent events trigger depressive thought patterns, which were latent and possibly learned in childhood. The exaggerated quality of depressed persons' thoughts do resemble some childhood thought patterns. Implicit in the behavioral theory is that depressed persons are more vulnerable to losses and other life changes because they initially have fewer behavioral and social skills for eliciting positive responses from the environment.

Applications to the older population have been interesting, although still limited. Many factors associated with aging might contribute to decreased opportunities for engaging in reinforcing activities. They include lower income, forced retirement, chronic health problems, and the deaths of spouses or friends. Lewinsohn and MacPhillamy (1974) report that older persons and depressed patients are similar in that both groups engage in fewer potentially pleasant activities than young, non-depressed controls. They differ, however, in that non-depressed elders perceive many more potentially pleasant activities than do the depressed. Cognitive factors in late life depression might be activated by the generally unfavorable view most people hold of aging and older persons. Depressed older persons have been found to make negative appraisals of their abilities, which reflect stereotypes about the aging process (Kahn, Zarit, Hilbert et al., 1975).

The relation of losses to cognitive dimensions has been investigated in a sample of older persons with significant visual impairments. Severity of vision loss was not related to depressive symptoms. Rather, a cognitive dimension, how impairing they believed the vision problem to be, was associated with depressive complaints (Center for the Partially Sighted, 1980).

In another study that focused on the relation of depression and illness (Cole, 1981), two groups of medically ill, hospitalized patients were compared. While the groups were approximately equal in severity of illness, one group had significant depressive features, meeting the criteria for major depressive disorder, while depressive symptoms were absent in the second group. Subjects differed behaviorally and cognitively: the depressed group had fewer social interactions, rated those that occurred as less enjoyable, and also reported their health status to be more impaired than the other subjects with similar illnesses. Cognitive differences have also been found in comparing recently widowed persons and patients with major depressive disorders (Gallagher, Dessonville, Breckenridge et al., 1982). While both groups endorsed affective distress items on the Beck Depression Inventory, the depressed patients also reported self-deprecatory thoughts (e.g., feeling like a failure, feeling disappointed in oneself, blaming oneself for bad things that happen).

ASSESSMENT PROCEDURES

Assessment for depression should assume both a threshold and continuum model of depression. With respect to thresholds, there is widespread agreement that depression is different from sadness and that treatment for occasional feelings of sadness is inappropriate. Clinicians should use some operational criteria, such as those found in the DSM III or the Research Diagnostic Criteria, which determine that a clinically significant problem is present. Once determined, the focus should shift to assessment of individual differences to identify factors that might be relevant to treatment planning.

The assessment of depressed persons includes determining the presence, frequency, and severity of typical symptoms. Lewinsohn, Biglan, and Zeiss (1976) suggest evaluation of five categories of symptoms: dysphoric mood, behavioral deficits, behavioral excesses, somatic symptoms associated with depression, and cognitive manifestations.

Assessment of older persons also should include differential diagnosis for dementia and evaluation of health status and current medications. Assessments can be made by interviewing the patient or by using a depression inventory. Areas for assessment and commonly used measures of depression are reviewed below.

Symptoms of Depression

A summary of symptoms of depression such as those described by Lewinsohn et al. (1976) provides an overview of the types of problems that should be assessed. At the core of depression, of course, is dysphoric mood: its frequency, severity, and any fluctuations should be determined. Behavioral deficits can include the patient's current activities, as well as the clinician's observations of behavior and appearance. Suicidal thoughts are crucial complaints to assess. Because of high suicide rates among the aged, especially older men, determination of risk is important (Zarit, 1980). Somatic symptoms are common in depression, with the most frequent being headaches, sleep disturbances, and fatigue. The negative thoughts discussed by Beck (1976; Beck, Rush, Shaw et al., 1979), are cognitive manifestations that include hopelessness, helplessness, and worthlessness.

An important consideration in the assessment of symptoms is whether older depressed people differ from younger ones in typical presenting complaints. Some authors have stressed that depressed mood is not as pronounced in the elderly, who instead tend to be apathetic and listless (Blumenthal, 1975; Epstein, 1976; Zung & Green, 1972). In contrast to complaints about mood, somatic problems tend to be higher among older persons (Blumenthal, 1975; Gurland, 1976; Zung, 1967; Zung & Green, 1972). The question has been raised as to whether these problems are due to chronic health problems that are more common in later life, or actually reflect normal age changes. The sleep cycle is altered with aging, for instance, as well as by many common illnesses.

A recent study (Dessonville, Gallagher, Thompson et al., 1982) provides some clarification on this issue. Older persons seeking treatment for depression were compared to normal community controls. All subjects were administered the Schedule of Affective Disorders and Schizophrenia (SADS), a structured interview for differential diagnosis of depression (Endicott & Spitzer, 1978). Depressed subjects met the previously discussed Research Diagnostic Criteria for having a major depressive disorder. Subjects also rated their current health status. The results indicated that on most scales derived from SADS, the older depressed patients could be readily distinguished from normals. Overlap occurred only on insomnia and weight-loss items when depressed subjects were compared to normals who rated themselves as being in poor health. Comparisons with norms on the SADS established for younger patients indicate that older depressives report more anxiety and less frequent thoughts of suicide.

The notion that major depression can be differentiated readily from normal aging has been supported by other research (Raskin & Rae, 1981; Steuer, Bank, Olsen & Jarvik, 1980). There has been less attention paid to the assessment and significance of minor depression. One other caution should be noted. Some authors have suggested that there are masked depressions, in which somatic or other complaints are prominent but the patient denies a depressed mood (Beck, 1967; Epstein, 1976). It has been suggested that a depressed patient may even present with symptoms of senile dementia (Kiloh, 1961). There are, unfortunately, few clinical descriptions to guide the assessment process for these masked depressions.

A number of measures of depression exist that are useful for confirming the findings of a clinical interview, as well as providing an index of symptoms against which treatment can be evaluated. Among the most widely used are the Zung Depression Scale (Zung, 1965; 1967), the Beck Depression Inventory (Beck, Ward, Mendelson et al., 1961), the Depression Scale of the Minnesota Multiphasic Personality Inventory [MMPI] (Hathaway & McKinley, 1943), and the Hamilton Depression Scale (Hamilton, 1967). The first three are self-reports, while the Hamilton Scale is completed by a trained interviewer. Each measure has its strengths and weaknesses, and it is likely that a certain amount of error will occur in estimating depression using any procedure. A major problem is that these measures have been developed with younger persons and there is evidence that both the meaning and intercorrelations among items change with age (Blumenthal, 1975; Gallagher, Thompson, & Levy, 1980). Adequate reliabilities with older patients have been reported for the Beck Depression Inventory (Gallagher, Nies, & Thompson, 1982), although the complex structure of this measure, where the respondent chooses among four statements, makes it difficult to administer to some older patients. Yesavage and his associates (1982) recently have developed a measure of depressive symptoms specifically for older persons that has a simplified, true–false format and minimizes the influence of somatic complaints. Clinical applications of the SADS are limited, since this measure is lengthy and often requires one-and-a-half to two-hours or more to complete.

Depression or Dementia?

It frequently has been noted that depression and dementia are difficult to distinguish. Depressed persons often complain about loss of memory and other intellectual impairment, while dementia patients, especially in the earlier stages of the disease, also may have depressive symptoms. In practice, however, the distinction is usually clear and can be made by examining current cognitive functioning as well as the history of the problem. While depressed persons complain of memory loss, they usually do not have an obvious deficit (Kahn, Zarit, Hilbert, & Neiderehe, 1975; Raskin & Rae, 1981). In contrast to dementia patients they rarely make errors on mental status tests. More extensive testing may reveal subtle intellectual impairments associated with depression, but they are not as global or profound as in cases of dementia (Friedman, 1964; Miller, 1975; Weingartner, Cohen, Murphy et al., 1981). A second consideration is history. With dementia, onset is usually insidious and symptoms progress gradually. Depression, in contrast, is typically episodic (Gurland, 1980). Even for persons with longstanding depression, there is usually no history of progressive cognitive impairment.

It is likely that assessment of some cases will result in ambiguous findings. Early stages of dementia, for instance, can be marked by a relatively minimal intellectual impairment and would not be revealed by mental-status testing. Depression has sometimes been reported as causing cognitive symptoms indistinguishable from dementia. When history cannot clarify, the clinician should err on the side of overdiagnosing depression (Kahn & Miller, 1978). Since there are currently no effective treatments for primary degenerative dementia, an error of omission in diagnosis has no serious consequences, but treatment of the symptoms of depression in the patient with dementia may have some benefits (Epstein, 1976).

Medical and Pharmacological Assessment

An important consideration with older patients is that many common illnesses and medications can cause symptoms of depression. Illnesses which can present with depressive symptoms include neurological disorders (Parkinson's disease, brain tumors, especially metastases from other sites, intracranial aneurisms, and meningitis), endocrine disorders, pernicious anemia, abdominal neoplasia, especially pancreatic cancer, and urinary tract disorders (Salzman & Shader, 1978a). Among medications which can cause depressive symptoms are antihypertensive drugs, antiparkinsonian drugs, anticancer medications, neuroleptics, and antianxiety drugs (Salzman & Shader, 1978b). Combinations of medications can also result in depressive symptoms.

SUMMARY

Depression is the most prevalent mental disorder of old age. While basic questions remain unanswered about the etiology of depression, proper assessment will greatly increase the likelihood of positive outcome, clearly improving the quality of life of elder patients. Assessment should consider depression as both a threshold phenomenon and as a continuum. Depression should be distinguished from normal fluctuations in mood, and individual differences in mood, thoughts, and behaviors should be highlighted.

REFERENCES

Akiskal, H.S., & McKinney, W.T. Depressive disorders: Toward a unified hypothesis. *Science,* 1973, *182,* 20–29.

Baffa, G.A. *Age comparisons of the effects of cognitive and behavioral mood elevating tasks.* Unpublished doctoral dissertation, University of Southern California, 1981.

Baldessarini, R.J. Biogenic amine hypothesis in affective disorders. In F.F. Flach & S.C. Draghi (Eds.), *The nature and treatment of depression.* New York: John Wiley, 1975.

Beck, A.T. *Depression: clinical, experimental and theoretical aspects.* New York: Harper & Row, 1967.

Beck, A.T. *Cognitive therapy and the emotional disorders.* New York: International Universities Press, 1976.

Beck, A.T., Rush, A.J., Shaw, B.F., & Emery, C. *Cognitive therapy of depression.* New York: Guilford Press, 1979.

Beck, A.T., Ward, C.H., Mendelson, M., Mock, J.E., & Erbaugh, J. An inventory for measuring depression. *Archives of General Psychiatry,* 1961, *4,* 561–571.

Bibring, E. The mechanics of depression. In P. Greenberg (Ed.), *Affective disorders.* New York: International Universities Press, 1953.

Blazer, D.G., *Depression in late life.* St. Louis: C.V. Mosby, 1982.

Blazer, D.G., & Williams, C.D. The epidemiology of dysphoria and depression in an elderly population. *American Journal of Psychiatry,* 1980, *137,* 439–444.

Blumenthal, M.D. Measuring depressive symptomatology in a general population. *Archives of General Psychiatry,* 1975, *32,* 971–978.

Bowlby, J. Attachment and loss. In *Separation: Anxiety and anger.* (Vol. 2) New York: Basic Books, 1973.

Burns, D. *Feeling good.* New York: William Morrow, 1980.

Butler, R.N. Toward a psychiatry of the life cycle: Implications of socio-psychologic studies of the aging process for the psychotherapeutic situation. In S.H. Zarit (Ed.), *Readings in aging and death: contemporary perspectives.* New York: Harper & Row, 1977.

Butler, R.N., & Lewis, M. *Aging and mental health* (3rd Ed.). St. Louis: C.V. Mosby, 1982.

Cath, S. Beyond depression: the depleted state: A study in ego psychology in the aged. *Canadian Psychiatric Association Journal,* 1966, *11* (special suppl.), 329–339.

Center for the Partially Sighted. *A comprehensive community care system for partially sighted older persons.* Unpublished manuscript, Santa Monica, California, 1980.

Cheah, K.C., & Beard, C.W. Psychiatric findings in the population of a geriatric evaluation unit: Implications. *Journal of the American Geriatrics Society,* 1980, *28,* 153–156.

Chiriboga, D.A., & Cutler, L. Stress and adaptation: Life span perspectives. In L. Poon (Ed.), *Aging in the 1980's: Psychological issues.* Washington, D.C.: American Psychological Association, 1980.

Cole, K.D. *Psychological features of depression among medically ill older men.* Unpublished doctoral dissertation, University of Southern California, 1981.

Copeland, J.R.M., Kelleher, M.J., Kellett, J.M., Fountain-Gourlay, A.J., Cowan, D.W., Barron, C., & DeGruchy, J. (U.K.), with Gurland, E.J., Sharpe, L., Simon, R.J., Kuriansky, J.B., & Stiller, P. (U.S.). Diagnostic differences in psychogeriatric patients in New York and London. *Canadian Psychiatric Association Journal,* 1974, *19,* 267–271.

Dessonville, C., Gallagher, D., Thompson, L.W., Finnel, C., & Lewinsohn, P.M. Relation of age and health status to depressive symptoms in normal and depressed older adults. *Essence,* 1982, *5,* 99–118.

Diagnostic and statistical manual of mental disorders—DSM III. (3rd Ed.) Washington, D.C.: American Psychiatric Association, 1980.

Diethelm, O. The evolution of the concept of depression. In F.F. Flach & S.C. Draghi (Eds.), *The nature and treatment of depression.* New York: John Wiley, 1975.

Dovenmuehle, R.H., & Verwoerdt, A. Physical illness and depressive symptomatology. *Journal of the American Geriatrics Society,* 1962, *10,* 932–947.

Endicott, J., & Spitzer, R.L. A diagnostic interview: The schedule for affective disorders and schizophrenia. *Archives of General Psychiatry,* 1978, *35,* 837–844.

Epstein, L.J. Depression in the elderly. *Journal of Gerontology,* 1976, *31,* 278–282.

Erikson, E.H. *Childhood and society* (2nd Ed.). New York: Norton, 1963.

Fenichel, O. *The psychoanalytic theory of neurosis.* New York: Norton, 1945.

Finch, C.E. Neuroendocrine and autonomic aspects of aging. In C.E. Finch & L. Hayflick (Eds.), *Handbook of the biology of aging.* New York: Van Nostrand Rinehold, 1977.

Foster, J.R., Gershell, W.J., & Goldfarb, A.I. Lithium treatment in the elderly. I. Clinical usage. *Journal of Gerontology,* 1977, *32,* 299–302.

Freud, S. Mourning and melancholia. In *Collected papers* (Vol. 4). London: Hogarth Press, 1950.

Friedman, A.S. Minimal effects of severe depression on cognitive functioning. *Journal of Abnormal and Social Psychology,* 1964, *69,* 237–243.

Gallagher, D., Dessonville, C., Breckenridge, J.N., Thompson, L.W., & Amaral, P. Similarities and differences between normal grief and depression in older adults. *Essence,* 1982, *5,* 127–140.

Gallagher, D., Nies, G., & Thompson, L.W. Reliability of the Beck Depression Inventory with older adults. *Journal of Consulting and Clinical Psychology,* 1982, *50,* 152–153.

Gallagher, D., Thompson, L.W., & Levy, S.M. Clinical psychological assessment of older adults. In L.W. Poon (Ed.), *Aging in the 1980's: Psychological issues.* Washington, D.C.: American Psychological Association, 1980.

Gerner, R., Estabrook, W., Steuer, J., Waltuch, L., Kakkar, P., & Jarvik, L. A placebo controlled double-blind study of imipramine and trazadone in geriatric depression. In J.C. Cole & J.B. Barrett (Eds.), *Psychopathology in the aged.* New York: Raven Press, 1980.

Goodwin, F.K., & Bunney, W.E., Jr. Psychobiological aspects of stress and affective illness. In J.P. Scott & E.C. Senay (Eds.), *Separation and depression: clinical and research aspects*. Washington, D.C.: American Association for the Advancement of Science, 1973.

Gurland, B.J. A broad clinical assessment of psychopathology in the aged. In C. Eisdorfer & M.P. Lawton (Eds.), *The psychology of adult development and aging*. Washington, D.C.: American Psychological Association, 1973.

Gurland, B.J. The comparative frequency of depression in various adult age groups. *Journal of Gerontology*, 1976, *31*, 283–292.

Gurland, B.J. The assessment of the mental status of older adults. In J.F. Birren & R.B. Sloane (Eds.), *Handbook of mental health and aging*. Englewood Cliffs, N.J.: Prentice-Hall, 1980.

Gurland, B.J., Dean, L., Cross, P., & Golden, R. The epidemiology of depression and dementia in the elderly: The use of multiple indicators of these conditions. In J.C. Cole & J.E. Barrett (Eds.), *Psychopathology in the aged*. New York: Raven Press, 1980.

Hamilton, M. Development of a rating scale for primary depressive illness. *British Journal of Social and Clinical Psychiatry*, 1967, *6*, 278–296.

Hathaway, S.R., & McKinley, J.C. *The Minnesota Multiphasic Personality Inventory*. Minneapolis: University of Minnesota Press, 1943.

Heinicke, M. Parental deprivation in early childhood: a predisposition to later depression. In J.P. Scott & E.C. Senay (Eds.), *Separation and depression: Clinical and research aspects*. Washington, D.C.: American Association for the Advancement of Science, 1973.

Kahn, R.L. The mental health system and the future aged. *Gerontologist*, 1975, *15* (No. 1, pt. 2), 24–31.

Kahn, R.L., & Miller, N.E. Assessment of altered brain function in the aged. In M. Storandt, I.C. Seigler, & M.F. Elias (Eds.), *The clinical psychology of aging*. New York: Plenum, 1978.

+ Kahn, R.L., Zarit, S.H., Hilbert, N.M., & Niederehe, G. Memory complaint and impairment in the aged. *Archives of General Psychiatry*, 1975, *32*, 1569–1573.

Kay, D.W.K., Beamish, P., & Roth, M. Old age mental disorders in Newcastle upon Tyne: A study of prevalence (Part I). *British Journal of Psychiatry*, 1964, *10*, 146–158.

Kay, D.W.K., Cooper, A.F., Garside, R.F., & Roth, M. The differentiation of paranoid from affective psychoses by patients' premorbid characteristics. *British Journal of Psychiatry*, 1976, *129*, 207–215.

Kay, D.W.K., Roth, M., & Hopkins, B. Affective disorders arising in the senium. I. Their association with organic cerebral degeneration. *Journal of Mental Science*, 1955, *101*, 302–314.

Kiloh, L.G. Pseudo-dementia. *Acta Psychiatria Scandinavia*, 1961, *37*, 336–351.

Klerman, G.L. Clinical research in depression. *Archives of General Psychiatry*, 1971, *24*, 305–319.

Klerman, G.L., Rounsaville, B., Chevron, E., Neu, C., & Weissman, M.M. *Manual for short-term interpersonal psychotherapy (IPT) of depression*. Unpublished manuscript. New Haven, Conn.: New Haven–Boston Colloborative Depression Project, 1979.

Kramer, M., Taube, A., & Redick, R.W. Patterns of use of psychiatric facilities by the aged: Past, present and future. In C. Eisdorfer & M.P. Lawton (Eds.), *The psychology of adult development and aging.* Washington, D.C.: American Psychological Association, 1973.

Leff, M.J., Roatch, J.F., & Bunney, W.E. Environmental factors preceding the onset of severe depressions. *Psychiatry,* 1970, *33,* 293–311.

Lewinsohn, P.M., Biglan, A., & Zeiss, A.M. Behavioral treatment of depression. In P.O. Davidson (Ed.), *The behavioral management of anxiety, depression and pain.* New York: Brunner/Mazel, 1976.

Lewinsohn, P.M., & Lee, W.M.L. Assessment of affective disorders. In D.H. Barlow (Ed.), *Behavioral assessment of adult disorders.* New York: Guilford Press, 1981.

Lewinsohn, P.M., & MacPhillamy, D. The relationship between age and engagement in pleasant activities. *Journal of Gerontology,* 1974, *29,* 290–294.

Lewinsohn, P.M., Mischel, W., Chaplin, W., & Barton, R. Social competence and depression: The role of illusory self-perceptions. *Journal of Abnormal Psychology,* 1980, *89,* 203–212.

Lewinsohn, P.M., Munoz, R.F., Youngren, M.A., & Zeiss, A.M. *Control your depression.* Englewood Cliffs, N.J.: Prentice-Hall, 1978.

Lipton, M.A. Age differentiation in depression: Biochemical aspects. *Journal of Gerontology,* 1976, *31,* 293–299.

Loeb, A., Beck, A.T., & Diggory, J. Differential effects of success and failure on depressed and nondepressed patients. *Journal of Nervous and Mental Disease,* 1971, *152,* 106–114.

Mendlewicz, J. The age factor in depressive illness: Some genetic considerations. *Journal of Gerontology,* 1976, *31,* 300–303.

Miller, W.R. Psychological deficit in depression. *Psychological Bulletin,* 1975, *82,* 238–260.

Morris, J.B., & Beck, A.T. The efficiency of anti-depressant drugs: A review of research 1958-1972. *Archives of General Psychiatry,* 1974, *30,* 667–674.

Paykel, E.S. Recent life events and clinical depression. In E.K.E. Gunderson & R.H. Rahe (Eds.), *Life stress and illness.* Springfield, Ill.: Thomas, 1974.

Peak, D. Psychiatric problems of the elderly seen in an outpatient clinic. In E. Pfeiffer (Ed.), *Alternatives to institutional care for older Americans: practice and planning.* Durham, N.C.: Center for the Study of Aging and Human Development, 1973.

Post, F. *The significance of affective symptoms in old age.* London: Oxford University Press, 1962.

Post, F. The management and nature of depressive illness in later life: A follow through study. *British Journal of Psychiatry,* 1972, *121,* 393–404.

Prange, A.J. Pharmacology of depression. In F.F. Flach & S.C. Draghi (Eds.), *The nature and treatment of depression.* New York: Wiley, 1975.

Raskin, A., & Rae, D.S. Psychiatric symptoms in the elderly. *Psychopharmacology Bulletin,* 1981, *17,* 96–99.

Redick, R.W., & Taube, C.A. Demography and mental health care of the aged. In J.E. Birren & R.B. Sloan (Eds.), *Handbook of mental health and aging.* Englewood Cliffs, N.J.: Prentice-Hall, 1980.

Roth, M. The natural history of mental disorder in old age. *Journal of Mental Science,* 1955, *101,* 281–289.

Rubenstein, B., Zaidi, Q., & Kahn, R.L. *Factors affecting the relationship of stress and depression in older persons.* Paper presented at the meetings of the Gerontological Society, New York, 1976.

Rush, A.J., Beck, A.T., Kovacs, M., & Hollon, S. Comparative efficacy of cognitive therapy and imipramine in the treatment of depressed outpatients. *Cognitive Therapy and Research,* 1977, *1,* 17–37.

Salzman, C., & Shader, R.I. Depression in the elderly. I. Relationship between depression, psychological defense mechanisms, and physical illness. *Journal of the American Geriatrics Society,* 1978a, *26,* 253–260.

Salzman, C., & Shader, R.I. Depression in the elderly. II. Possible drug etiologies. Differential diagnostic criteria. Journal of the American Geriatrics Society, 1978b, *26,* 303–308.

Salzman, C., & Shader, R.I. Clinical evaluation of depression in the elderly. In A. Raskin & L. Jarvik (Eds.), *Psychiatric symptoms and cognitive loss in the elderly: evaluation and assessment techniques.* New York: Hemisphere Publishing, 1979.

Seligman, M.E.P. *Helplessness.* San Francisco, Freeman, 1975.

Spitzer, R.L., Endicott, J., & Robins, E. Clinical criteria and the DSM III. *American Journal of Psychiatry,* 1975, *125,* 341–347.

Spitzer, R.L., Endicott, J., & Robins, E. Research diagnostic criteria: Rationale and reliability. *Archives of General Psychiatry,* 1978, *35,* 773–782.

Steuer, J., Bank, L., Olsen, E., & Jarvik, L. Depression, physical health and somatic complaints in the elderly: A study of the Zung self-rating depression scale. *Journal of Gerontology,* 1980, *35,* 683–688.

Velton, E. A laboratory task for induction of mood states. *Behavior Research and Therapy,* 1968, *6,* 473–482.

Vickers, R.V. The therapeutic milieu and the older depressed patient. *Journal of Gerontology,* 1976, *31,* 314–317.

Weingartner, H., Cohen, R.M., Murphy, D.L., Martello, J., & Gerdt, C. Cognitive processes in depression. *Archives of General Psychiatry,* 1981, *38,* 42–47.

Weissman, M.M., & Myers, J.K. Affective disorders in a U.S. urban community. *Archives of General Psychiatry,* 1978, *35,* 1304–1307.

Yesavage, J.A., Brink, T.L., Rose, T.L., Lum, O., Huang, V., Adey, M., & Leirer, V.O. Development and validation of a geriatric depression screening scale: A preliminary report. Unpublished manuscript. Palo Alto, California: Veterans Administration Medical Center, 1982.

Zarit, S.H. *Aging and mental disorders: Psychological approaches to assessment and treatment.* New York: Free Press, 1980.

Zung, W.W.K. A self-rating depression scale. *Archives of General Psychiatry,* 1965, *12,* 63–70.

Zung, W.W.K. Depression in the normal aged. *Psychosomatics,* 1967, *8,* 287–291.

Zung, W.W.K., & Green, R.L. Detection of affective disorders in the aged. In C. Eisdorfer & W.E. Fann (Eds.), *Psychopharmacology and aging.* New York: Plenum, 1972.

3

DEPRESSION IN LATER LIFE: TREATMENT

Judy M. Zarit
Steven H. Zarit

Depression is the most prevalent and important mental health problem of later life. Called the "common cold" of psychiatric disturbances, depression is more like the flu in its impact. It leaves the depressed person drained, and family and friends angry or bewildered. When coupled with health problems, as is often the case for older patients, depression can be a barrier to effective medical treatment.

There are some reasons for optimism, however. Unlike the dementias, depression often résponds to treatment. Sometimes, depressed people even get better on their own. Not enough is known about depression generally, and specific depression in later life, to provide effective treatment in every case. From clinical experience, there appears to be a substantial number of persons for whom no current treatment helps. Thus, making treatment for depressed elders more readily available will have a paradoxical effect: some individuals will indeed benefit markedly, while for others current models and treatments for depression are inadequate.

TREATMENT OF DEPRESSION

Treatment needs to be conducted on a pragmatic basis. Research has not differentiated which approach is better for a patient. When someone does not respond to one kind of regimen, it is important to try a different

GERIATRIC MENTAL HEALTH
ISBN 0-8089-1657-2

approach. It is disheartening to see patients switched from one antidepressant medication to another when there is no apparent response and no attempt to treat the problem in other ways. Likewise, therapists sometimes persist in the same approach even when the patient apparently makes no progress. The pragmatic approach for the professional is to define operational goals for treatment and to conduct continuing evaluations in order to determine the extent to which goals have been met.

Medication is the most frequently used treatment with older patients (Blazer & Williams, 1980). Because many elders do not respond and others cannot tolerate antidepressant drugs, it is important to be able to offer other treatment approaches. Even when medications can be used, a combination of therapy and medication promises better and perhaps longer term results (Rush, Beck, Kovacs et al., 1977; Weissman, Klerman, Prusoff et al., 1981).

Brief, structured psychotherapies have been developed in recent years for treatment of depression. These include the behavioral therapy of Lewinsohn and his associates (Lewinsohn, Biglan, & Zeiss, 1976; Lewinsohn, Munoz, Youngren et al., 1978), Beck's cognitive behavioral therapy (Beck, Rush, Shaw et al., 1979), and interpersonal psychotherapy developed by Klerman and associates (1979). Though developed primarily with younger patients, the behavioral and cognitive–behavioral approaches have had promising trials with older patients (Gallagher, 1981; Gallagher & Thompson, 1982). Although interpersonal psychotherapy will not be described in detail in this chapter, there is every reason to believe that it would have similar success with older persons.

BEHAVIORAL THERAPY FOR DEPRESSION

The treatment program developed by Lewinsohn and his associates (Lewinsohn, Biglan, & Zeiss, 1976; Lewinsohn, Munoz, Youngren et al., 1978) is based on the observed relationship between pleasant, reinforcing activities and mood. Depressed people, it has long been noted, have lower levels of activities. A common-sense remedy for occasional feelings of sadness is to become more active, but that kind of advice does not work for persons who are clinically depressed. Lewinsohn's approach, however, differs in two critical ways.

First, through a series of studies, Lewinsohn and his associates (Lewinsohn & Graf, 1973; Lewinsohn & Libet, 1972; MacPhillamy & Lewinsohn, 1974) have determined that it is not activity per se, but engaging in an activity that the person perceives as pleasant. A key assessment instrument is the Pleasant Events Schedule (PES), which consists of 320 items of potentially enjoyable activities. Clients are asked to indicate what activities they engaged in during the past month and which they perceive as pleasant. This allows the therapist to personalize treatment. Instead of telling someone to become more active, the therapist instructs the client to increase those activities that are perceived as pleasant. Preliminary results indicate findings on the PES are related to depression in older populations as well the younger age groups on which it was developed (Lewinsohn & MacPhillamy, 1974). Samples of items which are found to be pleasant by various different clients can be found in Lewinsohn et al. (1978).

The second aspect of the treatment program is sophisticated behavioral interventions to help a depressed, inactive individual to increase activities. The first step is to convince clients of the relationship between activities and depression, which is done by gathering information on mood and activities during a baseline period. Clients write down their daily activities and give a daily mood a score on a scale from 1 to 10, with "1" indicating very depressed mood and "10" very happy mood. Because there generally will be some daily variations, the therapist can use that information for demonstrating that activity affects mood. The next step is to increase the activities that are associated with less depression. Lewinsohn and his colleagues (1978) provide examples of record-keeping done by clients in order to ascertain a relationship between mood and pleasant activities.

Another aspect of therapist intervention is to break assignments down into a series of small, manageable steps. Most depressed clients cannot suddenly resume their previous level of activity and may feel overwhelmed by the idea. It is important for clients to take some small steps to see where they lead rather than continuing to be inactive. However, if goals are set too high, clients may not succeed, which would reinforce their negative self-evaluation. Clients also may be reluctant to make small changes, saying that they do not see how it will make a difference. The therapist provides the rationale that they did not become depressed overnight and it will take some time to overcome habits that are keeping them depressed. Assignments for activities need to be practical and manageable, and the therapist should help the client anticipate potential problems in carrying out a particular assignment.

The therapist also can increase compliance by developing an explicit plan for increasing activities, such as working out a schedule of activities for the next week with the client. There can be a contract between the client and therapist for following this plan, including contingencies for completing each part of it. Clients can reward themselves for compliance or the therapist can reward them. One very potent reinforcer for compliance is to reduce the fees of the therapy session when tasks have been completed (Lewinsohn, Biglan, & Zeiss, 1976).

While the major thrust of behavioral treatment is to increase pleasant events, other factors are considered also. Depressed persons sometimes have a moderate level of activities or events in their lives that tend to be aversive. The therapist may intervene in several ways, one possibility being to generate a plan that creates a balance between unpleasant activities the client has to do and more rewarding events. More effective management of aversive events can also be helpful. Certain types of reality-based problems, such as those involving money or health, may require the therapist to become an advocate for the client. For instance, one severely depressed and potentially suicidal older woman was troubled by her lack of income, among other things. Putting her in touch with agencies that place elders in jobs was a key to successful outcome.

Other aspects of the therapy include relaxation training, social-skills training, and cognitive interventions (Lewinsohn, Munoz, Youngren, & Zeiss, 1978). Relaxation is useful in providing some immediate relief from emotional tension and also may assist in controlling related problems such as insomnia. While relaxation has not yet been used widely with older persons, clinical impressions are that the response is generally good (Zarit, 1980). Because many potentially pleasant activities involve interpersonal situations, the therapist must assess social skills of clients for implementing planned activities. Some depressed persons have been found to have deficits in interpersonal skills (Lewinsohn, Biglan, & Zeiss, 1976; Lewinsohn & Lee, 1981). The therapist can use a variety of approaches to build social skills, including shaping, modeling, behavioral and cognitive rehearsal, and assertion training. The interpersonal therapy of Klerman et al. (1979) has additional suggestions. Finally, cognitive procedures are used to identify and modify self-defeating and negative thoughts similar to the methods of Beck and his associates (1979). These are decribed below.

Outcome studies with both younger and older persons have been promising (Lewinsohn, Biglan, & Zeiss, 1976; Gallagher & Thompson, 1981). Besides overall improvement by patients, the hypothesis of a relationship between increasing pleasant events and improving mood has been consistently supported.

COGNITIVE THERAPY OF DEPRESSION

In contrast to the emphasis on behavioral treatment of activities, the cognitive–behavioral treatment of depression considers the role of thoughts in determining feelings of depression (Beck, 1976; Beck, Rush, Shaw, & Emery, 1979). Although the depressed person may have experienced some losses, it is the tendency to exaggerate the negative implications and maintain a depressed mood that distinguishes depressed from nondepressed persons suffering similar setbacks. The cognitive–behavioral approach consists of procedures to assist clients in identifying the thoughts that are associated with depressed mood and learn to substitute more adaptive ways of thinking about themselves or others.

As with the behavioral approach, cognitive–behavioral treatment begins with recording daily activities and mood. After establishing this baseline recording, the first therapeutic intervention is usually to increase the client's daily activities, with emphasis placed on activities that are pleasant or involve mastery. Beginning by increasing activities is useful in providing some initial relief to the depressed patient (Beck, Rush, Shaw, & Emery, 1979). There is also considerable planning within treatment sessions to ensure compliance, including working-out a daily plan or schedule and identifying obstacles ahead of time that might prevent carrying out the schedule.

Activities also have a different purpose in cognitive–behavioral treatment. As the therapist discusses a plan with a client or the results of previous assignments, some of the client's negative thoughts are likely to be expressed, which gives the therapist the opportunity to demonstrate the relationship between negative thoughts and feelings and how they prevent clients from engaging in potentially positive behaviors. For instance, when scheduling an activity such as cleaning the house, a client may state that she cannot possibly do it. The therapist will then determine if the client can perform some portion of the activity (e.g., cleaning one room or cleaning for a specific period of time). Clients can usually find some part of a task they can complete, at which time the therapist can point out how the client's negative thinking resulted in both feeling more depressed and stopping herself from taking action.

The formal quality of depressed persons' thoughts involves distortions of reality. For instance, depressed persons may exaggerate negative experiences or infer negative consequences when none are present. Another belief, that one cannot do anything, is an instance of absolutist, "all-or-nothing," thinking. Sometimes the depressed person perceives the world through extremes of perfection and imperfection and reacts to any imperfection by being disappointed in oneself or others. Beck et al. (1979), Burns (1980), and others have discussed in detail the thought-patterns of depressed persons.

As the therapist is able to help clients identify some of the specific thoughts they are having, an assessment procedure called *thought records* is introduced. Clients use the thought records to identify situations in which they feel depressed and, if possible, to note what they are thinking. Initially, they may not be able to capture their thoughts, but the therapist can bring these out by careful questioning during sessions. In time, clients learn to identify what they are thinking in daily situations and generate an alternative, rational response to their dysfunctional thoughts. Examples of thought records can be found in Beck et al. (1979) and Burns (1980).

The crucial aspect of treatment is to teach clients how to evaluate their thoughts and generate alternatives. Clients will initially report that they believe their interpretation of events to be correct and that they are depressed because of deficiencies in themselves or others that they insist are "real." They do not believe that they have any alternatives and may regard attempts to get them to look at positive aspects of themselves or their situations as merely positive thinking. Cognitive–behavioral therapy is not treatment through optimistic thinking, however. Rather, the major emphasis is teaching clients to elicit evidence for supporting the beliefs they hold (Beck, et al., 1979).

The process of changing beliefs is done through an inductive method. In contrast to other cognitive therapies, such as Rational Emotive Therapy (Ellis & Harper, 1973), the therapist does not challenge the client's thoughts. Rather the therapist asks questions which enable clients to examine their beliefs and to develop alternative responses. In an example from Beck, *et al.* (1979), a patient reported that her adolescent children did not want to socialize with her. Instead of assuming that the patient's conclusion about her children was correct, the therapist first questioned her about how she had determined it. He then elicited evidence from her that suggested an alternative interpretation of those events, which more closely fit the evidence. By the therapist's provocative questioning of her beliefs, the patient was able to ask her son to go to the movies with her, and, in fact, he was willing to do so.

A case example with an older client illustrates how questioning clients about their thoughts both improves their moods and leads to more adaptive behaviors:

> A 60-year-old woman wanted to get a job as one of her goals, so that she could have more money than the meager amount she received from her husband's Social Security. She believed, however, that no one would hire her because of her age and that she would never find a job. With some help from her therapist, she was willing to risk finding out if her belief would be confirmed and went out on some interviews. She liked one job very much and reported that the interview went well, but when she did not hear from them in over a week, concluded that they must have hired someone else who was younger. Through questioning, the therapist helped her consider other alternatives ("They had an applicant who was more qualified." "I can do a good job." "It just would take more time to find someone who would recognize me.") and then encouraged her to call the company during the session to find out what happened. When she called, they replied that they had been trying to reach her because they liked her and wanted her to come for a second interview. She subsequently got the job.

This example illustrates how depressed persons react to ordinary disappointments by negatively exaggerating the results, as well as how negativity interferes with more adaptive behaviors.

Gradually, clients learn how to examine thoughts on their own and to provide alternative, rational responses. In effect, they learn to monitor their own thoughts and feelings, and to head off problems using the strategies they have learned in therapy. Studies of outcome are positive (Beck, Rush, Shaw et al., 1979; Rush, Beck, Kovacs et al., 1977), including those with elderly patients (Emery, Gallagher, Thompson et al., in press).

COMMON FEATURES OF THERAPIES FOR DEPRESSION

Although differing in their emphasis, both the behavioral and cognitive–behavioral treatments share similar components of how the therapy is structured and presented to clients. These common features may be as important to successful treatment of depression as the specific behavioral or cognitive–behavioral interventions. Among the important components are a structured and collaborative approach to therapy, emphasis on daily events, socialization to therapy, and teaching clients to monitor themselves.

A STRUCTURED AND COLLABORATIVE APPROACH. Both the behavioral and cognitive–behavioral treatments of depression are highly structured, brief, and time-limited. The therapist works within a time framework of approximately 16 sessions. These sessions are weekly, although Beck and his associates (1979) often begin with twice-weekly sessions for the first month. Clinical experience with older persons indicates a somewhat longer period may be desirable, perhaps 20 sessions (Emery, Gallagher, Thompson et al., in press; Gallagher & Thompson, 1981).

Therapy sessions are goal-oriented and structured. Both the behavioral and cognitive-behavioral approaches are composed of a series of assessment and treatment techniques, which are introduced in a recommended order, although the therapist can be flexible in responding to the needs of a particular case. Each treatment session will have relatively specific objectives. These may be introducing a particular treatment concept, such as the relation between mood and engaging in certain behaviors, or teaching the client how to use a personal assessment procedure.

The therapist's role is that of collaborator and requires active participation in the therapy session. In one sense the therapist is a teacher, instructing the client in the rationale for treatment. While the therapist is the "expert" in techniques, the client is the "expert" in his or her own activities and idiosyncratic thought patterns. Elevating clients from passive recipients of treatment to the role of collaborator allows them to regain their self-esteem.

The amount of structure, as well as the high activity of the therapist, is undoubtedly important in generating the rapid improvements that have been observed. Because depressed persons are lethargic and often feel hopeless, they might have difficulty mobilizing themselves to make changes in an unstructured therapy session. The behavioral or cognitive–behavioral therapist continually challenges the client in a supportive way in order to generate changes to reduce depression.

FOCUS ON EVERYDAY BEHAVIORS. Another major feature of both therapies is the emphasis on behaviors, thoughts, and feelings that occur between sessions, rather on the interaction of client and therapist. This represents a major difference from dynamic and client-centered therapies. The relationship of the treatment to the client is important, of course, and Beck et al. (1979) specifically discuss how to create positive psychotherapeutic rapport with empathy, warmth and a nonjudgmental attitude. While these attitudes are facilitative, they are not the core of the treatment. Rather, the therapist actively guides clients toward certain changes.

There are times when the therapist will use occurrences within the therapy session to demonstrate a therapeutic principle. Beck particularly cites examples of how the exchanges in the session can be used to illustrate to the client the relationship between thoughts and feelings. The ultimate goal is for the client to generalize learning in the therapy session to everyday behavior, not to work through the relationship with the therapist.

Despite the active role of therapists, both treatments are client-centered in that they work toward clients' goals. The overriding aims are to reduce the clients' feelings of depression and to make specific changes clients choose.

Socialization to therapy. Since both therapies stress the active collaboration of clients, it is important that clients have an understanding of the therapy process. Socialization to therapy has generally received very little attention. Clients are likely to have a relatively naive view of what occurs in therapy, views that have been gleaned from novels and movies or television. Popular writings about psychology do not consistently provide an understanding either, and may, in some cases, even act as a hindrance. Outcome in dynamic therapy has been found to improve considerably by spending from one-to-three sessions with clients explaining how the therapy will operate (Orne & Wender, 1968). In behavioral treatments, training clients to be an active part of their own therapy has taken on increasing importance (Thoreson & Mahoney, 1974).

Socialization to therapy may be even more important for older persons, whose understanding of psychological constructs can be limited. Beliefs sometimes encountered are that talking cannot make a difference and/or that only someone who is severely disturbed should get professional help. Unless identified early, these beliefs can contribute to the client's dropping out of treatment. By discussing the goals and procedures of treatment openly with clients, these obstacles can be overcome.

Both therapies for depression explain to clients how the therapy works and how the client can use treatment to reduce feelings of depression. Lewinsohn and his associates (1978) stress the relationship between activities and depression, using concrete examples. Clients can often relate to a vignette involving someone else. The example of the women felt depressed whether the therapist was early, on time, or late, can be used to demonstrate how thoughts affect feelings. Clients are also given the booklet, *Coping with*

Depression (Beck & Greenberg, 1974), which provides a rationale for the therapy.

Telling clients how therapy works also creates a situation in which they might reject the proposed course of treatment. Because of their pessimistic beliefs, depressed patients are especially likely to be skeptical about therapy. Rather than an obstacle to treatment, this situation represents an opportunity to examine barriers to accepting the rationale and gives the client fewer opportunities to passively subvert the direction of treatment.

For both treatments, the general approach to reluctant clients is to develop a contract with them whereby they try certain procedures and judge for themselves whether or not they are effective. In cases of severely depressed persons, Beck (1976) will sometimes challenge them directly in an initial session in order to engage them in treatment. For instance, when a patient complains that he cannot do anything, the therapist may hand that person a pencil and paper and ask him to draw a line. This task helps the therapist demonstrate that the client's original thought of being unable to do anything was an exaggeration and to suggest that treatment will involve finding out how many other things the patient can do. Clients do not have to be convinced completely that a treatment will work, but they should have some, however small, expectation of success. They can even be encouraged to view treatment as an experiment, in which they try different things to remediate their depression.

SELF-MONITORING BY CLIENTS. An integral part of both therapies is for the therapist to teach clients to monitor their moods, thoughts and behaviors. As noted earlier, both approaches begin by determining current activities. Clients complete a daily record of activities as well as noting their mood on a 1 to 10 scale. A variety of other self-monitoring procedures are gradually introduced, such as thought records or charts to indicate the frequency with which clients engage in certain pleasant events.

Self-monitoring has several important functions. First, the records clients keep at the beginning of treatment provide a baseline. This serves to gauge the overall success of the treatment. These records also function to demonstrate the effectiveness of specific interventions. By reviewing their records, clients are able to recognize that their moods do fluctuate because of certain behaviors or thoughts. Typically, they would be unable to make that connection if they relied only on memory. Sometimes the connection between behaviors or thoughts and mood will come as a surprise to the client, as he or she did not see how they were linked until the therapist pointed it out. What starts out as very mysterious determinants of mood will gradually turn out to be under the client's control. The important association of everyday events, whether thoughts or behaviors and moods, is made possible to a large extent by self-monitoring.

Self-monitoring can have an immediate therapeutic effect for some clients. Typical depressed patients report sweeping and global states of dysphoria. When asked if they ever feel a little better, they may say no. Once they monitor their moods, however, they will discover that there are fluctuations and this can create a sense of hopefulness. In recording daily activities, they may similarly discover that they are more active than they first thought. In controlled studies, self-monitoring by clients has been found to have a significant treatment effect, even when no other interventions are done (Harmon, Nelson, & Hayes, 1980).

Along with the collaborative relationship between the therapist, self-monitoring places depressed clients in an active role. They learn that they are not helpless in determining mood, but instead, there are things they can do to identify immediate causes of depression and how they can intervene. Learning how they can monitor themselves gives them a strategy for solving problems after therapy ends.

COMMON PROBLEMS IN THERAPY WITH OLDER CLIENTS

Both cognitive and behavioral treatment for depression require some modification for use with the elderly. As noted previously, treatment may take a few more sessions. Most often this is because it takes longer to establish rapport needed by allowing the client to relate relevant history. One or two sessions may be spent on history with a young client, but it may take three or four sessions to cover the events of sixty, seventy, or eighty years. Similarly, older clients may have been practicing maladaptive thoughts or behaviors for much longer than younger clients, so it sometimes requires more patience on the therapist's part because the client clings to well-established patterns. Clients often reflect the therapist's worst fears when they say, "I'm too old to change." This dysfunctional thought is dealt with directly in cognitive therapy because the therapist helps set up an experiment to see whether or not the client is capable of *any* change or may elicit examples of recent small changes the client has made. In behavioral terms, the client is shown that becoming depressed required a change in behavior and that the aim of the therapy is to use that ability to change in a positive way.

Chronic and acute medical problems and normal physiological changes that occur with age often play an important role in the etiology of depression in older clients. Very often the issue must be one of adjusting to limitations and maximizing remaining strengths rather than clinging to the hope of a return to youth and vigor. This concept must be understood thoroughly and accepted by the therapist if the client is going to be convinced of it in therapy.

Therapists who work with the elderly should have a firm understanding of the aging process so that they can view age as an asset to be enhanced rather than a degenerative process. This requires some exposure to well-functioning elders who differ from the depressed elderly only in mood, *not* in the extent of disability or age-related changes.

Older persons who have experienced multiple losses, such as death of loved-ones, health limitations, loss of income and employment, and forced relocation are particularly vulnerable to depression. If these changes come in close proximity to each other, poor decisions may be made and the person may be overwhelmed by the cascade of events. Sometimes therapists may need to become advocates for depressed elder clients to ensure that they receive the benefits they are entitled to, especially when they clearly are not able to understand the labyrinth of regulations that must be understood to successfully navigate the Social Security and Medicare systems. Though it is important not to infantilize older clients by doing too much for them, the therapist must recognize in which situations it is appropriate to intervene.

WHEN TREATMENT FOR DEPRESSION MAY NOT WORK

There is a small group of older clients who initially present with classic symptoms of depression, but who do not respond to therapy as one would expect. Using the Schedule of Affective Disorders and Schizophrenia (SADS) in conjunction with the Research and Diagnostic Criteria, this group of clients will be diagnosed with a major depressive disorder. A very careful history will reveal that they have poor relationship skills and that their social adjustment always have been marginal. Often they are quite intelligent and were physically attractive when younger. They had relied on these two qualities to attract people and get jobs, but lacked the skills to develop lasting relationships. Consequently they are likely to have changed jobs and marriages frequently. Now confronted with physical changes, they feel less attractive and experience a reduced capacity for finding new employment. Their style of coping has been seriously undermined by age and they respond with anger and depression. There may be a paranoid flavor to their thoughts as well.

During therapy this type of client may appear to pick up the rationale very quickly and can master the technique with little effort. But each time a negative behavior or thought is changed it is down-graded in importance and replaced by another. While the depressed person may appear to be responding to treatment the fundamental problem remains the same. Some authors feel that this type of person has a characterological or personality disorder. When this is found to be the case, short-term treatment for depression may have to be reconsidered and longer term therapy for the client may be indicated. The problem becomes most evident at the termination of short-term treatment when the client will become angry and/or dependent and will sometimes threaten suicide. It is important to try to identify this type of disorder early, but it is not always possible. Indeed, their very intelligence and sophistication about psychotherapy allows these clients to initially mask the quality of their thoughts.

SUMMARY

Psychotherapies that are time-limited and structured have had promising results with depression in later life. Common features include placing the client in an active, collaborative role, socializing clients to therapy, focusing on everyday behaviors and thoughts that are associated with greater or lesser feelings of depression, and training clients to monitor their own mood and behaviors. Applying the psychotherapeutic techniques to depressed elderly patients very frequently results in significant improvement in mood and functioning.

REFERENCES

Beck, A.T. *Cognitive therapy and the emotional disorders.* New York: International Universities Press, 1976.

Beck, A.T., & Greenberg, R.L. *Coping with depression.* New York: Institute for Rational Living, 1974.

Beck, A.T., Rush, A.J., Shaw, B.F., & Emery, C. *Cognitive therapy of depression.* New York: Guilford Press, 1979.

Blazer, D.G., & Williams, C.D. The epidemiology of dysphoria and depression in an elderly population. *American Journal of Psychiatry,* 1980, *137,* 439–444.

Burns, D. *Feeling good.* New York: William Morrow, 1980.

Ellis, A., & Harper, R.A. *A guide to rational living.* N. Hollywood, California: Wilshire Book Co., 1973.

Emery, G., Gallagher, D.E., Thompson, L.W., Bisno, B., Kahn, J., & Zarit, J.M. *Cognitive therapy of depression in older adults.* New York: Guilford Press, in press.

Gallagher, D. Behavioral group therapy with elderly depressives: An experimental study. In D. Upper & S. Ross (Eds.), *Behavioral group therapy, 1981.* Champaign, Ill.: Research Press, 1981.

Gallagher, D., & Thompson, L.W. *Depression in the elderly: A behavioral treatment manual.* Los Angeles: University of Southern California Press, 1981.

Gallagher, D., & Thompson, L.W. Cognitive therapy for depression in the elderly: A promising model for treatment and research. In L. Breslau & M. Haug (Eds.), *Depression in the elderly.* New York: Springer, 1982.

Harmon, T.M., Nelson, R.O., & Hayes, S.C. Self-monitoring of mood versus activity by depressed clients. *Journal of Consulting and Clinical Psychology,* 1980, *48,* 30–38.

Klerman, G.L., Rounsaville, B., Chevron, E., Neu, C., & Weisman, M.M. *Manual for short-term interpersonal psychotherapy (IPT) of depression.* Unpublished manuscript. New Haven, Conn.: New Haven–Boston Colloborative Depression Project, 1979.

Lewinsohn, P.M., Biglan, A., & Zeiss, A.M. Behavioral treatment of depression. In P.C. Davidson (Ed.), *The behavioral management of anxiety, depression and pain.* New York: Brunner/Mazel, 1976.

Lewinsohn, P.M., & Graf, M. Pleasant activities and depression. *Journal of Consulting and Clinical Psychology,* 1973, *41,* 261–268.

Lewinsohn, P.M., & Lee, W.M.L. Assessment of affective disorders. In D.H. Barlow (Ed.), *Behavioral assessment of adult disorders.* New York: Guilford Press, 1981.

Lewinsohn, P.M., & Libet, J. Pleasant events, activity schedules, and depression. *Journal of Abnormal Psychology,* 1972, *79,* 291–295.

Lewinsohn, P.M., & MacPhillamy, D. The relationship between age and engagement in pleasant activities. *Journal of Gerontology,* 1974, *29,* 290–294.

Lewinsohn, P.M., Munoz, R.F., Youngren, M.A., & Zeiss, A.M. *Control your depression.* Englewood Cliffs, N.J.: Prentice-Hall, 1978.

MacPhillamy, D.J., & Lewinsohn, P.M. Depression as a function of levels of desired and obtained pleasure. *Journal of Abnormal Psychology,* 1974, *83,* 651–657.

Orne, M.T., & Wender, P.H. Anticipatory socialization for psychotherapy: Method and rationale. *American Journal of Psychiatry,* 1968, *124,* 1202–1212.

Rush, A.J., Beck, A.T., Kovacs, M., & Hollon, S. Comparative efficacy of cognitive therapy and imipramine in the treatment of depressed outpatients. *Cognitive Therapy and Research,* 1977, *1,* 17–37.

Thoresen, C.E., & Mahoney, M.J. *Behavioral self-control.* New York: Holt, Rinehart & Winston, 1974.

Weissman, M.M., Klerman, G.L., Prusoff, B.A., Sholomskas, D., & Padian, N. Depressed outpatients. *Archives of General Psychiatry,* 1981, *38,* 51–55.

Zarit, S.H. *Aging and mental disorders. Psychological approaches to assessment and treatment.* New York: Free Press, 1980.

4

RECENT DEVELOPMENTS IN THE ASSESSMENT OF SENILE DEMENTIA*

Steven H. Ferris
Barry Reisberg
Mony de Leon
Thomas Crook

Cognitive deterioration in the elderly represents an immense medical and sociological burden. It has been estimated that at least 10 percent of the aged, a total of more than 3 million persons, will eventually suffer severe mental deterioration. A much larger number will experience sufficient cognitive decline which will impede their activities and compound the normal problems of aging. More than half the residents in nursing homes have been classified as senile, and the major form of dementia is now thought to be the fourth major cause of death. The true cost to society, in terms of loss of skilled labor, nursing and medical care, and institutional requirements, is difficult to estimate. The cost to individuals and their families is incalculable and often tragic.

The Diagnostic and Statistical Manual of the American Psychiatric

*Supported in part by grants MH 29590, MH 36969, AG 03051, and NS 15638

GERIATRIC MENTAL HEALTH
ISBN 0-8089-1657-2

Association (DSM III) defines dementia as a loss of intellectual abilities that may include, in addition to impairment of memory, deficits in abstract thinking, judgment, and other higher cortical functions. The diagnosis and detailed assessment of senile dementia is often a complex and lengthy process. The purpose of this chapter is to review the recommended clinical assessment procedures, as well as to discuss some recent research concerning the development of improved assessment measures.

CLINICAL DIAGNOSIS OF SENILE DEMENTIA

The three primary subtypes of dementia should be familiar to all professionals dealing with geriatric patients. The major subtype is a progressive degenerative brain disease known by several names: Senile Dementia of the Alzheimer's type (SDAT), Alzheimer's disease, or in terms of DSM III, primary degenerative dementia (PDD). Several fairly consistent autopsy studies have shown that approximately 50 percent of dementias can be categorized as being due to this degenerative disease of unknown etiology. The second major category erroneously has been called cerebral arteriosclerosis, or "hardening of the arteries of the head." As recently as 15 years ago, this syndrome was generally thought to be the usual cause of dementia. This vascular type of dementia is related to stroke pathology and is now called Multi-Infarct Dementia (MID). In its pure form, MID is actually relatively rare, accounting for only about 15 percent of cases. There is also a mixed patient group that on autopsy shows evidence for both SDAT and MID. The mixed group accounts for about 25 percent of cases. Finally, about 10 percent are in the "other" category. This miscellaneous group includes *pseudodementia,* which is really a manifestation of depression. It also includes a wide variety of other potentially treatable illnesses that can lead to dementia-like symptomatology. A good clinical workup for dementia must focus on excluding these many possible etiologies.

Since SDAT and MID may have quite different prognostic and treatment implications, it is important to differentiate the vascular type of dementia from the Alzheimer's type. In terms of clinical history, MID tends to have an abrupt onset and a step-wise course, whereas Alzheimer's disease has an insidious onset and its course generally tends to be very gradual. A rating instrument, known as the Modified Ischemia Scale (Rosen, Terry, Fuld et al., 1980), that can be helpful in making this differential diagnosis has now come into common use. Some limited data is available concerning the validity of this scale, that is, its correlation with postmortem diagnosis. The scale contains a variety of items given relative weights with respect to their likelihood of predicting a multi-infarct diagnosis. The items include abrupt onset, stepwise deterioration, actual history of stroke, and focal neurological signs and symptoms. There are cutoff scores that are somewhat arbitrary, but that seem to have predictive value for identifying a multi-infarct etiology.

In general, the diagnosis of Alzheimer's disease is made by excluding other possible causes. Since the ultimate diagnosis is based upon postmortem findings (senile plaque and neurofibrillary tangles), there is no positive clinical diagnosis. But a diagnosis of Alzheimer's disease by exclusion can be made by ruling out numerous other possible causes of cognitive decline. These include MID, depression or pseudodementia, as well as a wide variety of medical conditions (Cummings, Benson, & LoVerme, 1980). For example, there are various toxic agents, drug effects, nutritional deficiencies, infections, endocrine problems, and a variety of other kinds of cerebral diseases that can temporarily or permanently produce symptoms that could lead to a misdiagnosis of senile dementia. A thorough medical evaluation is essential to rule out some of these many possible causes. The components of a good medical workup should include a thorough medical and psychiatric history, a physical and neurological exam, an electrocardiogram (EKG), an electroencephalogram (EEG) (spectrally analyzed, if available), a computerized tomographic scan (CT), and a complete clinical laboratory battery (SMA–18, CBC with differential, urinalysis, thyroid function tests, B_{12}, and folate levels). None of these assessments provide a positive diagnosis of Alzheimer's disease, but they assist in ruling out MID or various other potential etiologies or contributory conditions.

CLINICAL EVALUATION OF COGNITIVE SYMPTOMS

With respect to the clinical presentation of age-associated cognitive decline, or its more serious manifestation, primary degenerative dementia, it is useful to divide the clinical course of cognitive decline into three general broad phases. Reisberg, Ferris, de Leon et al. (1982), have called these the *forgetfulness phase,* the *confusional phase,* and the *dementia phase.* Those who work with elderly patients on a day-to-day basis will recognize many of the descriptive criteria for these phases.

Forgetfulness phase

The initial forgetfulness phase, which may or may not progress to a full dementia, involves complaints of misplacing objects, forgetting names, and having trouble with concentration. To a slight degree, these are complaints all individuals occasionally experience, but in aging and very early dementia, these symptoms occur more frequently. However, basic cognitive abilities remain intact and there is really no overt loss of functional capacity. One remains capable of maintaining a job and social relationships, and there are no significant psychiatric symptoms.

Confusional Phase

As the syndrome progresses to the confusional phase, one begins to see more significant changes that are objectively measurable. A good clinician or a psychometrician can quantitate, either in an interview or with psychometric tests, the presence of significant memory impairment. Deficits in recent memory are most evident, as demonstrated by a reduced knowledge of current events. There may be a change in affect at this point. However, the impairment of these individuals is still relatively mild. Such patients can certainly recognize family members, their ability to give a personal history is quite good, they are reasonably well oriented to place and person, and by and large, their activities of daily living are reasonably intact despite a significant performance deficit.

Dementia phase

Finally, the syndrome progresses to the severe dementia phase. It begins at the point at which the patient, if left entirely on his own, would not be able to survive. There is very little, if any, memory retention for recent events at this stage, and there is a definite loss of knowledge about their past as well. They may begin to fail to recognize a spouse, even though that is the person they are dependent on for staying alive. At this stage, or perhaps a little earlier, there also may be serious psychiatric symptoms. These may include delusions and hallucinations.

A rating scale is now available for evaluating these various stages of symptomatology and for precisely staging the course of the illness. It is called the Global Deterioration Scale (GDS) (Reisberg, Ferris, de Leon et al. 1982). The scale involves seven rating points covering the full range of severity from normal to very severe. There are very precise, detailed criteria that anchor each rating point. The GDS allows clinicians to define the global severity of any cognitively impaired patient.

A clinical rating scale, called the Brief Cognitive Rating Scale (BCRS), and specifically designed for the detailed evaluation of various components of the cognitive symptoms of PDD, is also now available (Reisberg, Schneck, Ferris, et al., 1983). Separate ratings, on a seven-point scale, are obtained for concentration, recent memory, past memory, orientation, functioning and selfcare. Detailed criteria are provided for the rating points of each category.

PSYCHOMETRIC TESTING

It is important to realize that in the very early phases of dementia, there are some difficult diagnostic issues. To some extent, there is a normal, slowly developing deficit in certain areas of cognitive function with the normal aging process. There is also Kral's (1978) notion of "benign senescent forgetfulness" which is quite mild and does not progress very much with time. On the other hand, in Alzheimer's disease or PDD, there clearly is a progressive, downhill course over a number of years. The difficult problem is to distinguish between the very early stages of dementia and normal or benign decline. For example, if a patient appears with subjective complaints of poor memory, how can a clinician distinguish between the benign or normal age changes and the malignant changes of primary degenerative dementia? Assuming that a thorough medical evaluation has ruled out the various possible causes discussed previously, it becomes important to properly define in detail the nature and extent of cognitive impairment in order to help make this distinction.

To properly assess cognitive impairment, it is essential to do objective cognitive evaluations, also known as psychometric or neuropsychological testing. One value of these tests is that they can verify whether there is, in fact, some mild impairment. For example, depressed patients often complain of cognitive impairment, but data suggest that they do not show gross impairment despite their serious complaints. However, in documenting whether or not there is mild impairment, the catch is that such decisions require tests that have a very good normative data base. This is a serious problem in the field of assessing geriatric patients, since there are not very many, if any, good tests that have adequate norms.

Tests are also helpful for grading the severity of impairment. In a research environment, there may be certain criteria for the severity of patients required for a research protocol. Cognitive tests can be very helpful for meeting these criteria. They also assist in comparing populations between different clinical or research centers. Finally, tests are useful for documenting change in cognitive symptoms due to treatment or the longitudinal course of the illness.

The importance of cognitive tests for diagnosis decreases as the severity of symptoms increases. On the other hand, clinical mental status instruments such as the Mental Status Questionnaire (MSQ) (Kahn, Goldfarb, Pollack et al., 1960) tend to be insensitive in testing the severity for patients with very mild impairment, but become more useful as severity increases. These conclusions are illustrated in Figure 4-1, with the seven-point GDS levels of global severity indicated at the bottom. For the very mild stages (GDS 1–3), the ten mental status questions of the MSQ show few, if any, errors. As a result, this type of instrument shows no discrimination regarding different levels of severity. On the other hand, at the more severe end of the severity continuum (GDS 4–7), the MSQ is a sensitive instrument, as demonstrated by the ascending graph. The descending graph represents the results for an objective psychometric test, the Guild Memory Test (Gilbert, Levee, & Catalano, 1968). For GDS 1–3, the Guild clearly delineates different levels of impairment. But for GDS 4–7, there is floor effect (zero

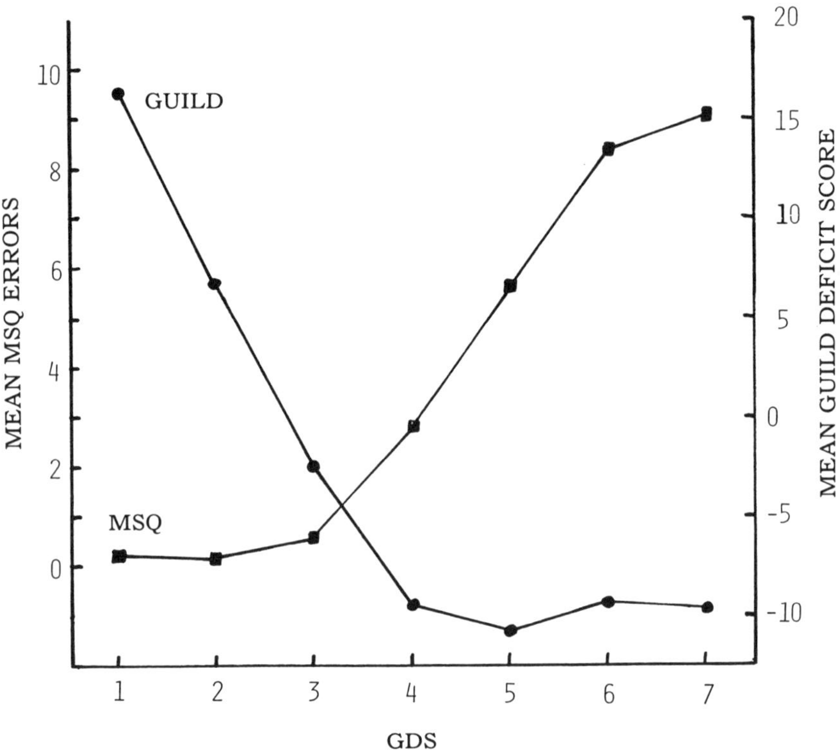

Figure 4-1. Mean Mental Status Questionnaire (MSQ) errors and mean Guild Memory Test deficit scores for the seven levels of severity on the Global Deterioration Scale (GDS). The number of subjects for each GDS level were: 1 = 27, 2 = 62, 3 = 41, 4 = 28, 5 = 19, 6 = 11, 7 = 19.

scores) and the Guild no longer discriminates among levels of severity. Thus, the clinical evaluation is certainly useful at the more severe end of the spectrum, but objective cognitive tests can be very helpful at the mild end of the spectrum. The gap between the MSQ and cognitive tests has been narrowed by the use of extended mental status evaluations such as the Mini Mental State (Folstein, Folstein, & McHugh, 1975). This scale is much more useful since it is a hybrid between the standard clinical interview questions and some objective cognitive assessment measures.

For diagnostic purposes, several cognitive tests are available that evaluate memory. Wechsler's (1945) well-known Wechsler Memory Scale has some significant limitations, including a lack of adequate norms. The Guild Memory Test has some advantages (Crook, Gilbert, & Ferris, 1980), but the norms are also not adequate. There is also the Fuld Object Memory

Test (Fuld, 1980), for which there is some normative data, as well as the extended mental status evaluations such as the Mini Mental State.

Table 4-1 illustrates the ability of cognitive tests to differentiate three groups of subjects: a young normal group, an elderly normal group (GDS = 1), and a mildly impaired elderly group (GDS = 3–4). The vocabulary function of the impaired elderly group on the WAIS Vocabulary test is not particularly impaired. There also is not much change on digit span, a result that has been reported extensively in the past. Digit Symbol does show a substantial deficit in the elderly impaired group as well as in normal aging. On the memory measures of the Guild Memory Test, there is a consistent, statistically significant, normal aging deficit and a much more dramatic impairment in the mildly impaired dementia group.

The results for the rather limited psychometric battery described above, illustrate a somewhat typical pattern of deficit found in patients with early to moderate Alzheimer's disease, namely, marked impairment on tests of recent memory (the cardinal symptom) and on integrative tasks such as the Digit Symbol Substitution Test (DSST), but relative sparing of immediate memory and overlearned functions such as vocabulary. However, exam-

Table 4-1.

Mean Scores of the Three Subject Groups on Standardized Psychometric Tests.

Measure	Elderly Impaired (N = 60)	Elderly Normal (N = 44)	Young Normal (N = 63)
WAIS			
Vocabulary*	13.7 (3.3)	15.4 (2.9)	14.7 (2.9)
Digit symbol*	6.3 (2.7)	8.6 (2.0)	13.3 (2.5)
Digit span			
Forward	6.8 (1.4)	7.2 (1.3)	7.3 (1.3)
Backward	4.5 (1.1)	5.5 (1.5)	5.7 (1.3)
Guild memory test			
Paragraphs:			
Immediate	5.3 (2.9)	9.7 (2.3)	11.1 (3.1)
Delayed	5.0 (3.5)	12.3 (3.0)	14.6 (3.8)
Paired associates:			
Immediate	1.4 (1.3)	4.6 (1.8)	6.7 (1.9)
Delayed	1.4 (1.4)	5.4 (1.9)	8.1 (2.1)

Note: SD's are in parentheses.
* Standard scaled scores

ination of mean scores for groups tends to mask the considerable individual differences between patients in the pattern of deficits.

In order to fully describe the pattern of deficits in individual cases, a more complete psychometric battery for clinical assessment of dementia is recommended. An optimal battery should include measures of attention, spatial ability, language ability (aphasia), constructional ability (apraxia), abstract thinking, and problem solving. In some of these areas, there may be considerable variability among patients with respect to degree of deficit. For example, many but not all patients have some degree of aphasia, and a smaller proportion of patients have apraxia. However, the issue of the typical versus individual symptom profile tends to be confounded with the issue of disease severity. In severe Alzheimer's disease, all aspects of cognitive function are profoundly impaired.

Although an optimal psychometric battery for clinical assessment of dementia should include measures for all areas of deficit discussed above, test selection is often restricted by time considerations and by limited availability of valid measures with adequate normative data. Since the test scores of "normal" elders and patients with dementia generally lie on a continuum, the distinction between normal for age and impaired, even with good test norms, is somewhat arbitrary. References must always be made to the actual functioning of the individual in routine daily activities. The normal or benign deficits of aging may be said to be exceeded when the decline in psychometric performance is reflected in genuine impairments in activities of daily living. The strategy of following patients longitudinally also may help to distinguish true Alzheimer's patients from those with benign changes, since deficits in this progressive disease should worsen significantly over a period of several years.

DEVELOPMENT OF IMPROVED COGNITIVE TESTS

The development of an improved cognitive assessment battery for use in diagnosis and for evaluating change is a difficult task. Figure 4-2 provides a conceptual model of cognitive impairment illustrating that cognition is a very complex process, and that various components mutually interact with one another. Thus it is almost impossible to develop a pure measure of any one aspect of cognition. With respect to memory, there are a variety of ways to subdivide components of the memory process. The usual components include immediate memory (i.e., primary or short-term memory), recent memory (i.e., secondary or long-term memory), which can be subdivided in various ways, and remote memory (i.e., tertiary memory) that includes aspects of language function. If one is to develop a battery to evaluate in a more microscopic way the aspects of mental decline in dementia, one

CONCEPTUAL MODEL OF COGNITIVE IMPAIRMENT

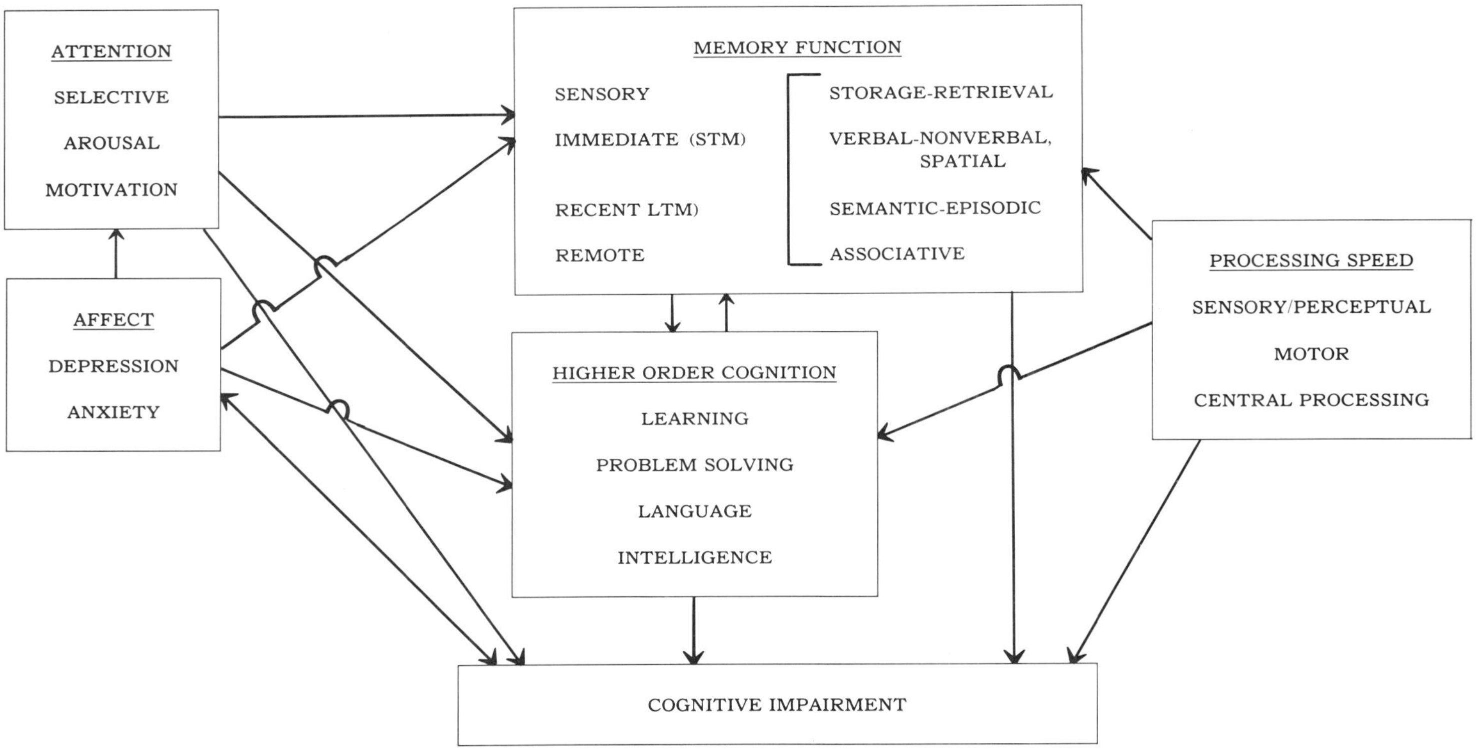

Figure 4-2. Diagram of an "idealized" conceptual model of cognitive impairment. Alterations in various mutually interacting components of mental function combine to produce clinically observable, global cognitive impairment.

should be aware of the ways in which these different processes at least can be separated in an artificial experimental sense.

In developing new instruments, we were concerned with the issue of ecological validity. More specifically, we were concerned with *face validity,* since it may be assumed that face-valid tasks have some ecological validity. By face validity we mean that the nature of the task appears to closely resemble an actual kind of difficulty the patients are having in their day-to-day life. Does a task administered in the laboratory make sense to the patient? If not, patients may react negatively to an experimental paradigm and become antagonistic, uncooperative, or anxious. The results may be a diminished or unreliable performance. Thus, our goal is to develop measures that minimize those possibilities and also have good face validity.

One such task for evaluating immediate memory involves remembering telephone numbers (Crook, Ferris, McCarthy et al., 1980). In this elaboration of the digit-span test, both the digit lengths (3, 7, or 10 digits) and the way in which the subject responds (verbal recall or dialing the number on a telephone) are varied. Even though the young, the normal elderly, and impaired elderly subject groups did not differ in standard digit span (see Table 4-1), when they were given 10 digits (area code + telephone number) that exceed somewhat the usual digit-span capability, there was a significant decline in verbal recall performance in normal elderly subjects, and a further decline in impaired subjects. When the situation was made even more difficult by having the subjects dial the number on an ordinary telephone, there were even larger differences between the three groups of subjects.

A common problem of recent memory involves putting things away and later not remembering their location. The Misplaced Object Task (Crook, Ferris, & McCarthy, 1979) evaluates that kind of difficulty, which is quite severe in dementia patients. In this task, a patient is presented a board showing the various rooms of a house. There is also a group of ten common objects, such as keys, a book, eyeglasses, a wallet, etc. The subject is asked to place these objects in various rooms, but not to put more than two objects in any one room. After about thirty minutes, in which the subject is engaged in other activities, we ask the subjects to indicate where the various objects had been placed. We find a small normal aging deficit in this task, but a very dramatic deficit in the performance of relatively mild dementia patients.

Another face-valid task we developed involves remembering a grocery shopping list (McCarthy, Ferris, Clark et al., 1981). Instead of using lists of nonsense syllables or other verbal materials, we used shopping lists composed of ten very common grocery store items that people actually have to remember to buy when they go to the store. The results for our three subject groups provided three distinct learning curves. The normal elderly took more trials to learn the list than the young normals, but most could remember all ten items. However, the elderly impaired subjects were not only slower learners, but most were unable to remember all the items on the list after five trials.

What about visual memory, such as remembering people's faces? In our Memory for Faces Task (Ferris, de Leon, Wolf et al., 1980), a long series of individual faces appear on a screen. The subject has to push a "yes" or a "no" button depending on whether the face was previously seen. The amount of time between the first and second presentation varies between 30 seconds and 4 minutes. What we found is that even young subjects have greater difficulty in remembering whether the face was seen previously or not as time-delay increases. But both of our elderly groups had significantly greater difficulty with this task. In this visual recognition memory task, however, the mildly impaired patients did not perform significantly worse than our normal elderly subjects.

Finally, we utilized classic paired-associate learning by having subjects remember either first and last names or the association between names and faces (Clark, Ferris, Crook et al., 1982). A sequence of faces with names is shown, and then subjects are asked to remember the name when they are shown the face alone. As the length of the list was gradually increased from one to seven pairs, the performance of the three groups was dramatically different. The maximum recall performance for the young normals occurred for a list length of seven, for the normal elderly a list length of five, and for the impaired elderly a list length of three. For both elderly groups, recall actually deteriorated when the subjects were overloaded with too much to remember.

In addition to memory function, there are other components of cognition that are important to evaluate. These include motor function, sensory-motor speed, attention, and the ability to maintain attention or vigilance. For example, finger-tapping speed (Lehman & Ban, 1970) is a very simple test of motor speed. The classic reaction time (RT) task is a good measure of sensory motor speed and attention that has long been known to slow gradually with age. RT is much slower in dementia, particularly if the subject's response involves a choice or decision. For example, if the subject is asked to respond to a red light, but not to a green light, there is a dramatic slowing with dementia as compared to normal elderly subjects (Ferris, Crook, Sathananthan et al., 1976). Thus, "disjunctive" RT is potentially a good diagnostic measure.

Finally, there is a good test of maintenance of attention and vigilance known as the continuous performance task, or CPT (Kornetsky, 1972). This task, as well as many of the memory tests discussed above, can be administered and scored using a computer. The computer automation of cognitive testing increases standardization and reliability, and greatly facilitates the handling of data. However, computers have to be introduced into the testing environment very carefully, since computerization can create a very artificial situation and reduce face validity. But if the tasks are designed and presented carefully, and interaction with a human tester is retained, face validity can be maintained.

The cognitive measures discussed above are currently being used in our studies of normal aging and senile dementia. They are valuable for the detailed characterization of individual patterns of cognitive decline and for relating these patterns to other measures, such as rating scales or physiologic measures (EEG, CT, or PET). They are also useful for assessing longitudinal changes or changes due to pharmacologic treatment. However, none of these measures have sufficient normative data to permit their use for diagnostic purposes, or for reliably distinguishing "normal" from "abnormal" cognitive performance.

ELECTROPHYSIOLOGICAL ASSESSMENT

In addition to behavioral evaluations such as clinical rating scales and cognitive tests, there are several potentially valuable physiologic approaches for assessing elderly patients who may have one of the several forms of dementia. One technique is the use of electrophysiological measurements. The classical brain wave recording called the electroencephalogram (EEG) is well-known. It is possible to evaluate the EEG objectively by using computers to obtain various EEG measures. In addition, sensory evoked potentials can be obtained. These represent the pattern of brain-wave activity that occurs in response to some event in the environment, such as repetitive clicks or flashes or more complex stimuli. There has been much work in recent years studying the effects of aging on electrophysiological measures and attempting to determine to what extent these measures may be of diagnostic value.

In a collaborative project with the Brain Research Laboratories at New York University, we have been using the technique of *Neurometrics* (John, Karmel, Corning et al., 1977) to study the clinical utility of these electrophysiological parameters. Neurometrics is a technique that extracts quantitative features of diagnostic utility from the EEG, cortical sensory-evoked responses, and brainstem-evoked responses. These features are evaluated statistically, relative to a normative data base, yielding the objective probability of abnormality for each measure in each brain region examined. Using multiple neurometric measures, individual profiles provide an assessment of the status of various brain regions and functional systems. Initial studies with dementia patients (John, Karmel, Corning et al., 1977) indicate that neurometrics can discriminate mild to moderately impaired patients from age-matched normals with a high degree of accuracy. In addition, cluster analysis revealed several distinct neurometric subgroups within the heterogeneous patient population.

In our current project, we studied several hundred individuals composed of both normal elderly control subjects and mildly to severely impaired elderly patients. We found that neurometric measures discriminated well among a variety of diagnostic groups that, in addition to patients with dementia, included alcoholics, head trauma victims, and depressed patients. The simple discrimination between dementia patients and age-matched normal controls was very accurate. It was even possible to separate subjects with very mild impairment from the normals. These discriminations were based on measures that included slowing in EEG frequencies, reductions in evoked potential amplitudes or latencies, and increased asymmetries.

Using the technique of cluster analysis, we also have been able to replicate the previous findings of several neurometric subgroups among the impaired population. Members of a particular neurometric subgroup share a common profile of neurometric abnormalities. By relating these clusters to a broad array of clinical assessment measures, we are now seeking to characterize the nature of these subgroups. When these groups are better understood, it may be feasible to develop treatment strategies that are specific to each group.

COMPUTED TOMOGRAPHY

The computed tomography (CT) scan is among the recommended procedures for a complete dementia evaluation. Figure 4-3 shows scans from two individuals: (A) one normal elderly subject and (B) one patient with moderately severe SDAT. These pictures of "brain slices" represent computer reconstructions of the density of brain tissue based upon x-ray attenuation. Although the CT scan is a noninvasive, painless procedure done on an intact individual, these images simulate what we might see if, on autopsy, actual slices of brain were made. The upper images show the typical appearance of a slice through the ventricular system. Most notable is the marked enlargement of the ventricles in the severely impaired SDAT patient as compared to the normal subject. There is also a greater degree of cortical atrophy in the SDAT patient, which is illustrated by the greater prominence of the cortical sulci. The cortical changes are even more obvious in the bottom images, showing slices taken above the ventricular system. The marked prominence of the cortical sulci is quite apparent for the SDAT patient. The degree of sulcal prominence is related to cortical atrophy, since the dark areas represent cerebral spinal fluid (CSF) that has filled the spaces left by the shrinkage of brain tissue.

What is the clinical utility of CT scans? Although most severe Alzheimer's patients show the typical abnormal pattern illustrated in Figure 4-3, and the majority of elderly normal subjects do not, there is considerable overlap. Thus by merely looking at CT pictures, it is not possible to make

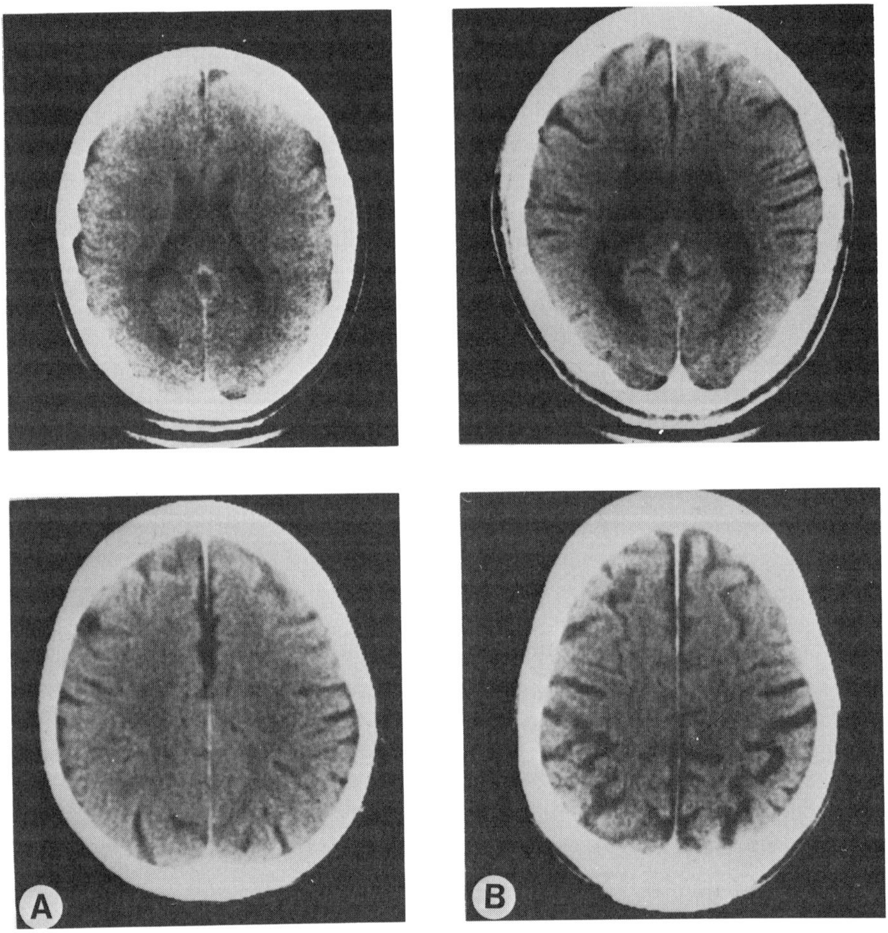

Figure 4-3. Representative CT scans from an **(A)** elderly normal subject and **(B)** an Alzheimer's patient with moderately severe symptomatology. The upper slices were taken at the level of the lateral ventricles, and the bottom slices above the ventricular system at the level of the centrum semiovale.

a reliable positive diagnosis. However, the CT scan is extremely useful for uncovering other causes of dementia-like symptoms, such as tumors, infarcts, or other focal lesions.

Although initial attempts to use CT scans for obtaining a positive diagnosis of dementia based on *structural* brain changes in dementia had been unsuccessful, the potential utility now has markedly improved with the use of new-generation CT scanners and more sophisticated objective CT assessment techniques. Our recent CT studies have demonstrated both ventricular and cortical changes associated with increasing cognitive decline in SDAT (de Leon, Ferris, Blau et al., 1979; de Leon, Ferris, George et al.,

1980). We reported subsequently that changes in grey and white matter are associated with increasing cognitive deficits and also with ventricular dilatation (George, de Leon, Ferris et al., 1981). These initial findings were determined either by objective linear measures of brain structure or by subjective assessments of CT.

More recent studies using computer techniques have replicated and extended these results. For example, it is possible to use the CT computer to measure the total volume of cerebral ventricles. We have found that ventricular volume is significantly increased in SDAT, and the degree of increase correlates with the degree of cognitive impairment (George, de Leon, Rosenbloom et al., in press). Similarly, we can determine the "density" of the tissue (the CT attentuation numbers) in various brain regions. For many regions the density is reduced in SDAT and the change in density is correlated with the degree of impairment on cognitive tests (de Leon & George, 1983). These ventricular and density changes occur to some extent in normal aging, but to a significantly greater extent in SDAT. In the future, we expect that improved CT analysis techniques will lead to new CT measures that have reliable diagnostic significance.

POSITRON EMISSION TOMOGRAPHY

Another new technology for the assessment of dementia is positron emission tomography, or the PET scan. PET scans are somewhat analogous to CT scans in that a computer is used to reconstruct tomographic images at different brain levels. A major difference is that rather than producing an image of the structure of the brain, the PET image relates to the *functioning* activity of the brain. Currently, PET generally is used to measure metabolic activity, but, as the technique is refined and new tracers are developed, it will eventually be possible to measure in vivo a wide variety of physiological processes in the brain. It is likely that PET will be a powerful tool not only for studying brain changes in aging and dementia, but also for diagnosis.

We are currently involved in a large collaborative PET project with Brookhaven National Laboratory. We have used ^{18}F-2-deoxy-2-fluoro-D-glucose (FDG) as a positron-emitting tracer for rate of glucose utilization in brain tissue. When a PET scanner is used following an intravenous injection of FDG, in vivo quantitative measurements of regional glucose utilization in humans can be obtained. We have applied this technique to study changes in regional brain metabolism in normal elderly subjects and in senile dementia outpatients, including both Alzheimer's type and multi-infarct etiologies, who have mild to moderately severe cognitive impairment.

We have also studied a few nondemented elderly patients with depression, as well as a large group of young normal subjects. Regional rates of glucose utilization in normal elderly groups were not significantly lower than in young controls (Ferris, de Leon, Wolf et al., 1983a; de Leon, Ferris, George et al., 1983). However, the SDAT patients showed a marked diminution in metabolism (20–30 percent) as compared to the age-matched controls (Ferris, de Leon, Wolf et al., 1980; Ferris, de Leon, Wolf et al., 1983b; de Leon, Ferris, George et al., 1983). Furthermore, the degree of diminution in SDAT was correlated highly with measures of cognitive impairment. Representative PET scans for an SDAT patient and an elderly normal subject are shown in Figure 4-4.

It is significant that there is a clear difference between the structural brain changes shown by CT and the functional changes shown by PET. For CT, there are changes with normal aging and further changes in SDAT. However, the structural changes in aging are not paralleled by metabolic changes. Only in SDAT is there a marked change in metabolism. With

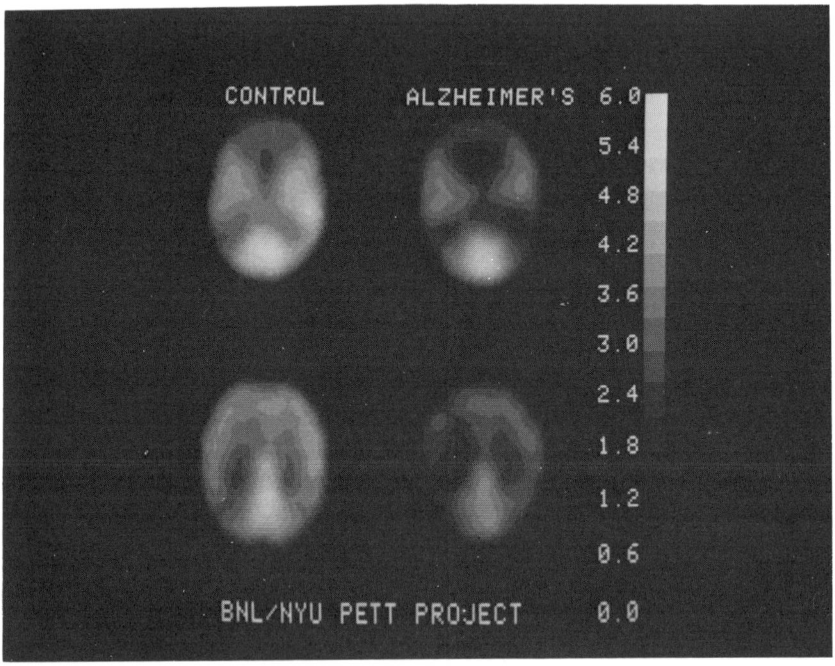

Figure 4-4. Representative PET scans from (left) an elderly normal subject and (right) a moderately severe Alzheimer's (SDAT) patient. The top scans were taken at the level of the basal ganglia, about 4 cm above the canthomeatal (ear–eye) reference plane. The bottom scans are above the ventricular system at the level of the centrum semiovale (7 cm above the reference plane). The grey scale at right indicates the rate of glucose utilization. It is apparent that the metabolic rates are lower for the SDAT patient.

respect to diagnosis, individual PET measures can discriminate between SDAT patients and elderly normals with about 70–80 percent accuracy. With further refinement and improved scanners, this modest diagnostic utility should improve.

CONCLUSIONS

There have been major advances in basic knowledge about senile dementia in the last fifteen years. Coupled with these developments, there also have been great improvements in our ability to diagnose dementias accurately and to characterize clinical symptomatology in detail. As discussed previously, there have been significant advances in the behavioral assessment of dementia using clinical rating scales and objective cognitive tests. Technologic advances, such as neurometrics, CT scans, and PET scans also show great potential. What remains is to find effective treatments that will reverse or even prevent senile dementia. The newer assessment techniques will be extremely useful for evaluating the efficacy of new treatments as they become available.

REFERENCES

Clark, E., Ferris, S.H., Crook, T., & McCarthy, M. Paired-associate span and learning in aging and dementia. Unpublished manuscript, 1982.

Crook, T., Ferris, S.H., & McCarthy, M. The misplaced objects test: A brief test for memory dysfunction in the aged. *Journal of the American Geriatrics Society,* 1979, *27,* 284–287.

Crook, T., Ferris, S.H., McCarthy, M., and Rae, D. The utility of digit recall tasks for assessing memory in the aging. *Journal of Consulting and Clinical Psychology,* 1980, *48,* 228–233.

Crook, T., Gilbert, J.G., & Ferris, S.H. Operationalizing memory impairment in elderly persons: The Guild Memory Test. *Psychological Reports,* 1980, *47,* 1315–1318.

Cummings, J., Benson, D.F., & LoVerme, S. Reversible dementia. *Journal of the American Medical Association,* 1980, *243,* 2434.

de Leon, M.J., Ferris, S.H., Blau, I., George, A.E., Reisberg, B., Kricheff, I.I., & Gershon, S. Correlations between CT changes and behavioral deficits in senile dementia. *Lancet,* 1979, *Oct. 20,* 859–860.

de Leon, M.J., Ferris, S.H., George, A.E., Reisberg, B., Kricheff, I.I., & Gershon, S. Computed tomography evaluations of brain-behavior relationships in senile dementia of the Alzheimer's type. *Neurobiology of Aging,* 1980, *1,* 69–79.

de Leon, M.J., & George, A.E. Computed tomography in aging and senile dementia Alzheimer's type. In R. Mayeux and W. Rosen (Eds.), *The dementias.* New York: Raven Press, 1983.

de Leon, M.J., Ferris, S.H., George, A.E., Christman, D.R., Fowler, J., Gentes, C., Reisberg, B., Gee, B., Emmerlich, M., Yonekura, Y., Brodie, J., Kricheff, I.I., & Wolfe, A. Positron emission tomography (PET) studies of aging and Alzheimer's disease. *Advances in Neurology,* 1983, *38,* 123–129.

Ferris, S.H., Crook, T., Clark, E., McCarthy, M., and Rae, D. Facial recognition memory deficits in normal aging and senile dementia. *Journal of Gerontology,* 1980, *35,* 707–714.

Ferris, S.H., de Leon, M.J., Wolf, A.P., Farkas, T., Christman, D.R., Reisberg, B., Fowler, J.S., MacGregor, R., Goldman, A., George, A.E., & Rampal, S. Positron emission tomography in the study of aging and senile dementia. *Neurobiology of Aging,* 1980, *1,* 127–131.

Ferris, S.H., de Leon, M.J., Wolf, A.P., George, A.E., Reisberg, B., Brodie, J., Gentes, C., Christman, D.R., & Fowler, J.S. Regional metabolism and cognitive deficits in aging and senile dementia. In P. Samuel, S. Algeri, S. Gershon, V.E. Grimm, & G. Toffano (Eds.), *The aging of the brain.* New York: Raven Press, 1983a.

Ferris, S.H., de Leon, M.J., Wolf, A.P., George, A.E., Reisberg, B., Cristman, D.R., & Fowler, J.S. Positron emission tomography in dementia. In R. Mayeux and W. Rosen (Eds.), *The dementias.* New York: Raven Press, 1983b.

Folstein, M.F., Folstein, S.E., & McHugh, P.R. Mini-mental state: A practical method for grading the cognitive states of patients for the clinician. *Journal of Psychiatric Research,* 1975, *12,* 189–198.

Fuld, P.A. Guaranteed stimulus-processing in the evaluation of memory and training. *Cortex,* 1980, *16,* 255–271.

George, A.E., de Leon, M.J., Ferris, S.H., & Kricheff, I.I. Parenchymal CT correlates of senile dementia (Alzheimer's disease): Loss of grey-white matter discriminability. *American Journal of Neuroradiology,* 1981, *2,* 205–211.

George, A.E., de Leon, M.J., Rosenbloom, M.D., Ferris, S.H., Gentes, C., Emmerich, M., & Kricheff, I.I. The relationship of CT ventricular volume to cognitive deficit. *Radiology,* 1984, in press.

Gilbert, J.G., Levee, R.F., & Catalano, F.L. A preliminary report on a new memory scale. *Perceptual and Motor Skills,* 1968, *27,* 277–278.

John, E.R., Karmel, B.Z., Corning, W.C., Easton, P., Brown, D., Ahn, H., John, M., Harmony, T., Prichep, L., Toro, A., Gershon, I., Bartlett, F., Thatcher, R., Kaye, H., Valdes, P., & Schwartz, E. Neurometrics. *Science,* 1977, *196,* 1393–1410.

Kahn, R.L., Goldfarb, A.I., Pollack, M., & Peck, A. Brief objective measures for the determination of mental status in the aged. *American Journal of Psychiatry,* 1960, *117,* 326–328.

Kornetsky, C. The use of a simple test of attention as a measure of drug effects in schizophrenic patients. *Psychopharmacologia,* 1972, *24,* 99–106.

Kral, V.A. Benign senescent forgetfulness. In R. Katzman, R.D. Terry, & K.L. Bick (Eds.), *Alzheimer's disease: Senile dementia and related disorders.* New York: Raven Press, 1978.

Lehman, H.E., & Ban, T.A. Psychometric tests in evaluation of brain pathology responsive to drugs. *Geriatrics,* 1970, *25,* 142–147.

McCarthy, M., Ferris, S.H., Clark, E., & Crook, T. Acquisition and retention of categorized material in normal aging and senile dementia. *Experimental Aging Research,* 1981, *7,* 127–135.

Reisberg, B., Ferris, S.H., de Leon, M.J., & Crook, T. The Global Deterioration Scale (GDS): An instrument for the assessment of primary degenerative dementia (PDD). *American Journal of Psychiatry,* 1982, *139,* 1136–1139.

Reisberg, B., Schneck, M.K., Ferris, S.H., Schwartz, G.E., & de Leon, M.J. The brief cognitive rating scale (BCRS): Findings in primary degenerative dementia (PDD). *Psychopharmacology Bulletin,* 1983, *19,* 47–50.

Rosen, W.G., Terry, R.D., Fuld, P.A., Katzman, R., & Peck, A. Pathological verification of Ischemia Score in differential dementias. *Annals of Neurology,* 1980, *7,* 486–488.

Wechsler, D.A. A standardized memory scale for clinical use. *Journal of Psychology,* 1945, *19,* 87–95.

5

LONG-TERM CLINICAL MANAGEMENT OF THE DEMENTIA PATIENT

Robert Barnes
Murray Raskind

The dementia syndrome is manifested by marked impairment of intellect and personality that usually has a prolonged course of many years. Whether due to gradually progressive disorders, such as Alzheimer's disease, or more stable disorders, such as multi-infarct dementia, the dementia syndrome is a psycho-social-biological phenomenon (Kahn, 1975). At the present time, specific treatments for reversing the biological component of most dementing illnesses are not available. For this reason, the long term treatment of dementia focuses primarily on modification and improvement of secondary behavioral and social problems caused by the disorder.

Most dementia patients live in the community with family members or other care providers (Bergman, Foster, Justice et al., 1978) and enter extended care institutions only late in the course of their illness. Unfortunately, home care of the dementia patient places great psychological and physical stress on families or other care providers (Brocklehurst, 1977). While the patient is still residing at home, the objectives of therapeutic interventions are to maximize patient function and reduce the burden and stresses on care providers in order to enable the patient to continue to reside in the community (Godber, 1977). As such, treatment must involve not only

GERIATRIC MENTAL HEALTH
ISBN 0-8089-1657-2

the patient but also those providing care. Once the burden of care becomes too great for the family, the patient must be managed in extended care institutions. However, even in these settings, the objectives of treatment remain maximizing patient function and minimizing problem behaviors that bring distress both to the patient and to persons in the patient's environment.

TREATMENT OF SOCIAL COMPLICATIONS OF DEMENTIA

Problems of Care Providers

Some of the most common problems described in studies of family members or other persons caring for the dementia patient at home include poor understanding of the illness, depression, social isolation, stress related to role changes, and difficulty managing such secondary behavioral problems as agitation, sleep disturbance, and assaultiveness (Barnes, Raskind, Scott et al., 1981; Fuller, Ward, Evans et al., 1979; Godber, 1977; Lazarus, Stafford, Cooper et al., 1981; Lezak, 1978; Rabins, Mace, & Lucas, 1982). One of the most frequent problems for care providers is the lack of an adequate understanding of the nature of dementing illnesses. Progressive dementing disorders, such as Alzheimer's disease, are particularly hard to understand. Care providers have difficulty relating such character changes as irritability, lack of initiative, impulsivity, and emotional lability to the disease process. They may become hostile towards the patient, whom they perceive as consciously choosing to have their symptoms rather than as being affected by the illness. Some family care providers actually feel guilty and blame themselves for causing behavioral problems that in fact are the result of the disease. Anxiety and denial on the part of care providers, as well as inadequate explanations by physicians, often contribute to poor understanding of the illness.

A sense of isolation is frequently a problem for caregivers. If the patient has one of the progressive dementing disorders, care providers gradually assume almost total care for the patient and feel trapped by the time and effort required. Social isolation develops when caring for the patient prevents initiating independent social activities, and worsens if the care provider deliberately avoids social contacts because of embarrassment about the patient's behavior. Friends also may be uncomfortable around the patient and decrease the frequency of their visits. The sense of isolation is heightened for spouses because the interpersonal and affectional needs formerly met inside the marriage by the demented partner are left unsatisfied.

Caring for a demented family member is associated with a variety of conflicting emotional reactions. Many care providers, particularly spouses, feel a deep sense of loss and depression. Spouses provide care for a person who looks the same, but who no longer acts the same as the person they married. Family members experience the paradox of grieving for the loss of a "dead" companion who is still present physically and demanding increasingly burdensome care. Anger towards the patient can lead to fantasies and wishes of their early death. Such thoughts often provoke intense guilt.

Even though intellect and personality deteriorate in the dementia patient, physical strength remains intact for much of the illness. The combination of intact physical strength and regressed, impulsive, even belligerent behavior, creates many difficulties. Some care providers, especially women, can be physically abused by patients, often while physically struggling to prevent inappropriate or dangerous behavior. Agitated behaviors, especially at night, are particularly stressful (Sanford, 1975).

Level of Burden and Stress of Care Providers

Along with the stresses of providing day-to-day care, the primary care providers usually assume household and financial chores previously performed by the patient. For some care providers, these new roles may be even more stressful than daily care of the patient. In addition, caring for the patient frequently creates severe financial stress and uncertainty due to such expenses as day care, respite care, visits to physicians, and the prospect of the tremendous financial cost of long-term nursing home care.

Individuals may experience very different levels of burden and stress while caring for a patient at home. Behavioral changes produced by dementing illnesses vary greatly from patient to patient. At any given stage of the illness, some dementia patients can be easily managed relative to others who are restless, irritable, and hostile. Care providers have widely varying resources and coping skills to manage behavioral and social changes produced by the disease.

Several studies have investigated the determinants of the level of burden for families caring for demented geriatric patients. Sainsbury and Gard de Alarcon (1970) found that caregivers were especially stressed by potentially harmful behaviors, restlessness, and agitation in the evening (Sanford, 1975). Among dependent geriatric patients, many of who had senile dementia, Sanford reported that night-time restlessness in the patient and restriction of social life for the care provider were the two most difficult problems to tolerate (Sainsbury & Gard de Alarcon, 1970). In a study by Rabins, Mace, & Lucas (1982), family care providers described physical violence, emotional outbursts, and incontinence as the most difficult problems to manage. Zarit, Reever, & Bach-Peterson (1980) found that the level of burden and stress for caregivers of senile dementia patients was less when the household had more social contacts (Zarit, Reever, & Bach-Peterson, 1980). In this study, the extent of burden reported by primary caregivers was not related to behavioral problems caused by the dementing illness, but was associated with the social supports available, specifically the number of visitors to the household.

Treatment of Care Providers' Problems

Given the absence of specific medical treatment for the underlying cause of dementia, strengthening the morale, emotional well-being, and treatment skill of the care-providing family is an important factor in providing optimal care to the patient with early- and middle-stage dementia. Excessive stress on the care providing family is a major factor in institutionalization of the elderly (Krause, Spasoff, Beattie et al., 1976). Successful intervention to reduce stresses and level of burdens for care providers frequently makes continued home care possible and can greatly reduce the need for institutionalization. Institutional care poses financial hardship for most families and transfer to a long term care institution can have direct negative effects on the patient, such as increased confusion or even increased risk of mortality (Blenkner, 1967; Borup, Gallego, & Hefferman, 1979, 1980). For these reasons, it is wise to maintain demented patients in familiar surroundings in the community as long as it is practical and safe to do so.

Treatment techniques such as education, emotional support, social support, and problem solving can address the problems of care providers, and decrease their levels of stress and burden. Providing information about the biology, behavioral effects, and course of dementing illness can be very helpful. It is particularly important for families to know how the illness affects the patient's behavior and personality. Understanding that problems such as passivity, wandering, or emotional lability are not deliberate acts, but the results of a brain illness, often helps dispel the caregiver's anger and fosters more appropriate expectations. Many families will need information about the illness repeated many times. Educational pamphlets, books, and films about dementia are often helpful. In the case of Alzheimer's disease, families frequently appreciate accurate information about the effectiveness of medical treatment, the communicability of the disease, and the inheritability of the illness. Even though the causes of this disorder remain unknown, a helpful approach is to communicate to families that there is research currently being conducted that offers hope for the future. However, the promise of a cure should not be made and the fact also emphasized that no currently known treatment is effective in restoring memory or preventing deterioration of the patient. While it can be explained that patients gradually deteriorate over a period of 5-to-10 years, it should be stressed that the time course of the disease varies from person to person and many patients do well for long periods of time.

Care providers also benefit from an emotionally supportive psychotherapeutic relationship that allows them to ventilate their feelings. The ventilation process helps discharge tension and allows exploration and resolution of some of the frustration and grief created by the illness. Family members find it helpful to learn that their feelings and reactions are normal responses to a difficult situation.

Since social contact is an important determinant of level of burden, family members usually benefit from increased social support. Caregivers should be encouraged to have frequent contact with family and friends. Whether through the help of other family members, friends, or even hired "dementia sitters," care providers need to find ways to create time away from the patient for their own social outlets and personal activities. It is important that caregivers understand that attention to their own needs improves their mental well-being and thereby improves their ability to care for the patient.

Many care givers also need help in solving practical problems created by the dementing illness. Care givers vary greatly in problem-solving skills. Some are creative and effective problem solvers who experience little stress as they provide care for the dementia patient. Unfortunately, most care providers are repeatedly faced with situations for which they have little preparation or understanding. Practical advice about behavioral treatment strategies or pharmacologic management of behavioral problems can greatly reduce the stresses on family members. The use of medications as well as behavioral treatment strategies in the demented patient are also beneficial and will be discussed later in greater detail.

Many care providers can benefit from referral to community services that can help with specific problems. Referrals to geriatric day treatment centers, home health workers, chore services, or dementia self-help groups are often helpful. The need for information about legal and financial problems such as guardianship, power of attorney, or wills may require the assistance of an attorney familiar with the problems created by dementing illness. Some caregivers need social service help to understand Medicare and Medicaid forms and rules surrounding nursing home placement.

Individual counseling, family meetings, and support groups have all been reported as useful treatment modalities capable of providing information, emotional support, social support, and problem solving for care providers (Blumenthal, 1979; Reifler & Eisdorfer, 1980). Depending on the needs of the care providers, any one or combination of these treatment modalities may be appropriate. Family meetings are useful if the primary caregiver is not utilizing available family resources or if there are conflicts within the family about the care of the patient. Such meetings can increase the caregivers' social support and improve the entire family's understanding of the burden of caring for the patient.

Support groups for care providers are now widely available and are a particularly useful treatment modality (Barnes, Raskind, Scott et al., 1981; Lazarus, Stafford, Cooper et al., 1981). Most support groups described in the literature have consisted of 8-to-12 family members who met weekly for a prescribed length of time, usually 2 to 3 months. These groups were typically led by individuals with a knowledge of both dementia and group process. Lazarus has reported that support groups help family members separate themselves from the patient and feel more in control of their own lives (Lazarus, Stafford, Cooper et al., 1981). Participants report that they find education and emotional support in such groups beneficial (Godber, 1977). The Zarits have suggested that support groups are especially effective in allowing care givers to learn new strategies of responding to the dementia patient by hearing what other members have done in similar situations (Zarit & Zarit, 1982). Such modeling can be an important source of new learning, particularly for care givers who have had trouble making changes. Many communities now have ongoing groups organized and led by the care providers themselves. Such groups are also capable of providing support and education, especially on community resources. It may be preferable for care providers to participate initially in support groups that are professionally led, but such groups are not always available.

Individual counseling of family members can be done by the primary physician or through referral to therapists with experience in working with dementia families. The individual counselor needs a good knowledge about dementia, an understanding of the social support services available in the community, and some creativity at solving day-to-day problems created by dementia. Most families find it helpful to have an identified health care provider to contact for emergencies or advice.

Single Patient Living Alone

The dementia patient who lives alone and has no care provider presents especially difficult management problems (Aronson & Lipkowitz, 1981). These patients usually come to attention during an acute situational crisis. They frequently do not have adequate social support or financial resources, and cannot comprehend and organize community support services available to help maintain them at home. Their poor judgment makes them especially vulnerable to accidents or even criminal abuse. Treatment planning must center on deciding if the patient still has the cognitive skills to allow him or her to live safely in the community if given a reasonable level of support. If memory impairment, poor judgment, and poor impulse control make the patient a danger to himself or the community, placement in an extended care facility is often the wisest treatment alternative.

TREATMENT OF BEHAVIORAL COMPLICATIONS IN DEMENTIA

The secondary behavioral features of dementia are the most treatable aspects of this disorder. Paranoid states, agitation, hostility, depression, sleep disturbances, and many other behaviors are frequently responsive to treatment. Management of behavioral problems associated with dementia includes psychopharmacologic as well as psychosocial treatment approaches.

Antipsychotic Drugs

Antipsychotics are widely used in treating older patients with dementia. In summarizing data from 9 nationwide surveys, Prien reported that 20 percent of nursing home patients, many of whom had dementing illness, received antipsychotic drugs (Prien, 1980). Among Tennessee Medicaid nursing home patients, Ray et al. found that 38 percent received antipsychotics continuously for more than one month (Ray, Federspiel, & Schaffner, 1980). This survey suggested that antipsychotic drugs are overprescribed to nursing home patients.

Unfortunately, the majority of past clinical trials of antipsychotic medications in geriatric patients are difficult to interpret because of inadequacies of experimental design, confusion in the psychiatric diagnostic nomenclature, and the frequent inclusion of patients with psychiatric diagnoses other than dementia (Veith & Horita, 1984). While uncontrolled trials of these agents have usually reported positive effects, the results of placebo-controlled trials have been less consistent. Several studies found low dosages of halperidol, chlorpromazine and trifluorperazine more effective than placebo for controlled symptoms such as hallucinations, hostility, excitement, anxiety, agitation, and hyperactivity (Hamilton & Bennett, 1962; Seager, 1955; Sugarman, Williams, & Alderstein, 1964). At the same time, other studies have reported no significant positive behavioral effects for thiothixene and chlorpromazine compared to placebo in older patients with dementia (Abse & Dahlstrom, 1960; Barton & Hurst, 1966; Rada & Kellner, 1976; Robinson, 1959).

In one of three negative studies (Robinson, 1959), treatment of demented elderly female patients with chlorpromazine was actually associated with a higher rate of behavioral deterioration than was treatment with placebo. Most of this deterioration was attributed to increased inertia in the active drug group. An uncontrolled trial of antipsychotics among psychogeriatric patients in a state hospital demonstrated clinical improvement in many patients previously on psychotropics during the initial 6-week "clearance period" (Altman, Mehta, Evanson et al., 1973). This clearance period was the time prior to entering the drug study during which all previously prescribed psychotropic medications were discontinued. The findings in these latter two studies suggest that side effects of antipsychotics such as lethargy, central anticholinergic toxicity, and extrapyramidal effects may adversely affect the function and behavior of dementia patients.

Two recent placebo-controlled studies of antipsychotic medications in carefully selected dementia patients provide more specific information about the efficacy of these drugs. Among behaviorally disturbed demented nursing home patients treated with either loxapine, thioridazine, or placebo, Barnes, Veith, Okimoto, et al. (1982) found that antipsychotics were more effective than placebo in reducing anxiety, excitement, emotional lability, and uncooperativeness (Barnes et al., 1982). The patients most likely to benefit from ongoing treatment with antipsychotics were those with the most severe behavioral symptoms at baseline, but response to antipsychotics did not appear related to the cause of dementia. Petric et al. found that loxapine and haloperidol were both more effective than placebo in improving the symptoms of suspiciousness, hallucinatory behavior, excitement, hostility, and uncooperativeness among behaviorally disturbed demented patients residing in a state hospital (Petric, Ban, Berncy et al., 1982). However, among 77 patients receiving antipsychotics in these two studies, only 35 percent clearly improved, while 46 percent did not improve substantially and 10 percent were actually worse with treatment. These results suggest that antipsychotics are much less effective in this population of older demented patients than among individuals with schizophrenia.

Both studies reported a high incidence of adverse effects. The most frequently reported side effect was sedation with 38 percent of subjects, and which, in these patients, was often associated with increased incontinence, confusion, and withdrawal. The second most common side effects were extrapyramidal reactions, in 32 percent of subjects. These two studies provide clinical guidelines for the use of antipsychotics in dementia patients. The behavioral symptoms most drug-responsive include suspiciousness, hostility, anxiety, excitement, hallucination, and emotional lability. Patients with more severe symptoms are those most likely to benefit from treatment.

Antipsychotics are not helpful for symptoms such as impaired memory, unsociability, poor self-care, or indifference to surroundings. In fact, side effects of antipsychotics, particularly sedation, may make many of these symptoms worse. The high frequency of adverse effects associated with antipsychotic use underscores the need for close monitoring of a patient's clinical condition. Because both studies demonstrated a significant placebo effect, improvement may not always be due to specific drug efficacy; thus, even in symptomatically improved patients, antipsychotic medications should be periodically withdrawn to determine the need for continued treatment.

There is no evidence that any one antipsychotic drug is more effective than any other for treatment of dementia patients. The choice of an antipsychotic medication for an individual patient should be based on the side-effect profile for a particular drug, and the behavioral and medical status of the individual being treated. Common adverse effects of the antipsychotic drugs include peripheral and central anticholinergic toxicity, extrapyramidal signs and symptoms, sedation, and orthostatic hypotension. Anticholinergic effects include urinary retention, constipation, dry mouth, blurry vision, and delirium with exacerbation of cognitive impairment. High-dosage antipsychotics, such as chlorpromazine and thioridazine are more anticholinergic than low-dosage antipsychotics, such as haloperidol, thiothixene and loxapine. One of the latter medications would be preferable in a patient susceptible to anticholinergic drug effects.

In contrast, the low-dosage antipsychotic medications such as haloperidol, thiothixene, and loxapine are more likely to cause extrapyramidal signs and symptoms than are the high-dosage medications such as thioridazine and chlorpromazine. Extrapyramidal side effects commonly seen in elderly patients include a reversible Parkinsonian syndrome, akathisia, akinesia and tardive dyskinesia. Akathisia, a syndrome of motor restlessness with a subjective sense of discomfort, can be confused with agitation and motoric hyperactivity secondary to the underlying cognitive disorder. In the patient with pre-existing Parkinsonism or a low threshold for developing extrapyramidal toxicity, a drug such as thioridazine would be preferable.

Thioridazine and chlorpromazine are more sedating than low dosage medications. This effect can be helpful in a severely agitated patient or in one with sleep disturbance, but may cause problems in the patient with social withdrawal or lethargy. Although overdoses of antipsychotic medication have been associated with disturbances of cardiac rhythm and conduction, these effects are uncommon in the relatively low dosages used in dementia patients (Petric, Ban, Berncy et al., 1982).

The dosage of antipsychotic medication in dementia patients is usually much lower than that in patients with schizophrenia. For more potent agents such as haloperidol or thiothixene, reasonable starting dosages would be 1 or 2 mg at bedtime; for less potent agents such as thioridazine, the starting dosage is commonly 25 mg at bedtime. Some patients with behavioral problems can be helped by dosages even lower than these. Once medication is started, the dosage can be increased gradually according to therapeutic effect, sedation or other adverse effects. Since these drugs have long half-lives, they frequently can be used once daily, most commonly at bedtime.

Sensible use of the antipsychotics in demented patients can greatly reduce the chance for adverse effects. Guidelines to minimize side effects include:

1. Selecting a drug with side effects that will likely be tolerated by the individual patient (e.g., patients with symptoms of benign prostatic hypertrophy should be started on an agent with low anticholinergic side effects).
2. Avoiding, if at all possible, parenteral administration, which greatly increases the likelihood of side effects.
3. Starting with very low doses that are then increased gradually while monitoring for side effects.
4. Making the goals of antipsychotic treatment realistic; i.e., making the patient and persons in the environment more comfortable rather than creating a symptom-free situation.
5. Medication on a brief—as needed—basis may be all that is necessary if episodes of agitation are infrequent.

While medications are frequently the correct treatment for the agitated demented patient, it is important to remember causes and environmental causes *(vide infra)* for agitation. The demented patient is especially prone to developing a superimposed delirium that may result in further cognitive deterioration and episodes of agitation. In order to decrease the likelihood of delirium, it is wise to avoid the use of medications that are not absolutely necessary. Other concurrent medical conditions can be difficult to diagnose in the demented patient and may be manifested only by agitated behavior. Pain is of particular importance in this regard because more severely impaired patients are often unable to verbalize pain sensation and may express it only as a behavioral disturbance. A careful search for conditions such as arthritis, fractures, constipation, or even silent myocardial infarction, is in order.

Sleep Disturbance

Sleep disturbance in the elderly demented patient is often treatable, and control of this problem is of critical importance in maintaining elderly dementia patients at home (Rabins, Mace, & Lucas, 1982). Increasing daytime activity and limiting napping are general approaches that should be instituted if possible. Educating family and patient to the fact that sleep in the elderly normally contains increased awakening episodes and decreased deep sleep (stage IV slow-wave sleep) can be reassuring to those disturbed by any change in sleep pattern (Prinz, 1980). Otherwise, treatment of sleep disturbance secondary to pain, congestive heart failure, or pulmonary insufficiency, should be addressed by the appropriate medical regimen. If sleep disturbance is a symptom of major depression, the more sedating tricyclic antidepressants such as amitriptyline or doxepin may be indicated. If night-time agitation (so-called "sundown syndrome") is the cause of impaired sleep, low-dosage antipsychotic medication is the treatment of choice. The traditional hypnotics and sedatives, such as the barbiturates or benzodiazepines, are of limited usefulness; they will improve sleep during acute episodes of situational anxiety but usually lose their effectiveness with chronic administration. Unfortunately, these agents can paradoxically increase agitation and confusion in the susceptible patient. The sedative antihistaminic drugs such as diphenhydramine or hydroxazine also may be useful and are relatively free of side effects.

Depression

Depression has been thought to be more common in patients with multi-infarct dementia (Barnes & Raskind, 1980; Busse, 1973), but also has been found to be a problem among patients with Alzheimer's disease (Reifler, Larson, & Hanley, 1982). Symptoms of emotional lability with crying episodes—the pseudobulbar palsy of multi-infarct dementia—should not be confused with depression. Patients with unhappiness and mild symptoms of depression, related to worry about their cognitive impairment, may benefit from supportive psychotherapy which gives them an opportunity to ventilate their feelings. Major depression also can occur in patients with dementia. Accurate diagnosis of depression in the presence of dementia may be difficult because depressive symptoms can be confused with those of dementia or the depressive symptoms may have unusual presentations. Unfortunately, there are no clear diagnostic criteria for depression in the presence of significant dementia. Early escape from dexamethasone suppression may occur in 50 percent of patients with major depression and has been suggested as a helpful diagnostic test for depression in the demented patient (Carroll, Curtis, & Mendels, 1976). Unfortunately, nondepressed patients with dementia, especially those with Alzheimer's disease, also commonly have early escape from dexamethasone suppression (Raskind, Peskind, Rivard et al., 1982; Spar & Gerner, 1982). For this reason, the dexamethasone suppression test currently cannot be considered useful for diagnosis of depression in patients with dementia.

Pharmacologic treatment of depression in the demented patient is more difficult than in the nondemented patient, but clinical case reports suggest that tricyclic antidepressants and even electroconvulsive therapy (ECT) can be helpful in carefully selected patients (Demuth & Rand, 1980; Post, 1976). Tricyclic antidepressants have been demonstrated effective in depressed patients and are widely used in the elderly. Unfortunately, data from placebo-controlled clinical studies of tricyclic antidepressant therapy in depressed dementia patients are not available. Indications for using these medications in such patients rest on inferences from their use in young and elderly nondemented patients. The tricyclics are most effective in depression manifested by decreased appetite, weight loss, psychomotor retardation, and sleep disturbance with early morning awakening (Bielski & Friedel, 1976). Insidious onset also favors the use of these medications. In the case of dementia, treatment with tricyclic antidepressants would appear most appropriate in cases where depression was clearly accompanied by these vegetative signs and symptoms.

The various tricyclic antidepressants have equal therapeutic efficacy but profiles of adverse effects differ. Of particular importance are differences in anticholinergic and sedative activity. As with the antipsychotic drugs, selection of a tricyclic antidepressant should be guided by matching the side effect profile of the drug with the clinical and medical condition of the individual patient. A reasonable starting dose of commonly used tricyclic antidepressants (doxepin, amitriptyline, imipramine, desipramine, or nortriptyline) in older depressed patients is 25 mg/day. The drug can be increased by 25 mg every 5-to-7 days until patients begin to show a therapeutic response, side effects become troublesome, or a total daily dosage of 150 mg/day (in divided doses) is reached. Higher doses are advisable only if low-plasma drug levels can be documented. In demented patients, the physician must be careful not to worsen the patient's confusion and disorientation through the anticholinergic and sedative effects of these drugs.

Environmental, Behavioral, and Social Therapies

In order to maximize the function of the patient with cognitive impairment, the environment should be supportive, i.e., not requiring new learning and geared towards those with low vision, poor hearing, and postural instability (Blumenthal, 1979). The more demanding the environment, the greater the degree of disability in the demented patient. Sensory isolation also can be the cause of decreased cognitive function and subsequent agitation in demented patients. To avoid sensory isolation, hearing and vision deficits should be corrected where possible and patients should be provided with consistent, warm interactions with other human beings, whether nursing staff or family.

A move to a new, unfamiliar environment frequently results in agitated behavior in the demented patient. Once a patient is familiar with a new setting, the agitation often subsides. However, acclimatization may take several weeks or longer. Knowledge of this common response to change and its subsequent resolution can reassure medical personnel and family members, and reduce the premature use of psychotropic medications.

Vigorous pacing which may last for hours often is associated with dementia, particularly Alzheimer's disease. This behavior is difficult to distinguish from agitation, and, if pacing is interfered with by physical restraint, agitation or hostility are the likely results. Short of excessive sedation, medication frequently does not control this behavior. Ideal management of pacing behavior is provision of a safe, controlled environment in which the patient can pace and wander without excessive risk or injury to self or others. Long-term care facilities should be designed to provide such an environment. Unfortunately, such settings usually are not available in the average private home.

A variety of specific behaviors such as wandering, asking frequent questions, emotional outburst, or bowel and bladder incontinence can cause distress on the part of care providers. If a care provider has difficulty managing a specific behavior, developing a managing plan first requires defining the problem as clearly as possible with the care provider. It is important to understand when the behavior occurs and if there are any specific antecedents that may be causal factors. If a specific task or event is likely to cause emotional outbursts, the caregiver can work to remove the precipitating stress as much as possible from the daily routine of the patient. It is also important to understand the caregiver's view of the identified problem behavior. Caregivers may become more tolerant of deviant behavior if it is seen as the result of a disease process rather than as a deliberate act. For instance, caregivers may be more willing to tolerate repetitive questions if these are viewed as the result of the patient's poor memory and as a way of interacting to obtain reassurance. Emotional and social support, as mentioned previously, can also decrease the level of stress on caregivers and make bothersome behavior seem less irritating.

Some problem behaviors can be reduced by environmental changes. Patients who leave home to wander about the neighborhood can sometimes be kept in the home through use of door locks that only the care provider can open. Such wandering patients also need identification bracelets with their phone numbers and addresses so that they can be returned if found by neighbors or police. An orderly, uncluttered house, or even signs pointing to an object's location, can reduce a patient's difficulty with misplacing or losing things. Patients who are disturbing their care providers at night may be less bothersome if they are in their own separate rooms. Dangerous firearms or tools should be removed from the house. If use of major appliances is inappropriate, the care provider should have switches or circuit breakers installed in order to shut off the gas or electicity when the patient is likely to be left at home alone.

For specific, repetitive problems, behavioral treatment techniques may be helpful. Some behavioral treatment techniques are simple—such as not allowing daytime naps for the patient who does not sleep at night. However, because the dementia patient is not able to remember and has great difficulty learning new information, behavioral treatment of problem behaviors requires great ingenuity on the part of the caregiver. For instance, in patients who ask the same question over and over, large timers with bells have been used to signal the patient when the next question can be asked. The time between questions is initially short, but is gradually increased so that the interval between questions is progressively lengthened. In other cases, behavioral solutions are found in a more serendipitous fashion. One care provider discovered that reading to the patient for a half-hour in the morning and in the afternoon greatly reduced the number of repetitive questions.

In some cases, the caregiver's response to the patient's behavior also has to be modified. The caregiver who frequently corrects or criticizes memory deficits may cause increased frustration and agitation. For the patient who is irritable and who has outbursts of temper, sometimes the situation can be defused by having the care provider leave the room and not reciprocate angry feelings. In other cases, care providers may be successful in learning to divert the patient's attention to another topic and thereby defuse the sense of agitation.

In cases of moderate to advanced dementia, incontinence is a problem that many families find difficult to manage at home (Rabins, Mace, & Lucas, 1982). Once a specific, reversible cause of incontinence, such as urinary tract infection, has been ruled out, specific information about bowel and bladder training can be helpful. Adult incontinent briefs can reduce patient discomfort and minimize the soiling of clothing, and incontinent bedpans can reduce the soiling of linen at night. While briefs and bed pans do not solve the problem of incontinence, they can reduce the workload that it creates for families.

Reality Orientation

Reality orientation therapy (RO) was developed by Taulbee and Folsom at the Veterans Administration Hospital in Tuscaloosa, Alabama (Taulbee & Folsom, 1966). This treatment modality has been recommended for improving behavior and cognition in elderly patients residing in institutional settings who have confusion, disorientation, and memory loss (Stephens, 1966). As it has evolved over the years, RO utilizes two basic approaches.

Twenty-four hour RO utilizes institutional staff who are in contact with the patient to function as orienters. Nurses, aides, and other personnel throughout the day repeatedly present basic information during routine patient–staff interactions about the time, location, daily activities, and other current circumstances in hopes of enabling the patient to retain this information. Staff are encouraged to speak slowly and clearly and to use direct eye contact and touching to maintain the patient's attention.

Classroom RO is the second approach of this therapy and is a more intensive form that can be used alone or as a supplement to the 24 hour RO. Classes of 4 to 8 individuals meet for 30 minutes each day. The central tool in the classroom session is a large board with oversize letters that spell out information such as the date, time, place, patient's name, weather report, next meal, and other discrete every-day events. The leader utilizes visual and auditory reinforcement to gain the patient's attention and to elicit active responses indicating that the information has been memorized, even if only transiently. Taulbee has noted that mechanically presenting RO information to the confused patient will not in itself reduce confusion (Taulbee, 1976). The orienter genuinely and consistently must be concerned about the other person, and ideally should maintain a calm environment, have a set routine for the patient, and give clear responses to patient's questions.

Many anectodal reports in uncontrolled studies claim wide-ranging improvement in patient behavior and orientation after implementing RO programs. However, the result of controlled studies have produced less consistently positive results. Brook, Degun, Mather (1975) found improvement in ward-behavior rating scales in a small number of disoriented nursing home patients receiving RO classes compared to a control group who received only exposure to the RO setting. Of interest is the fact that improvement was demonstrated only for mildly-impaired patients. Numerous other controlled studies have reported that, compared to controls, reality orientation can significantly improve subjects' ability to answer questions relating to orientation, but these studies could not document improvement in ward behavior or in activities of daily living (Citrin & Dixon, 1977; Greene, Nicol, & Jamieson, 1979; Hanley, McGuire, & Boyd, 1981; Woods, 1979; Zepelin, Wolfe, & Kleinplatz, 1981). Because orientation items tested were similar to those rehearsed in RO classes, these results are not surprising.

Zepelin, Wolfe, & Kleinplatz (1982) reported that the least-impaired subjects benefited the most, although Hanley, McGuire, & Boyd (1981) could not demonstrate any effects of dementia severity on outcome. Hanley et al. also found that specific ward orientation training programs proved better than RO in actually getting confused residents to find places on the ward. Johnson, McLaren, & McPherson (1981) found that frequency and type of RO program had no effect on the results. Woods (1979) found that both RO and a socialization group were more effective than no treatment, but that RO was more effective than the socialization group. These results suggest the benefits of RO were more than just the nonspecific effects of doing something. Hogstel (1979) and Holden and Sinebruchow (1978) could not demonstrate that RO was significantly better than a control procedure at improving behavior or orientation.

Recent careful reviews of the RO literature by Schwenk (1979) and Powell-Proctor and Miller (1982) detail a number of problems and shortcomings in our knowledge of the efficacy of RO. Most RO studies have not carefully defined the extent, cause, or duration of dementia in their subject populations, making it impossible to determine which patients are most likely to benefit from this treatment. While most RO programs produce statistically significant improvement in accuracy of answers to questions about orientation, the practical value of this effect for residents of institutions is not clear. The great majority of studies do not suggest that this improvement generalizes to other ward behaviors or to the ability to perform activities of daily-living.

On balance, RO does appear to have an effect that is more beneficial than nonspecific consequences of performing some kind of treatment. Best results can be anticipated from programs in which the specific content of therapy is tailored to individual attributes of the patient. The greatest benefits of RO are likely to be seen in patients with mild dementia. Enthusiastic and regular interaction of staff members with patients probably contributes a great deal to the success of treatment. In fact, Citrin and Dixon (1977) have suggested that the beneficial effects of 24-hour RO consist of changing the institutional staff so that they communicate more effectively with elderly patients. Use of RO can certainly create and help maintain a positive, therapeutic approach to the care of institutionalized, demented elderly patients that has often been lacking in the past.

CONCLUSION

Providing long term care to the elderly demented patient is a major problem that will become even more compelling as the proportion of elderly persons in the population increases. Because treatments for preventing or reversing most dementing illness are not available now, and probably will not be available in the near future, optimal long-term care implies support and training of family care providers, treatment of secondary behavioral and medical problems, and providing environmentally sound long-term institutional settings when the patient can no longer be maintained in the community. Such an approach can relieve suffering and promote optimal quality of life for the dementia patient.

REFERENCES

Abse, W., & Dahlstrom, W. The value of chemotherapy in senile mental disturbances. *Journal of the American Medical Association,* 1960, *174,* 2036–2042.

Altman, H., Mehta, D., Evanson, R., & Sletten, I. Behavioral effects of drug therapy on psychogeriatric patients. Chlorpromazine and thioridazine. *Journal of the American Geriatrics Society,* 1973, *21,* 241–248.

Aronson, M., & Lipkowitz, R. Senile dementia, Alzheimer's type: The family and the health care delivery system. *Journal of the American Geriatrics Society,* 1981, *29,* 568–571.

Barnes, R., & Raskind, M. DSM III criteria and the clinical diagnosis of dementia: A nursing home study. *Journal of Gerontology,* 1980, *36,* 20–27.

Barnes, R., Raskind, M., Scott, M., & Murphy, C. Problems of families caring for Alzheimer patients: Use of a support group. *Journal of the American Geriatrics Society,* 1981, *29,* 80–85.

Barnes, R., Veith, R., Okimoto, J., Raskind, M., & Gumbrecht, G. The efficacy of antipsychotics in behaviorally disturbed dementia patients. *American Journal of Psychiatry,* 1982, *139,* 799–802.

Barton, R., & Hurst, L. Unnecessary use of tranquilizers in elderly patients. *British Journal of Psychiatry,* 1966, *112,* 989–990.

Bergman, K., Foster, E., Justice, A., & Matthews. Management of the demented elderly patient in the community. *British Journal of Psychiatry,* 1978, *132,* 441–449.

Bielski, R., & Friedel, R. Prediction of tricyclic antidepressant response. *Archives of General Psychiatry,* 1976, *33,* 1479–1489.

Blenkner, M. Environmental change and the aging individual. *Journal of Gerontology,* 1967, *7,* 101–105.

Blumenthal, M. Psychosocial factors in reversible and irreversible brain failure. *Journal of Clinical Experimental Gerontology,* 1979, *1,* 39–55.

Borup, J., Gallego, D., & Hefferman, P. Relocation: Its effects on health functioning and mortality. *Gerontologist,* 1980, *20,* 468–479.

Borup, J., Gallego, D., & Hefferman, P. Relocation and its effects on mortality. *Gerontologist,* 1979, *10,* 135–140.

Brocklehurst, J. Brain failure in old age—social implications. *Age and Ageing,* 1977, *6,* 30–34.

Brook, R., Degun, G., & Mather, M. Reality orientation, a therapy for psychogeriatric patients: A controlled study. *British Journal of Psychiatry,* 1975, *127,* 42–45.

Busse, E. Mental disorders in later life—organic brain syndromes. In E. Busse and E. Pfeiffer (Eds.), *Mental illness in later life.* Washington, D.C.: American Psychiatric Association, 1973.

Carroll, B., Curtis, G., & Mendels, J. Neuroendocrine regulation in depression. II. Discrimination of depressed from nondepressed patients. *Archives of General Psychiatry,* 1976, *33,* 1051–1058.

Citrin, R., & Dixon, D. Reality orientation: A milieu therapy used in an institution for the aged. *Gerontologist,* 1977, *17,* 39–43.

Demuth, G., & Rand, B. Atypical major depression in a patient with severe primary degenerative dementia. *American Journal of Psychiatry,* 1980, *137,* 1609–1610.

Fuller, J., Ward, E., Evans, A., Massam, K., & Gardner, A. Dementia: Supportive groups for relatives. *British Medical Journal,* 1979, *1,* 1684–1685.

Godber, C. Planning services for the elderly demented patient. *Age and Ageing,* 1977, *6,* 100–103.

Greene, J., Nicol, R., & Jamieson, H. Reality orientation with psychogeriatric patients. *Behavior Research and Therapy,* 1979, *17,* 615–618.

Hamilton, D., & Bennett, J. The use of trifluoperazine in geriatric patients. *Journal of American Geriatrics Society,* 1962, *10,* 140–142.

Hanley, I., McGuire, R., & Boyd, W. Reality orientation and dementia: A controlled trial of two approaches. *British Journal of Psychiatry,* 1981, *138,* 10–14.

Hogstel, M. Use of reality orientation with ageing confused patients. *Nursing Research,* 1979, *28,* 161–165.

Holden, U., & Sinebruchow, A. Reality orientation therapy: A study investigating the value of this therapy in the rehabilitation of elderly people. *Age and Ageing,* 1978, *7,* 83–90.

Johnson, C., McLaren, S., & McPherson, F. The comparative effectiveness of three versions of "classroom" reality orientation. *Age and Ageing,* 1981, *10,* 33–35.

Kahn, R. The mental health system and the future aged. *Gerontologist,* 1975, *15,* 24–31.

Krause, A. Spasoff, R., Beattie, E. et al. Elderly applicants to long-term care institutions: Their characteristics, health problems, and state of mind. *Journal of the American Geriatrics Society,* 1976, *24,* 117–124.

Lazarus, L., Stafford, B., Cooper, K. et al. A pilot study of an Alzheimer patients' relatives discussion group. *Gerontologist,* 1981, *21,* 353–358.

Lezak, M. Living with the characterologically altered brain injured patient. *Journal of Clinical Psychiatry,* 1978, *39,* 592–598.

Petric, W., Ban, T., Berncy, S. et al. Loxapine in psychogeriatrics: A placebo- and standard-controlled clinical investigation. *Journal of Clinical Psychopharmacology,* 1982, *2,* 122–126.

Post, F. Diagnosis of depression in geriatric patients and treatment modalities appropriate for the population. In D. Gallant, G. Simpson (Eds.), *Depression: Behavioral, biochemical, diagnostic and treatment concepts.* New York: Spectrum, 1976.

Powell-Proctor, L., & Miller, E. Reality orientation: A critical appraisal. *British Journal of Psychiatry,* 1982, *140,* 457–463.

Prien, R. Problems and practices in geriatric psychopharmacology. *Psychosomatics,* 1980, *21,* 213–223.

Prinz, N. Sleep changes with aging. In E. Fann & C. Eisdorfer (Eds.), *Psychopharmacology of Aging.* New York: Spectrum Books, 1980, 1–12.

Rabins, P.V., Mace, M.L., & Lucas, M.J. The impact of dementia on the family. *Journal of the American Medical Association,* 1982, *248,* 333–335.

Rada, R., & Kellner, R. Thiothixene in the treatment of geriatric patients with chronic organic brain syndrome. *Journal of the American Geriatrics Society,* 1976, *24,* 105–107.

Raskind, M., Peskind, E., Rivard, M. et al. The dexamethasone suppression test and cortisol circadian rhythm in primary degenerative dementia. *American Journal of Psychiatry,* 1982, *139,* 1468–1471.

Ray, W., Federspiel, L., & Schaffner, W. A study of antipsychotic drug use in nursing homes: Epidemiologic evidence suggesting misuse. *American Journal of Public Health,* 1980, *70,* 485–491.

Reifler, B., & Eisdorfer, C. A clinic for the impaired elderly and their families. *American Journal of Psychiatry,* 1980, *137,* 1399–1403.

Reifler, B., Larson, E., & Hanley, R. Coexistence of cognitive impairment and depression in geriatric outpatients. *American Journal of Psychiatry,* 1982, *139,* 623–626.

Robinson, D. Evaluation of certain drugs in geriatric patients. *Archives of General Psychiatry,* 1959, *1,* 41–46.

Sainsbury, P. & Gard de Alarcon, J. The psychiatrist and the geriatric patient: The effects of community care on the family of the geriatric patient. *Journal of Geriatric Psychiatry,* 1970, *1,* 23–41.

Sanford, R. Tolerance of debility in elderly dependents by supporters at home: Its significance for hospital practice. *British Medical Journal,* 1975, *3,* 471–473.

Schwenk, M. Reality orientation for the institutionalized aged: Does it help? *Gerontologist,* 1979, *19,* 373–377.

Seager, C. Chlorpromazine in treatment of elderly psychotic women. *British Medical Journal,* 1955, *1,* 882–885.

Spar, J., & Gerner, R. Does the desamethasone suppression test distinguish dementia from depression? *American Journal of Psychiatry,* 1982, *138,* 238–240.

Stephens, L. *Reality orientation.* Washington, D.C.: APA Hospital and Community Psychiatry Service, 1966.

Sugarman, W., Williams, B., & Adlerstein, A. Haloperidol in the psychiatric disorders of old age. *American Journal of Psychiatry,* 1964, *120,* 1190–1192.

Taulbee, L. Reality orientation and the aged. In I. Burnside (Ed.), *Nursing and the aged.* Hightstown, New Jersey: McGraw-Hill, 1976.

Taulbee, L., & Folsom, J. Reality orientation for geriatric patients. *Hospital and Community Psychiatry,* 1966, *17,* 135–137.

Veith, R., & Horita, A. Drugs for psychiatric disorders. In R.C. Adelman (Ed.), *Handbook Series on Aging,* West Palm Beach, Florida: CRC Press, Inc., 1984.

Woods, R. Reality orientation and staff attention: A controlled study. *British Journal of Psychiatry,* 1979, *134,* 502–507.

Zarit, S., Reever, K., & Bach-Peterson, J. Relatives of the impaired elderly: Correlates of feelings of burden. *Gerontologist,* 1980, *20,* 649–655.

Zarit, S., & Zarit, J. *Families under stress: Interventions for caregivers of senile dementia patients.* Paper presented at an NIMH Workshop for Directors of Clinical Training Programs in Mental Health of the Aging. Silver Springs, Maryland: 1982.

Zepelin, H., Wolfe, C., & Kleinplatz, F. Evaluation of a year long reality orientation program. *Journal of Gerontology,* 1981, *36,* 70–77.

PART III

Therapeutic Techniques

6

BRIEF PSYCHOTHERAPY WITH THE AGED: A CLINICAL APPROACH

Jerome M. Grunes

Brief psychotherapy with the aged was born of the necessity to give psychiatric services to aged individuals who were in congregate living arrangements. As a resident in psychiatry in 1954, and later as a consultant from 1955 to 1981, I utilized a brief dynamic psychotherapeutic approach to the institutional aged at Drexel Home. I shall describe the treatment which was undertaken in the home.

Drexel Home was a home for aged Jews founded after the Civil War as the "Israelitesche Altenheim." It maintained its essential German-Jewish tradition even after it became Drexel Home for Aged Jews in 1890, and the majority of the residents eventually were of Eastern European or American origin. When I arrived in 1954, there were approximately 250 residents living in the main home. (An apartment annex was later created for physically healthier residents.) At that time the average age for admission was 75 years, but by 1970, the average age of incoming residents was 84. The length of stay was approximately four years, and few residents left the home either to return to the community or transfer to another setting. Clearly, then, this was a "Home for Life," which was the title of a film made at the home to celebrate its 75th anniversary. The Psychiatric Service consisted of myself as consultant, who spent one half-day a week at the Home, and from 2-to-4 second-year residents in Psychiatry from Michael Reese Hospital and for some years from the University of Chicago. A clinical

GERIATRIC MENTAL HEALTH
ISBN 0-8089-1657-2

psychologist was available for psychological testing. There was a full-time social worker in the department.

The idea of having a Psychiatric Service came from the director of the home, Mr. Ben Grossman. He had pioneered in the development of professional administration of homes for the elderly, and was also psychoanalytically oriented and encouraged Dr. Marc Hollender, a psychoanalyst, to spend time at the home directly after World War II. Dr. Hollender remained as consultant and teacher until 1955, when he left Chicago.

Until Mr. Grossman's development of a special department, psychiatrists were used by institutions mainly on an emergency basis; i.e., to prescribe medications for problem patients or to commit patients to state hospitals. The ideal of prevention of psychiatric emergencies or help in the selection of residents for the home were part of the motivation for the new department. By having all the residents seen by psychiatrists either before admission or very soon after being admitted, the stigma that the aged at times attribute to psychiatric consultation was eased. To see a psychiatrist was part of the normal, expected routine of Drexel Home. Almost all the residents at some time or other during their stay at the home were seen in psychotherapy. Approximately half the referrals were made by administration, nursing staff, occupational therapy, or other departments and about half were self-referrals. It was quite rare that such services, once offered, were refused.

The psychiatric sessions were thirty minutes in duration, and residents could be seen in their rooms if they were too feeble or ill to come to the psychiatrists' offices. Although institutional populations are stereotyped as being similar, there was a wide spectrum of social and personality differences among the residents at the home. For those who were referred by the administration, the most common problems were difficulties with room mates, aggressive and/or negativistic behavior, the latter of which included refusing medication or surgery, cursing, being untidy in dress, and those who were noisily confused. Self-referred residents generally experienced loss of an adult child, were concerned about the feared physical or mental losses of their capacities, suffering from anxieties, phobias, or depressive symptomatology. This latter group clearly was not different in their concerns than the population of the same age who were in the community.

TECHNIQUES

With both groups, psychotherapy, consisting of ten-to-twenty sessions, was provided. As a psychiatric history was available on all patients from time of admission, the special conditions that had precipitated the need for treatment became the focus. A psychodynamic formulation was arrived at and a therapy strategy devised. A variety of technical procedures were utilized including active interpretation and confrontations that stated both sides of the conflict to which the patient was reacting. The following cases will illustrate the techniques.

Case One

One of my first patients was a 73-year-old man who had been a resident of the home for six years. He had entered the institution two years after his wife's death, when he had fallen into a depression after loss and was unable to maintain himself in the community. He was an elfin man, with bright eyes and rather abrupt and sudden movements. He could not tolerate the thirty-minute sessions and would terminate the interviews abruptly by leaving after smoking a cigarette. He refused to speak of his dead wife or of his children with whom he tried to live following her death. Instead, he spoke of his youth in Russia, of his early socialistic ideals, of his rebellion against his tyrannical father, and of his running away from home and joining a group of wild boys on the road. Eventually he made his way to the United States, learned a trade, married, and had two children. At the home, he was an isolate and participated in none of the activities that the institution provided. He slept poorly and refused all medications. He enjoyed the "intellectual discussion" he had with me. One day as he bounced up and was about to leave, I commented on his cracked, worn shoes and suggested that he see the housekeeper for a new pair. When I saw him a week later, he told me that he "had not slept for days and had wrestled with the idea of suicide." If he had come to so sorry a state so that his doctor had to tell him that he needed shoes, he did not need to live any longer, for he had lost the faintest semblance of self-observation and self-sufficiency. I realized that I had dealt him a severe narcissistic blow by a seeming off-handed comment about his shoes. He told me that he thought of suicide, but finally decided to live based on his youthful ideals, "to see what would happen to the world." Within a month, this patient organized himself to leave the home, found an apartment and job for himself, and continued to see me in my city office.

This case illustrates the importance of caution in treating the elderly. At the time, the narcissistic vulnerability of this man was not recognized. Fortunately, his positive transference and youthful ideals saved him from self-destruction. The ability of the therapist to recognize errors and correct them is an essential part of treatment. In this case a "screen" interpretation of the patient's regressive tendencies was reacted to by mobilizing the patient into activity.

Case Two

An 83-year-old male resident presented with symptoms of confusion and depression. I had known him for some years as a pleasant, rather superficial man who conducted tours for prospective residents or family members through the home.

He also served as a beadle at the religious services. He had asked to see me. His usual neat appearance had given way, his clothes were soiled, and he had even failed to shave for several days. He related that he was not feeling well, was sleeping poorly and had no appetite, and could not deliver the mail to the other residents. He told of his many symptoms and then, in passing, mentioned that his sister was ill. As I knew his history from his admission some years earlier, I asked about his sister. I knew that this man had never married, had been very attached to his mother until her death, and was very dependent on his older sister both for emotional and financial support. He had worked as a haberdasher. After his mother's death he went to live with his sister, who was married. He entered the home after a protracted illness when it became evident that his sister no longer could care for him. The patient was a somewhat effeminate man who preferred the company of women. The men at the home avoided him. I explored with him the nature of his sister's illness, and it became apparent that she was terminally ill with cancer. I told him that I thought he had reacted to her illness as if she was already dead, and that he seemed confused and lost as a result of the impending loss. He brightened considerably and by the next week was much improved. After nine additional sessions, we agreed to stop with the understanding that he was to see me if the depression recurred. As we ended, the patient took out a piece of paper upon which he had written some notes that he had gleaned from our sessions. They turned out to be homilies, none of which I ever delivered, for example, "It is always darkest before the dawn," "Every cloud has a silver lining;" etc. He kept this paper with him as long as he lived. In time his sister died, but his mourning reaction was not severe. Eventually, some four years later, he also died rather quietly. There were recurrences of acute depression and he remained on good terms with me until his end.

This case is a good example of confrontation, i.e., the feared death of the sister that helped the patient orient himself emotionally and consciously to the task of mourning that lay ahead. In time his sister died. Having worked through his ambivalence in his treatment with me, his mourning reaction was not severe. The paper on which he had written his homilies, and which he kept with him for the rest of his life, served as a transitional object, soothing him when he became anxious.

Case Three

Mr. S. was an 85-year-old man who had been in the home for about three years. He suffered from diabetes mellitus with peripheral vascular involvement. I was asked to see him by the internist of the home because he had refused surgery for gangrene of his toes. Mr. S. was a rather determined man who had great difficulty in his adjustment to the home. He insisted on defying everyone and was there only because of the care he required. He had made a bad marriage and was divorced. His only child lived in a distant city. When first seen, he was belligerent and angry. He denied that anything was the matter with him. He claimed his toes were dark because he was unable to bathe as frequently as he wished, and when we talked of his diabetes, he admitted that he had had the disease for some years but that it was well controlled. At 85, he felt that he did not want to be a "guinea pig" for the doctors. When I pointed out the fact that he was well within his rights to refuse surgery if he was fully aware of the consequences, he listened attentively to me. I further indicated that I would go the distance to stop the "harassment" by the surgeons. He left the session less angry and agitated. I did speak to the internist and surgeon, expressing my view that the patient should make the decision without being pressured. Over the next week, the gangrene worsened and there were signs of toxicity. In the next session, the patient recounted his need to be "his own boss" and of events in his life for which he had to make decisions. He stated that he had always been right.

At the end of the session, he decided to go ahead with the surgery, which involved a mid-thigh amputation, reminding me that it was his "decision." I followed the patient while in the hospital and after his return to the Drexel Home. He then insisted on having a prosthesis despite the skepticism of the Physical Therapy Department. Within a short time he was able to master the prosthesis. Two years later, he required a second amputation of the other leg, and eventually, he had to use a wheelchair. He died at age 89.

This case emphasized the need of patients to have someone on their side in institutional settings, where patients are frequently alone and without family.

Case Four

Mrs. Z. was an 87-year-old woman who entered the home reluctantly when her three daughters decided she could no longer care for herself. I saw her prior to her admission and decided to see her for brief psychotherapy for 15 sessions. Mrs. Z. was the youngest of 7 children. She came to America as a young woman, went briefly to school and then to work. At 21, she met and married a man considerably older. The marriage was a disaster: he was unreliable, not a good provider, and she was very critical of him. They had three girls and when the youngest daughter went to college, Mrs. Z. divorced her husband. She found a job as a seamstress and was still working, though with considerable difficulty, when she entered the home. Mrs. Z. was angry and resentful at being sent to the home. She blamed her sons-in-law rather than her daughters for this turn of events. It was their fault. If only her daughters had not married! She would have been smarter if she had not married, but became a professional like her daughter who had a Ph.D.. If she had such a degree, she would never need a man. Her rage at men eventually included her husband, father, sons-in-law, and the director of the home. She exempted me from this long list at the time. However, as we met for our sessions, her rage gave way to frank paranoid delusions. She was being poisoned. The poison was introduced into her food and at night as gas from pipes in her room. She could soon no longer contain the delusions and would be found in the stairwell of the building shouting and cursing her persecutors. The only interpretation which seemed to be received with some influence was my comment about her strength to withstand all the abuse that she was receiving and that she felt had always received from life. She smiled and said, "One should be grateful for what one has."

While psychotherapy did not relieve the late onset paraphrenia, it proved to be of use in helping the nursing and ancillary services in dealing with this woman. Although Mrs. Z. remained isolated from the residents of the home, her need to be alert and vigilant made her an excellent observer of what was happening in the institution. Some years later, I was informed by the nurses that Mrs. Z. had undergone a transformation; she was now pleasant and tractable and her delusions had disappeared. I immediately went to see her, for I suspected an undiagnosed physical illness. Such had been my experience with aged paranoid patients who suddenly lose their symptoms. Mrs. Z. was indeed quite pleasant. I asked about her physical health and went through a review of systems with her. She was constipated and her stools were "like peanuts," she told me. I insisted that she see the internist in the home, but she refused. Over the next few weeks, we had a battle of wills. Finally, it was arranged that she see a physician not associated with the home. He hospitalized her and it was discovered that she had a carcinoma of the colon. The patient refused surgery despite the entreaties of the attending surgeon. She returned to the home and resumed her paranoid state until she was about to die. Her last four days were marked by a serenity and acceptance of death that I have rarely seen. The paraphrenia of this lady helped her deal with the shame of being in an institution, i.e., of not being loved enough. She was well-liked by the staff, despite the fact that they were objects of her projections. This in part was due to their understanding of some of the mechanisms for her delusions.

This case represented the need for psychiatric consultation in long-term care facilities. The need for the staff to understand transferences, particularly negative ones of which they are the objects, and their own countertransferences is a prime necessity. The consultant can bring his understanding of the patient's problems and also help the staff understand their own reactions to patients.

Case Five

The patient, A.F., was 71 when she entered the home. She was the youngest resident at that time and had come from a stay of several months at a psychiatric hospital where she had undergone extensive electroshock (ECT) therapy for psychotic depression. When she was first seen, she presented with organic brain syndrome as a reaction to the 28 ECTs she had undergone. Her emotions were flat and superficial. She had no memory of the illness that had necessitated hospitalization. Her history that was obtained from her son and elder sister revealed that the patient's husband had died two years before her illness. She had done quite well and seemingly had mourned for him. In her second year following his death, she became immobilized and fearful of being alone. Her only son was married and although he tried to be of help, he was unable to. The patient wanted only to be with her elder sister. The sister was a wealthy woman who lived with her husband. The husband disliked the patient and openly denigrated her.

Past history revealed a woman who always appeared adequate. She was European-born, the second of two children and was ten years her sister's junior. The patient's father had come to the United States and left his wife and daughters in Russia. World War I intervened and the family was not reunited until 1920. She did not remember her father and was frightened of the stranger who met her in the United States. Her parents were divorced shortly after they arrived in the United States. The patient's major attachment was clearly to her mother. When her mother died, the patient had a normal mourning reaction and went to live with her sister who, by then, was married. She received a high school diploma and worked for a short while as a secretary until she married. Her husband was considerably older than she and was a good caretaker. She had only one child and did not like the role of mother. Nevertheless, she did the job as mother "good enough." She never returned to work when her son entered college, but enjoyed social activities.

As therapy progressed, it became clear that her major object relationship was her mother and later her sister. She chose a maternal man to marry, and when he died, turned once again to her sister for organizing her life. The failure of this attempt led to a profound and psychotic depression.

As might be expected, the patient did extremely well in the institution. She viewed herself as a very adequate resident of the home, more like an auxiliary staff member than a resident of the home. I had known her for some years when she asked to be seen again. She was afraid that she was becoming depressed again and feared being hospitalized and having to receive ECT again. Her sister's husband had died and this had stirred up all her old yearnings to live with her sister. Instead, the sister chose to stay with her daughter, the patient's niece, and her family. The patient's unexpressed rage at her sister's "betrayal" was intense and was worked on for about twenty psychotherapy sessions. The insights that had been previously obtained over the years about the patient were interpreted to her. A depressive reaction was prevented. The resolution of the patient's conflict took a curious turn when she began to "keep company" with a man who was also a prominent resident in the home. She further was "adopted" by his family, particularly by his daughter, and while she did not marry this man, they were constant companions.

In this case active interpretation of Mrs. F's rage and her understanding of her anger helped to avoid a depression. While psychotherapy benefitted this patient, this case also demonstrates the restorative power of life-long coping and compensatory behaviors.

Case Six

The patient, F.L., was an 85-year-old woman who entered the home following a series of physical illnesses, including coronary occlusion with congestive heart failure and generalized arthritis.

Mrs. L. was a childless widow who became known, without foundation, as the "whore" of the home. Although chronically ill and having great difficulty in ambulation, she was seen by most of the women in the home as sexually provocative and seductive. The male residents also avoided her but her reputation remained. It was based on two phenomena: one, her narcissistic interest in her own body; the second was her history. She had indeed utilized her sexuality in her survival during the Holocaust. She had been a successful businesswoman in Poland and had operated several beauty shops before the second World War. She had been widowed and had become the mistress of a Polish doctor, who was married. He was able to arrange false identity papers for her so that, throughout the German occupation, she was able to masquerade as a gentile. Sponsored by a cousin, she came to the United States as a cosmetician and worked for some years before her illnesses necessitated retirement and eventual institutionalization.

The course of her stay at the home was tumultuous. Her need to feel superior to the residents and her alienation from the women because of the jealousy she provoked, as well as the fear of her sexuality she elicited from the male residents made her a *persona non grata*. The nursing staff found her intolerable because she demanded their attention constantly, playing one nurse off against the other and causing dissention among the staff. I saw her intermittently for ten sessions or so over two years. This usually followed a referral by the nursing staff.

Therapy remained much the same. The patient would insist on her innocence for whatever offense she felt accused. She saw herself as a victim of the other residents. She idealized me and emphasized my power as her defender against the attacks of residents and staff. In this sense, she utilized the therapist much the way Goldfarb and Sheps (1954) described in their work with institutional aged. She consciously manipulated me to gain her own ends, that is, to remain in the home. This patient was terribly fearful of being ejected as an undesirable resident and, having nowhere else to go, was in fear for her life much as she was during the war. In fact, she was psychologically something of an imposter: her sexuality was a sham, as were her object-relationships, and her narcissism was in the service of her survival. She used the therapist to re-establish an equilibrium with the hostile environment. As therapist, I interpreted the patient's needs to the staff and things would go along smoothly for some time. When the patient lay dying of her chronic cardiac condition, she became frankly paranoid, and had hallucinations, among others, of being sexually misused by men who came through the walls at night.

Brief psychotherapy enabled this difficult and isolated narcissistic woman to remain in the home until her death some five years after her admission. This patient utilized the therapist as an ally to gain something of his power to ward off the feeling of helplessness that plagued her. The patient's narcissism was supported by the therapist.

DISCUSSION

Brief psychotherapy has its roots in psychoanalysis. In the early cases described by Breuer and Freud (1953) in *Studies on Hysteria,* patients were seen once, like Katherina, or for as long as one year, like Anna O. Many of Freud's earliest cases were of relatively short duration. For example, the classic case of Dora (1953) was treated by Freud for just 11 weeks. Bruno Walter, the famous conductor, described a successful six-session treatment with Freud in 1906, and the composer, Gustave Mahler, rid himself of a painful symptom in a single four-hour walk with Freud (Ferenczi and Rank, 1925).

As objectives of psychoanalysis became more ambitious and its theoretical structure grew more complex, the trend was to more lengthy analysis.

To counter this, Sandor Ferenczi (1926) published a series of papers whose thesis was to shorten psychoanalysis through conscious opposition to what he labeled "passivity" on the part of the analyst and regression in the patient. This has become a cardinal rule in all successive short-term psychotherapies.

The second dictum was enunciated by Ferenczi and Rank (1925) in *The Development of Psychoanalysis*. Using the experience of Freud, who had set a termination date in advance with his analysis of the "Rat Man," Ferenczi and Rank generalized on it to focus on separation anxiety by developing a time-limited treatment. It was their view that separation was the prototype of all later anxieties. By eliciting it early in treatment by having a limited number of sessions and having the patient know that therapy will be ending at a specific date, Ferenczi and Rank felt that analysis would be hastened. This dimension of brief psychotherapy has been adopted by all recent practitioners of the technique.

Ferenczi (1926) proposed, a third, more controversial point, emphasis on affective experience in treatment rather than intellectual understanding. This aspect of treatment has probably caused greater dissension than any other in this field. Many critics felt that Ferenczi proposed manipulating the transference of the patients to the therapist. Most brief therapists utilize interpretation as the major intervention (though differing on what aspect of the patient's problems should be the focus) rather than the more active treatment of Ferenczi. The concept of the "corrective emotional experience" of Alexander and French (1946) harkens back to Ferenczi's "active" treatment and became the cornerstone of the attack on Brief Psychoanalysis that the two developed in the 1940s.

All brief therapies involve early and rapid diagnosis and elucidation of basic conflicts that become the focus for therapeutic work. It is in this area that most brief therapies diverge. Malan (1963) at the Tavistock Clinic in London, adheres to the most classic analytic model by making transference interpretations the center of treatment as well as "the working through of anger and grief at the loss of the therapist at termination." At the other extreme, crisis intervention clinics, essentially brief psychotherapy, attempt anxiety-suppression therapy as a means of returning the patient to the premorbid state (Sifneos, 1972).

A major problem is selection of patients for the short-term psychotherapies. Criteria frequently are described in terms of onset of symptoms, focality of conflicts, intelligence of patient, capacity to experience anxiety, and "psychological mindedness." Nowhere is there a criterion on aging except in a negative sense, i.e., the aged as unacceptable for treatment. Recently, Sifneos (1982) has reported on short-term psychotherapeutic work with elderly patients: he seems to be the first to have worked intensively with this modality to include patients in their 60s and 70s. His experience indicates that, while using the same criteria and similar psychoanalytic techniques that he has evolved for treating younger patients, results with the aged were similar.

The one pioneer in using psychodynamic approach to the aged and who developed a specialized technique for treatment was Goldfarb (1954). Unfortunately, his work is forgotten by most therapists today. Like all innovators in this field, he developed a technique for treatment as well as one for learning about the aged—particularly the impaired elderly. In many facets it resembled the active treatment of Ferenczi (1926) and Ferenczi and Rank (1925).

Essentially, Goldfarb viewed the impaired, institutionalized aged as suffering from ego weakness that could be overcome by an alliance with a powerful person. In treatment, Goldfarb permitted himself to be used by the "impotent" elder who needed to feel strong through the therapist. The therapist thus would become the source of power for the previously weak patient. If not interfered with by premature interpretation, Goldfarb argued that the patient would struggle actively to be seen as worthwhile, useful, and potent as he or she established a sense of self with the therapist. Although Goldfarb wrote before the recent work on narcissism, his theory of technique can be translated into self-psychological terms. He postulated that the aged suffer from a dearth of self-esteem in the narcissistic area. Psychotherapy revives the grandiose self and re-equilibrium is restored. The therapist becomes the self-object in "mirror" transference as well as becoming an idealized object. In Goldfarb's treatment, idealization of the therapist is not worked through by interpretation because the therapist's implied power is necessary for the maintenance of the "grandiose self" of the impaired elderly.

In the sixth case I reported, the "whore" of Drexel Home, the technique of treatment was essentially that of Goldfarb. The impoverished self of this lady sought power from me in her effort to struggle with an environment that appeared malevolent to her, but upon which she was dependent for her sustenance.

CONCLUSION

Brief psychotherapy was used by this author for many years at Drexel Home for the Aged. Based on psychodynamic principles, it was a technique that was individualized to fit the patient. Using the patient's history and current problems, the focus was on age-specific issues. Confrontation and interpretation were the major instruments of change, although in cases four and six, the staff of the home played a significant role in treatment. Selection of those cases for brief psychotherapy was based on focal issues that could be formulated within the first session. Transference interpretations, particularly negative ones, as in cases one and three, enabled the work to proceed. Separation and termination issues did not emerge for special effort except when it was part of the focal conflicts. Follow-up studies of treatment results were easily obtainable, as the patients generally remained in the setting until death.

At present there is a general reaction among geropsychiatrists and geropsychologists against use of the institutionalized aged as representatives of normal aging. While there is validity in such a view, it must not be forgotten that people in institutions have their own personalities that are not destroyed by pressures of congregate living. It should be further noted that as the researcher becomes more familiar with an institution, he or she can learn that variety in adaptation, rather than mere superficial conformity, is the rule.

Looking back on the people in the cases included in this chapter, I am not impressed with my therapeutic "correctness" but remember instead a group of people who taught me to respect their individuality and defensive struggles to maintain their sense of self despite intrapsychic conflicts, losses of significant others, and the inexorable march of time that undermined their bodies.

REFERENCES

Alexander, F., & French, T.M. *Psychoanalytic therapy.* New York: Ronald Press, 1946.

Breuer, J., & Freud, S. *Studies on hysteria 1895* (S.E. Vol. II). London: The Hogarth Press, 1953.

Ferenczi, S. The further development of an active therapy in psychoanalysis. In S. Ferenczi (Ed.), *Further contributions to the theory of psychoanalysis.* London: Hogarth Press, 1926.

Ferenczi, S., & Rank, O. *The Development of psychoanalysis.* New York: Nervous and Mental Disease Publishing Co., 1925.

Freud, S. *Fragment of an analysis of a case of hysteria 1905.* (S.E., Vol. VII) London: The Hogarth Press, 1953.

Goldfarb, A.I., & Sheps, J. Psychotherapy of the aged. *Psychosomatic Medicine,* May-June 1954, *XVI* (3), 24–29.

Malan, D.H. *A study of brief psychotherapy.* New York: Plenum Press, 1963.

Malan, D.H. *The frontier of brief psychotherapy.* New York: Plenum Press, 1976.

Sifneos, *P.E. Psychopathology and Treatment in Later Life,* Paper presented at the NIMH Conference on Psychodynamic Research Perspectives on Development, Rockville, Maryland, Nov. 6-8, 1982.

SELECTED READINGS

Hollender, M.H. Individualizing the aged. *Social Casework,* 1952, *33,* 337–342.

Hollender, M.H. Selection of patients for definitive forms of psychotherapy. *Arch. General Psychiatry,* 1964, *10,* 18–21.

Sifneos, P.E. *Short-term psychotherapy and emotional crisis.* Cambridge, Mass.: Harvard University Press, 1972.

7

GERIATRIC BEHAVIOR THERAPY

Richard A. Hussian

The development of assessment and therapy based upon an experimental analysis of behavior is a relatively new event in the history of psychotherapy. Concentrating on a functional analysis of problem behavior within the context of potentially quantifiable antecedent and consequence variables, the behavioral movement sought to offer a continuous view of the development of maladaptive behavior. In such a nondiscrete view of behavior, inappropriate responses (disorders) are seen as developing by the same laws that are at work for all behavior. The relationships between controlling events (stimuli), contingencies that effect response parameters, and behavior, are seen as being independent of the "appropriateness" of the output. In essence, a psychological or psychiatric disorder results, not from a qualitative disruption of normal learning processes, but rather from an independent process involving either a description of personal discomfort, labeling by observers, or the degree of interference with constructive behavior.

On the surface it appears as though behavioral assessment and therapy, given the continuity-of-development thesis, may have little to offer gerontologists, wherein the onset of many psychological disorders appear quite abruptly and often independently of learning processes. However, problematic behavior can evolve in two ways to present as operants, that is, behavior that may be modified through manipulation of antecedent or consequence variables (Hoyer, Mishara, Reidel, 1975). First, behavior that we label as inappropriate in elderly individuals may develop independent of

GERIATRIC MENTAL HEALTH
ISBN 0-8089-1657-2

organic involvement and present in much the same manner as behavior in other age groups. Therapeutic approaches for problems generated in this manner resemble treatment for younger persons, with only slight modifications in order to compensate for changes correlated with aging (e.g., sensory decrements, or memory impairment).

Second, inappropriate behavior may arise as a direct or indirect consequence of organic changes, resulting in a biobehavioral presentation which suggests "excessive dysfunction" beyond that accounted for by tissue pathology alone. Therapy designed to modify responses initially generated from organic changes will be dictated by the level of functioning of the impaired individual and the nature of the maladaptive behavior.

Baltes and Barton (1977) have derived an explanatory model based upon the interaction between biological or organic changes and environmental contingencies which, together, shape elderly responding. This *biobehavioral* view describes the prevalence of psychological disorders among the elderly as due to the following relationships, which tend to occur at high rates in later life:

1. The absence of positive consequences for adaptive behavior.
2. The presence of negative consequences for adaptive behavior.
3. The paucity of discriminative stimuli in the environment and/or a lessening of the ability of the elderly individual to discriminate among available stimuli.
4. The presence of discriminative stimuli in the environment that tend to inhibit adaptive responses.

The problems resulting from these relationships can be conveniently divided into three descriptive categories that may suggest the type of behavioral approach to alter the behavior.

The first category includes those behaviors that are present at *excessive* rates. The response itself may not be inappropriate in and of itself but rather labeled as inappropriate because of the high frequency of occurrence. Some of the behaviors that occur at disproportionately high rates among the elderly include chronic somatic complaints, frequent requests for analgesics and other medications in the absence of organic problems, repetitive vocalizations and other self-stimulatory behavior often associated with advanced dementia, hyperactivity, agitation, and self-injurious behavior. According to the Baltes–Barton model, these excesses may result from the presence of positive consequences (e.g., attention, or medication) or from the absence of positive consequences for alternative adaptive behavior. Through a careful functional analysis of target behavior the stimulus–response–consequence relationship can be determined and environmental adjustments made to effect the rate of responding.

The second category of behavior involves responses that occur at a frequency lower than that deemed adequate for functioning or lower than the baseline rate for the individual. The biobehavioral model explains the low occurrence or nonoccurrence of a particular response *(behavioral deficit)* as a result of deficient discriminative stimuli, the absence of positive consequences for the exhibition of the response, or the presence of negative consequences following the exhibition of the response. The loss of previously exhibited skills, low activity level, a decrease in social interactions, some aspects of depression, and reduced verbal behavior may be seen as common response deficits. Organic variables may interact with these contingencies as well. For example, if an event of an organic nature has occurred (e.g., cerebrovascular accident) and resulted in making a previously exhibited response (e.g., verbal behavior, or self-feeding) more difficult, and the positive consequences for these behaviors are not present or not enhanced sufficiently, the desired behavior will probably not be maintained.

The natural, albeit unfortunate, contingencies that are widespread in many settings in which the elderly find themselves, may make deficiencies in responding the most frequent reason for referral to clinicians. They contribute to a large extent to the picture of an unavoidable decline *due* to age-related changes. For instance, if minimal self-care behaviors are ignored by staff of a long-term care facility and basic care is provided routinely, it is not likely that independently generated self-care will be maintained. Negative consequences, in the form of reprimands or restraint, may even follow the occurrence of some adaptive behavior (e.g., independent ambulation). What develops may be inhibited responses due, not simply to physical limitation, but to functioning that is lower than would be accounted for by organic damage alone. Functional analysis, often through systematic observation, reveals the maintaining variables behind these deficits and suggests the therapeutic regimen.

The third category of problem behavior seen in the elderly involves *problems with stimulus control.* These problems exist quite frequently in the more impaired elderly individual who is experiencing a combination of sensory and central processing impairment. This category includes behavior that is not necessarily inherently inappropriate, nor does it occur at inappropriate rates, but rather it is occurring in the presence of inappropriate stimuli or appears to be occurring independently of the appropriate controlling stimuli. Problems of this nature would fit into the Baltes–Barton model as a lack of sufficient discriminative stimuli or, more likely, the inability of the individual to discriminate stimuli that are present (Baltes & Barton, 1977). The cause of this lack of discriminative ability is quite clearly organic, originating from either sensory deficits, central processing deficits, or a combination, and may result from acute organic difficulties or more chronic, irreversible involvement, or a combination of the two. Behavior that might fit into the designation includes wandering, inappropriate voiding, incontinence, and inappropriate sexual behavior.

It should be evident that behavior therapy techniques designed to change the rate of a response, either by increasing or decreasing the probability of its occurrence, would not be used when problems of stimulus control are involved. By designing our programs to increase the likelihood of a behavior occurring *in a different context* rather than to eliminate the behavior, we also avoid, in part, the ethical dilemma surrounding the reduction of a "normal" response in order to make other people more comfortable.*

A format for the analysis of behavioral problems and disorders from a behavior theory approach, which helps in the assessment of behavior and blends smoothly into the design and implementation of treatment, is desirable and useful. The treatments that may be applied to geriatric behavior problems are particularly well documented for their effectiveness when used with nonelderly groups. The list of such techniques includes shaping, token economies, successive approximation, systematic desensitization, extinction, flooding, self-instructional training, stress inoculation training, problem-solving training, skills retraining, modeling, response prevention, overcorrection, and assertiveness training, among others (Agras, 1978; Bandura, 1968; Mahoney, 1974; Rimm & Masters, 1974).

Though the application of many of these techniques to problems associated with the elderly is relatively new, a substantial body of literature verifying effectiveness already exists.

As early as 1964, Lindsley proposed the application of behavioral technology to problems of the elderly through the design of prosthetic living environments and the manipulation of contingencies that are often peculiar to the elderly (Lindsley, 1964). Cautela (1966), Cohen (1967), and Filer and O'Connell (1964) followed with descriptions of the application of behavior therapy to a variety of problems exhibited by geriatric clients. These early accounts of successful programs showed common themes that separated them from other approaches and developed logically from the theoretical bases of behavior therapy. These themes included a reduced emphasis on changing "personality," the use of more short-term therapies, functional analysis in assessment, descriptions of behavior of interest in easily quantifiable terms, a reliance on an experimental/clinical approach that emphasizes accountability through continuous data collection, the utilization of paraprofessionals and other mediators to reduce costs and increase the likelihood of maintainence, and the minimization of inferences drawn from the behavior sample (Hussian, 1981).

Outcome research on the clinical application of behavior therapy con-

---

*Purists might argue with the availability of effective stimulus control procedures: that all behavior which is deemed inappropriate by anyone other than the clients should be subject to a change in setting, therefore making response–reduction a less attractive clinical pursuit.

ducted since the initial studies has shown consistent success. This research will be reviewed briefly within the framework of behavioral excesses, deficits, and problems of stimulus control.

APPLICATION OF BEHAVIOR THERAPY IN GERIATRICS

The Reduction of Behavioral Excesses

Response–reduction techniques of behavior therapy have been successful in the reduction of a variety of negative behaviors that exist in many age groups. These same techniques also have been effective in reducing similar behavior in the elderly, including multiple verbalizations of dying (Hussian, 1979), screaming (Baltes, 1975), self-stimulatory behavior (Hussian, 1982), and drug-induced stereotypy (Jackson, Schonfeld, & Griffith, 1982; Palmer, Marshall, & Foster, 1980; Szekely, Turner, & Jacob, 1981; Taylor, Zlutnick & Hoehle, 1979). The methods employed attempted either to eliminate the long-standing positive events that follow the occurrence of the target behavior or attempt to reinforce and prompt alternative behaviors that are incompatible with the target response.

The first approach can be illustrated by attempts to reduce a client's multiple complaints in the absence of organic etiology. If staff or family time is limited, it is likely that the client receives intermittent positive reinforcement following some requests (either for attention or medication), thus making the behavior more difficult to eliminate. Those who come in contact with the client can make a concentrated effort to ignore such verbalizations while selectively reinforcing more appropriate statements. This should result in less time spent engaging in negative statements and more time engaging in neutral or positive statements. Carstensen and Fremouw (1981) utilized this type of selective reinforcement program for the reduction of paranoid delusions.

The second method, known as differential reinforcement of other behavior (DRO), is illustrated in a study by Hussian (1982). Three patients with Alzheimer's disease, who were exhibiting high frequencies of self-stimulatory behavior (average age = 74.67 years; average duration of symptoms = 39 months), were trained to differentially respond to two cues of different colors that were then used as cues to engage in more constructive but topographically similar behavior. Two of the patients spent large amounts of time manipulating their clothing (e.g., folding, rolling pants leg up and down, placing socks on their hands, etc.). By associating a previously reinforced cue with the alternative behavior of clay molding, the excessive stereotyped response was reduced by more than half (Patient I, 42% percent of the time observed to 8.4 percent; Patient 2, 56.8 percent to 6.4 percent). The third patient received reinforcement when her repetitive, nonsensical vocalizations were replaced by silence, which was the alternative response (from 60.2% of time observed during baseline to 34.2% after treatment). In these three cases, which involved extremely impaired individuals, differential reinforcement for alternative behavior was bolstered by a stimulus control enhancement procedure to reduce the excessive response.

Resolution of Deficit Responding

This area of response modification is the most well-researched in behavioral gerontology, probably because deficits in the behavioral repetoire tend to correlate more highly with deterioration. Treatment generally involves the gradual reshaping or retraining of absent or low-rate response by either providing more readily apparent or meaningful discriminative stimuli, by selectively reinforcing successive approximations toward the desired response, or a combination of the two. Behavioral treatment for deficits of response in the elderly have been evaluated in the areas of skill deficits, low activity level, low participation level, low levels of exercise, and deficient social interaction.

Skills that have been lost due to the interaction between organic dysfunction and a lack of reinforcement for exhibition of the skill can be retrained. Skills that have been re-established include self-feeding (Baltes & Zerbe, 1976), eating (Geiger & Johnson, 1974), social skills (Lopez, 1980), tooth care (Sachs, 1975), ambulation (MacDonald & Butler, 1974), exercise (Libb & Clements, 1969), bathing (Rinke, Williams, Lloyd et al., 1978), and verbal behavior (Green, Marlow, Briggs et al., 1980; Hoyer, Kafer, Simpson et al, 1974; MacDonald, 1978). Most of these studies utilized positive reinforcement delivered contingently upon the occurrence of the desired behavior or a small early component of such.

Low-activity level and withdrawal from interactions with environmental stimulation frequently have been targeted for modification. In 1975, McClannahan and Risley (1975), demonstrated that by making objects of interest available, prompting their use, and delivering reinforcement contingent upon their use, the number of such contacts increased significantly. Quattrochi-Tubin and Jason (1980) have reported similar results. Entire environments have been designed and studied that included elements of availability, selective prompting, and reinforcement, such as the Living Environments Group at the University of Kansas (Edwards, 1981; Risley & Edwards, 1978).

Recently, behavior therapists/experiments have begun to explore process variables involved in these programs, a logical step after outcome research yielded significant results. MacDonald et al. (1982) have examined how different aspects of the activity enhancement program work differentially depending upon the client's baseline rate of activity. They demonstrated that elders with relatively lower baseline rates of activity respond more to prompts, while persons with higher baseline rates of activity benefit mostly from availability of activities and reinforcement for active participation.

Berger and Rose (1977), Blackman et al. (1976), and other behavior therapists have used social interaction as a target. Observational studies have shown that, in many long-term care facilities, residents show low levels of social interaction with other residents and staff. Through the use of systematically delivered positive reinforcers contingent upon social contacts, researchers have been able to increase the number of contacts and, concomitantly, other adjunctive positive behaviors (e.g., activity level, or morale).

A related area of study may be viewed as an attempt to modify a deficit in responding. Decubiti or pressure areas are quite common among debilitated elders and result from continual contact between the fragile skin and other surfaces. The response of interest is continued skin contact, or, conversely, lack of sufficiently frequent breaks in contact (Malament, Dunn, & Davis, 1975). The authors increased the number of breaks in skin–wheelchair contacts through an avoidance procedure. In order to prevent the occurrence of an alarm, the aversive stimulus, patients learned to do five push-ups in their wheelchairs on a pre-determined schedule. The response was learned rapidly and the development of pressure sores was prevented.

Though this cursory summary of response enhancement techniques is far from complete (see Riedel, 1981), it should be clear that behavioral technology, as applied to problems frequently encountered in elderly clients, is well established.

Problems of Stimulus Control

MacDonald (1973) cited changes in sensory input as part of nonneurological causation of apparent senile dementia. Baltes and Barton (1977) cited the lack of discriminative stimuli or discriminative ability as a potential cause of age-related behavioral decline. Observers of low functioning geriatric patients will note the maintenance of intact stimulus–response chains (e.g., loosening of clothing–reclining–falling asleep) that nonetheless are inappropriate because of the location or timing of the completed chain. It appears to observers that the behavior is occurring independently of the stimulus (context) which previously had elicited the same pattern of response. In fact, frequent exhibition of such behavior in inappropriate settings often leads family members and care providers to become exasperated, labeling the exhibitor as "difficult," "purposely obnoxious," or "deviant."

More careful functional analysis, however, reveals that the behavior is not being effected by external consequences but that poor stimulus control is responsible. Three forms of behavior that are exhibited at relatively high frequencies by some debilitated elderly that may represent poor stimulus discrimination are inappropriate sexual behavior, incontinence, and wandering.

Stimulus control procedures traditionally have involved permitting access to sources of reinforcement (Quattrochi-Tubin & Jason, 1980). Stimulus control also technically involves the training of differential responding in the presence of different stimuli. This definition will be used for our purposes. In severely disoriented elderly patients, however, special stimulus enhancement or stimulus simplification may be necessary to effectively establish discriminative control. Written or verbal instructions that are intended to identify a restroom, for example, may be insufficient to shape selective and proper toilet usage. The impaired patient may not process the instructions, rapidly forget the association, or be incapable of discriminating among the available options at all. Though the patient may exhibit the complete array of urination behavior, if he or she is indiscriminate in "choosing" receptacles, the patient may be considered incontinent.

Even standard bladder-control programs that use such behavioral methods as shaping, conditioning, feedback, and contingent reinforcement (Pollack & Liberman, 1974), may be unsuccessful in changing the behavior since, not only have the appropriate stimulus response (SR) associations been interrupted, but "one stimulus looks as good as another." Therefore, it often is necessary to determine which stimuli can be discriminated before beginning retraining. The stimuli or stimulus components are then presented in a highly repetitive and routinized manner prior to placement on or near the appropriate objects in the environment.

The above technique is useful in control of wandering behavior. Snyder et al. (1978) and Hussian (1981) found that wandering, a behavior with potentially dangerous results, is a partial consequence of deficient stimulus control. It appears that elders exhibiting true wandering are not responding to those cues that control ambulation in less impaired individuals (e.g., written signs, indications of dangerous footing, structural barriers, or even simplified international warning symbols). Nevertheless, pilot data gathered in one study (Hussian, 1982) suggested that these individuals were discriminating among a variety of environmental events such as food trays, windows, and other residents, and could respond differentially to colors if the colors were associated with different consequences. This ability was then used to modify potentially dangerous wandering behavior, as is illustrated in the following case:

Three patients (mean age = 73.4 years) with diagnosis of Alzheimer's disease, who resided in a long-term care facility (mean length of institutionalization = 13 months), were presented with two sets of stimuli in a random manner. An orange cue when presented and attended to by fixed gaze for two consecutive seconds was accompanied by the presentation of a positive reinforcer such as candy or fruit. Another cue, a blue cardboard circle, when presented alternately with the orange cue, was accompanied by a loud noise when attended to by the patient. A total of 20 randomly alternating presentations for each patient were made and the average length of these training sessions was three and one-half minutes over a five day span.

After baseline data were collected which included the number of entries or attempted entries into potentially hazardous areas (i.e., kitchens, stairwells, other off-limit areas), the blue circles were placed in or on these areas while the orange cues were placed in other areas where ambulation was permitted. Other contingencies were included in this study, but for our purposes, the results show a substantial reduction in the mean number of entries in potentially hazardous areas. Patient 1 went from a baseline rate of nine entries per 30-minute observation time to two after training, patient 2 went from fifteen to three, and Patient 3 from two to zero.

It appears that cues occurring naturally and usually effecting ambulation patterns are not effective in modifying ambulation, but the simple color cues that are associated with naturally occurring environmental cues through training, are effective. With selective reinforcement for attending to these artificial cues, and with booster sessions utilizing the original training procedure, a potentially dangerous behavior can be brought under control without the use of a designated aide, restraints, or sedative medications.

The same principles may be applied to control other behaviors simply by the placement of a cue which has become associated with a positive reinforcer near the natural stimulus. Patients for whom traditional urinary control programs fail to work may be shaped to respond appropriately if toilets are marked with the training stimulus. If functional analysis suggests that episodes of inappropriate sexual behavior are due to poor stimulus discrimination, the same type of program, individually tailored to the patient and the target, may be used, to modify the site of occurrence without effecting the frequency or topography of the response.

The use of stimulus-control procedures requires more verification and variables involved require further analysis. In addition to stimulus control, behavior therapy should also play an important role in other areas of concern in the future of clinical geriatrics.

FUTURE APPLICATIONS OF BEHAVIORAL ASSESSMENT AND THERAPY

Behavior therapy is able to contribute uniquely to the field of geriatrics. Although the possibilities are limited only by the clinician's and researcher's interest and creativity, these contributions would involve three general areas: (1) brain-behavior relationships; (2) behavioral assessment; and (3) behavioral therapy.

Brain-Behavior Relationships

Behavioral methodology can be applied to questions concerning brain-behavior or physiology-behavior relationships within the field of gerontology. The bottom line to the behavior that clinicians see lies in tissues and neurochemicals. This is most strikingly evident in patients with Alzheimer's disease and related disorders, but is also a factor to many other age-related disorders. Explanations of the clinical manifestations of age-related disorders has been hindered by a lack of specific relationships between the more sophisticated diagnostic tools (e.g., the CT and PET scans) and behavioral symptomatology. Though this may be due in part to the true state of correlations between tissue pathology and behavior, it is also due to deficiencies in the quality of the behavioral measures used in correlational analysis. Behavioral descriptions of responses, such as frequency counts yielded by time-sampling, may prove to be objective and valid methods of gathering clinical data to compare with laboratory findings. By gathering sound quantitative data, discrimination between behavior correlated with Alzheimer's disease and other etiologies of dementia, along a yet unspecified dimension, may result. Measurements of speech and motor changes that occur, and correlations of these changes with CT scan changes, can be made. Mapping changes in speech process as dementia progresses and looking for correlations with the magnitude and site of tissue damage also may be valuable.

By objectively recording the nature and intensity of self-stimulatory behavior and then comparing this with measurements of tissue pathology, relationships between the type of self-stimulation (e.g., repetitive vocalizations, rocking, standing) and the site of maximal tissue impairment may be revealed. If this proves a valid relationship, a non-invasive diagnostic technique would then be available.

Other uses of behavioral assessment and therapy in the exploration of brain-behavior relationships might involve the correlation between delirium and underlying acute physical illness or imbalances. Since these states appear to have abrupt, discrete onsets, and the commonly encountered organic causes are generally easy to test, it might be possible to map an individual's behavior across selected responses and time graphically, which would thus lead to early treatment and management. In some cases, behavioral changes appear before clinical manifestations, and with careful monitoring and recording, these changes in response rates might even be useful in the diagnosis of underlying physical disorder.

A similar "mapping" procedure also would be effective for the evaluation of drug regimens. Clinical trials of lecithin, ergot alkaloids, and other potentially valuable drugs would be aided by the inclusion of behavioral methodology. Though group, double-blind, placebo designs are valuable in determining drug safety and efficacy, the variability in drug response and the unpredictable incidence of side effects suggest the use of single subject designs as well. Through the comparison of baseline rates of a target behavior with post-intervention rates, and the inclusion of a sample of motoric side-effects, the value of a particular drug could be determined *for a particular patient*. In practice this would entail more time spent in observation, but it would also mean the development of an individually tailored drug-response profile.

Trends in Behavioral Assessment

More research has been generated verifying the effectiveness of behavior therapy than has been generated in the description of sound assessment techniques with the elderly. A sensitive behavioral measurement is needed to measure changes across time, particularly in long-term care facilities, in order to alert the staff of potential problems early in the chain of response.

One recently developed assessment device, the Geriatric Assessment Inventory (GAI) (Schnelle & Traughber, 1982), may fill part of this need after further validation studies. This 70–item, two-point rating system has been shown to have an interrater reliability of 92.3 percent and was correlated significantly with direct independent observations. Discriminative validity of the inventory was suggested by the *GAI's* ability to differentiate between responders in a nursing home setting and elderly responders who lived in non-restrictive settings.

Behavioral methodology already has been applied to the assessment of several problem behaviors including wandering (Snyder, Rupprecht, Pyrek et al., 1978), the evaluation of drug side-effects (Hussian, Hill, & Ward, 1982), and self-stimulation (Hussian & Hill, 1980), as well as an attempt to find age-related reinforcers which may be most effective in modifying geriatric behavior (Wisocki, 1982). More such attempts are warranted.

Trends in Behavioral Therapy

There are two directions to go to validate treatment approaches in geriatrics. The same techniques used with younger patients can be utilized and their usefulness with age-related problems verified. One may also assume a more problem-oriented approach and test new techniques, or modifications of techniques, on problems that occur frequently with advanced years. Both approaches are valuable, though the latter approach suggests that one has taken the time to *observe* the behavior of elders; only after this observation can effective treatments be designed for behaviors observed.

Two problems areas already are quite evident and require attention immediately. First, one must attempt to discover the variables which are important to increase the probability of maintaining and generalizing treatment effects. One striking observation common among behavioral researchers and clinicians is that the significant gains made during and immediately following intervention do not often endure much beyond the termination of treatment nor do these gains hold up if the client faces different surroundings. It will be necessary to find ways to enhance maintenance and generalization with the elderly and to include these components into the treatment program. This might entail adding cognitive components, more extensive use of mediators, the use of multiple therapists, or other modifications in standard procedure. Second, the early successes of stimulus-control procedures dictates that an attempt be made to analyze more fully the processes involved in the establishment of behavior control. Experimental psychology may inform the clinicians of aspects of artificial cues that are most likely to be responded to, thus reducing wasted time and increasing the probability of successful training. Operant psychologists in their work on various schedules of reinforcement will help define those parameters that are particularly effective in working with different types of elderly clients.

Behavior therapists are just beginning to contribute to this cutting edge of mental health. New sources for publication and new opportunities to exchange ideas are now being developed that should provide sources of reinforcement for these clinicians to continue their pursuits. Behavior therapists are beginning to feel an extreme need to apply their skills to this new problem area. This development is quite heartening.

REFERENCES

Agras, W.S. *Behavior modification: Principles and clinical applications.* Boston: Little, Brown and Company, 1978.

Baltes, M.M., & Barton, E.M. New approaches toward aging: A case for the operant model. *Educational Gerontology,* 1977, *2,* 383–405.

Baltes, M.M., & Lascomb, S.L. Creating a healthy institutional environment for the elderly via behavior management: The nurse as a change agent. *International Journal of Nursing Studies,* 1975, *12,* 5–12.

Baltes, M.M., & Zerbe, M.B. Reestablishing self-feeding in a nursing home resident. *Nursing Research,* 1976, *25,* 24–26.

Bandura, A. *Principles of behavior modification.* New York: Holt, Rinehart, and Winston, Inc., 1968.

Berger, R.M., & Rose, S.D. Interpersonal skill training with institutionalized elderly patients. *Journal of Gerontology,* 1977, *32,* 346–353.

Blackman, D.K., Howe, M., & Pinkston, E.M. Increasing participation in social interaction of the institutionalized elderly. *Gerontologist,* 1976, *16,* 60–76.

Carstensen, L.L., & Fremouw, W.J. The demonstration of a behavioral intervention for late life paranoia. *Gerontologist,* 1981, *21,* 329–333.

Cautela, J.R. Behavior therapy and geriatrics. *Journal of Genetic Psychology,* 1966, *108,* 9–17.

Cohen, D. Research problems and concepts in the study of aging: Assessment and behavior modification. *Gerontologist,* 1967, *7,* 13–19.

Edwards, K.A. The nursing home environment. In F.J. Berghorn, D.E. Schafer, and Associates (Eds.), *The dynamics of aging: Original essays on the processes and experiences of growing old.* Boulder: Westview Press, 1981, 447–465.

Filer, R.N., & O'Connell, D.D. Motivation of aging persons. *Journal of Gerontology,* 1964, *19,* 15–22.

Geiger, O.G., & Johnson, L.A. Positive education for elderly persons: Correct eating through reinforcement. *Gerontologist,* 1974, *14,* 432–436.

Green, G.R., Marlow, C., Briggs, H., Linsk, N.L., & Pinkston, E.M. *Modification of dysfunctional verbal interactions in the elderly.* Paper presented at the Association for Behavior Analysis, Dearborn, Michigan, 1980.

Hoyer, W.J., Kafer, R.A., Simpson, S.C., & Hoyer, F.W. Reinstatement of verbal behavior in elderly mental patients using operant procedures. *Gerontologist,* 1974, *14,* 149–152.

Hoyer, W.J., Mishara, B., & Reidel, R.G. Problem behavior as operants: Application with elderly individuals. *Gerontologist,* 1975, *15,* 452–456.

Hussian, R.A. *The combination of operant and cognitive therapy with geriatric patients.* Paper presented at the Association for Behavior Analysis, Dearborn, Michigan, 1979.

Hussian, R.A. *Geriatric psychology: a behavioral perspective.* New York: Van Nostrand Reinhold, 1981.

Hussian, R.A. Stimulus control in the modification of problematic behavior in elderly institutionalized patients. *International Journal of Behavior Geriatrics,* 1982, *1,* 33–42.

Hussian, R.A., & Hill, S.D. Stereotyped behavior in elderly patients with chronic organic mental disorder. *Journal of Gerontology,* 1980, *35,* 689–691.

Hussian, R.A., Hill, S.D., & Ward, R.T. Assessment of drug-induced abnormal motor movements in institutionalized elderly patients. *International Journal of Behavioral Geriatrics,* 1982, *2,* 125–134.

Jackson, G.M., Schonfeld, L.I., & Griffith, K. Comparisons of visual feedback, instructional prompts and discrete promptings in the treatment of orofacial tardive dyskinesia. *International Journal of Behavioral Geriatrics,* 1982, *2,* 134–144.

Libb, J.W., & Clements, C.B. Token reinforcement in an exercise program for hospitalized geriatric patients. *Perceptual and Motor Skills,* 1969, *28,* 957–958.

Lindsley, O.R. Geriatric behavioral prosthetics. In R. Kastenbaum (Ed.), *New thoughts on old age.* New York: Springer, 1964.

Lopez, M.A. Social-skills training with institutionalized elderly: Effects of precounseling structuring and over-learning on skill acquisition and transfer. *Journal of Counseling Psychology,* 1980, *27,* 286–293.

MacDonald, M.L. The forgotten Americans: A sociopsychological analysis of aging and nursing homes. *American Journal of Community Psychology,* 1973, *1,* 272–294.

MacDonald, M.L. Environmental programming for the socially isolated aging. *Gerontologist,* 1978, *18,* 350–354.

MacDonald, M.L., & Butler, A.K. Reversal of helplessness: Producing walking behavior in nursing home wheelchair residents using behavior modification procedures. *Journal of Gerontology,* 1974, *29,* 97–101.

MacDonald, M.L., Davidowitz, J.J., Gimbel, B., & Foley, L.M. Physical and social environmental reprogramming as treatment for psychogeriatric patients. *International Journal of Behavioral Geriatrics,* 1982, *1,* 15–32.

Mahoney, M.J. *Cognition and behavior modification.* Cambridge: Ballinger Publishing Company, 1974.

Malament, I.B., Dunn, M.E., & Davis, R. Pressure sores: An operant conditioning approach to prevention. *Archives of Physical Medicine and Rehabilitation,* 1975, *56,* 161–164.

McClannahan, L.E., & Risley, T.R. Design of living environments for nursing home residents: Increasing participation in recreation activities. *Journal of Applied Behavior Analysis,* 1975, *8,* 261–265.

Mueller, D.J., & Atlas, L. Resocialization of depressed elderly residents: A behavioral management approach. *Journal of Gerontology,* 1972, *27,* 390–392.

Palmer, K.C., Marshall, P., & Foster, E. *A behavioral treatment approach to tardive dyskinesia.* Paper presented at the Association for the Advancement of Behavior Therapy, New York: 1980.

Pollack, D.D., & Liberman, R.P. Behavior therapy of incontinence in demented inpatients. *Gerontologist,* 1974, *14,* 488–491.

Quattrochi-Tubin, S., & Jason, L.A. Enhancing social interactions and activity among the elderly through stimulus control. *Journal of Applied Behavior Analysis,* 1980, *13,* 159–163.

Reidel, R.G. Behavior therapies. In C. Eisdorfer (Ed.). *Annual review of gerontology and geriatrics.* New York: Springer Publishing Company, 1981.

Rimm, D.C., & Masters, J.C. *Behavior therapy.* New York: Academic Press, 1974.

Rinke, C.L., Williams, J.J., Lloyd, K.E., & Smith-Scott, W. The effects of prompting and reinforcement on self-bathing by elderly residents of a nursing home. *Behavior Therapy,* 1978, *9,* 873–881.

Risley, T.R., & Edwards, K.A. *Behavioral technology for nursing home care: Toward a system of nursing home organization and management.* Paper presented at the Nova Behavioral Conference on Aging, Port St. Lucie, Florida, 1978.

Sachs, D.A. Behavioral techniques in a residential nursing home facility. *Journal of Behavior Therapy and Experimental Psychiatry,* 1975, *6,* 123–127.

Schnelle, J.F., & Traughber, B. A behavioral assessment system applicable to geriatric nursing facility populations. *Behavioral Assessment,* 1982, *3,* 21–28.

Snyder, L.H., Rupprecht, P., Pyrek, J., Brekhus, S., & Moss, T. Wandering. *Gerontologist,* 1978, *18,* 272–280.

Szekely, B.C., Turner, S.M., & Jacob, R.G. *Behavioral control of L-dopa induced dyskinesia in Parkinsonism.* Paper presented at the Association for the Advancement of Behavior Therapy, Toronto, 1981.

Taylor, C.B., Zlutnick, S.I., & Hoehle, W. The effects of behavioral procedures on tardive dyskinesias. *Behavior Therapy,* 1979, *10,* 37–45.

Wisocki, P.A. Actual and predicted responses of institutionalized elderly to the Psychiatric Reinforcement Survey Schedule. *International Journal of Behavioral Geriatrics,* 1982, *1,* 47–55.

8

CONDUCTING FAMILY THERAPY WITH ELDER CLIENTS

John J. Herr
John H. Weakland

This chapter addresses the assumption that family therapy is an accepted psychotherapeutic tool for treating behavioral and relationship problems presented by families with aging members. The validity, effectiveness, and techniques of therapeutic work with elders and their families has been discussed in detail by Brody (1966) and by Herr and Weakland (1979a). The present discussion will focus on some specific clinical differences in the conduct of family therapy in which an elder, rather than younger, member is the identified patient (IP). Particular attention will be paid to continuing cycles of problematic behavior within a given family or even an institutional system.

POSSIBILITY OF THE PRESENCE OF CHRONIC DEMENTING ILLNESS

The authors have written elsewhere of the uncanny resemblence between diagnosis and treatment of the dementias in elders and diagnosis and treatment of schizophrenia in young adults (Herr & Weakland, 1979b). It is fanciful, though, to assume that all problematic behavior in older adults can be understood by recourse to models of psychopathology and treatment

GERIATRIC MENTAL HEALTH
ISBN 0-8089-1657-2

appropriate to younger clients. Changing certain central elements of the family's interactional system may not significantly alter presenting problems, especially for those with irreversible dementias. This should not be construed as suggesting that significant benefit cannot be achieved through family therapy, even when the identified patient is suffering hopelessly from dementia. In such cases the whole family experiences significant distress. The experience of an American social worker living in England, who returned briefly to this country to study at the Mental Research Institute, is most illustrative. He had made a recent pilgrimage to visit his "hopelessly senile" grandfather in a convalescent hospital. Contrary to his expectations, which were based on letters from his mother, the old man was quite alert and curious as to our colleague's experiences in England. In general, his grandfather seemed quite in control of his mental faculties, though his cognitive skills and behavior deteriorated drastically into a state of apparent dementia when their private visit was interrupted by the colleague's mother and grandmother. This is clearly a case in which family therapy would have been most useful in delineating those features of the family relationship that apparently had great control over the elder's behavior. The absence of such intervention resulted in a very grave error in treatment planning and even diagnosis.

Because of the prevalence of this phenomenon in our clinical experiences, and the presence of an established theoretical model that stresses *family* therapy that includes the identified patient, we believe at least one interview must be held with *all* family members present, no matter how demented the patient's behavior might appear. In additional interviews our rule of thumb is simple: if in any doubt at all, include the elder in every session. After all, what is there to lose? The worst that can happen is that the "unspeakable" will at last be spoken, and if it can be talked about, it loses much of its paralytic power on the family. Families usually find great relief in this process because they no longer have to wait for "the other shoe to drop."

Another benefit resulting from sessions with all family members is that younger members facing personal difficulties get attention. A family therapist working with clients in this group should be prepared to make referrals to nonelders, particularly in problem areas of substance abuse (usually alcohol) and marital therapy.

However, in working with aging families, as opposed to families at the other end of the developmental continuum, the possibility is very real that the basis of a behavioral problem is primarily organic and progressive. As nonphysician therapists, it should be suggested routinely that new patients have a thorough physical, even though it would be most surprising and is not expected that the physician will uncover any pathology in younger patients. In working with elders, however, such expectations no longer hold.

It is too often seen, unfortunately, that the expectation of dementia in an elder by family, friends, and even professionals, is more damaging for the elder and the family than the organic impairment itself. It is often this situation in which family and professionals alike perceive significant behavioral problems as inevitable and essentially hopeless concomitants of growing older. With Alzheimer's disease, the problem is compounded in the sense that it is always the diagnosis of last resort when an elder displays problematic behavior, or behavior perceived as problematic. This diagnosis is basically a hopeless implication.

The interactional aspects that may be overlooked in making this diagnosis of last resort, and the human consequences of their neglect, are probably best summed up in a passage from the popular novel, *Heartsounds.** The context for the following passage is that the author's mother has mistakenly swallowed her denture-soaking solution during the night. Alarmed, she called for an ambulance. She is talking with her daughter about her experience from her hospital bed:

"It was *nothing*. I got scared, that's all. I thought maybe it was poison. And the policemen! All of a sudden, they're banging on the door. You know me: when I get scared, I get *a bissel meshugge* [a little crazy]. So they bring me here and then they bring a psychiatrist. And he asked me the *stupidest things*. 'What year did the war end?' I said, 'What war?' There have been *so many wars,* how am I supposed to know what war he means? He asks how old I was in 1933. *Azamin frage* [such a question]! Who remembers such things? Especially when you're scared. He says, 'Where were you born?' I said, 'I don't know.' Mashala, you *know* I don't know. Who knows, these days, if it was Poland or Russia?"

The psychiatrist was very young. He had an accent I could not place. He spoke almost in a whisper, as supply carts rattled past us in the hospital corridor, and I kept edging toward him to hear, and he kept edging backward.

". . . and sometimes they appear to get better, and there are no further episodes for a time," he whispered. "Or there may be steady deterioration . . . and certainly . . . she lives alone . . . I think you may have to start making plans. . . ."

"What makes you think its Alzheimer's Disease?"

"I did not say it was." Edging back. "That was a tentative diagnosis."

"On what basis did you arrive at this tentative diagnosis?"

"There were signs of a personality breakdown. She could not tell me the most basic facts: where she was born, her own telephone number. . ."

"Listen," I said, "imagine that you are elderly, you are all alone, you are very timid, you have had many bad illnesses, you don't see too well, you are frightened of authority, and you have a language problem, and in the middle of the night you think you have taken poison. Then the police come and put you in a car, and they take you to a place with bright lights, and strangers start throwing questions at you, and *you think you are going to die*. Can you imagine what that would be like? Tell me, Doctor *how old* were you in 1961? . . . *Where* did you live when you were nine? *Who* was the President during the Korean War?"

---

*Lear, Martha W. *Heartsounds*. New York: Simon & Schuster, 1980. Permission granted by Simon & Schuster, Inc.

He clicked his tongue reproachfully. "Madam, I am not from this country," he said.

I took her home the next day and stayed with her overnight, then telephoned her from New York.

"How are you feeling, Mom?" I said.

"Fine!" she said. "In the pinks."

And I knew in my bones there was no Alzheimer's Disease. But still, there were loneliness and fear. There was fragility. Things happen. I had friends who had come recently to that crisis with their parents, a broken hip, a fading memory, creeping depression; and the impossible guilt-laden alternatives—disruption of households, obscenity of nursing homes, that whole damned agonizing business; and no one had found a good way. What could be done? With her, frightened in her bed, and I, frightened in mine. . . .

When working with elders, the most obvious clinical consequence of the difference between working with other age groups is that the family therapists are apt to give up too soon or set their aspirations too low because of the possibility of a dementing illness. When an IP is an elder, this possibility is almost always raised, if only in the therapist's own mind. Sadly enough, it thus seems easier to call it quits when working with an elder having disturbed behavior than with a child or young adult. The two examples of familiar interactions presented thus far provide very clear indications of the positive and negative impact of various family members on the behavior of elder clients. Not only does therapeutic efficacy improve when all family members are part of treatment planning, but diagnostic accuracy improves as well.

An additional problem is that when an impairment is clearly organic in origin, many therapists, especially nonmedical therapists, believe such matters are out of their territory. Too often family therapists lose sight of the fact that even if the behavioral problem is the result of an organic impairment, the way in which the family and/or hospital staff handles that behavior may influence the impact of the impairment on all concerned. In this case, the family therapist, much like the geriatric physician, must be willing to settle for amelioration of difficulties rather than restoration of function.

Another consequence of the expectation of dementia in working with "disturbed" elders and their families is that the family therapist may have to become considerably more aggressive in collaborating with the elder's physicians. This will ensure that any behavioral problems the elder has are not the result of diseases, malnutrition, overmedication, or the interaction of drugs prescribed by different specialists, who may not know their patient is under treatment with another physician. In other words, even a nonmedical family therapist may be the one who first discovers that a *chronic* brain syndrome was really an *acute* brain syndrome induced by a number of sources.

Just as acute brain syndromes can be mistaken for true dementia, so can an endogenous depression that will respond favorably to antidepressants. In fact, so many elders diagnosed as suffering from "dementia" have improved when administered these drugs, that a new nondisease has been described: *pseudodementia of depression*. Pseudodementia, resulting from endogenous depression, may have its biomedical cure in the antidepressants, but obtaining patient and family compliance in taking a medication that seems to require two to four weeks to be effective and has some rather irritating side effects, is extremely difficult. It may require heroic efforts on the part of a family therapist when (1) *after three days* the elder complains about the side effects; (2) the family sees no improvement and may not believe the drug will work anyway; and (3) the elder's cardiologist or family practice physician has not yet collaborated on adjusting drug dosages, which must be accomplished in order to prevent ultimately and potentially grave iatrogenic effects to the elder.

In a sense, the effort required to introduce the possibility of change by the use of medication makes a good metaphor for the pivotal role of the family therapist. The therapist must be an aggressive "case manager" within a systematic ambiance, where hopelessness and helplessness are already firmly entrenched and are daily squeezing tighter on the elder, his or her family, and staff. Denial, guilt, and anger become the resultant verbal and nonverbal currency of communication for service providers and recipients of all ages. The family therapist may be the only professional who has not been willing to give up. Experienced observation has shown that a family therapist's interest and willingness to consider that there is still the possibility that something can be done can be an inspiration to a family to keep on trying. This care and tenaciousness can also inspire professional colleagues. Clearly, such pivotal case management requires a considerable amount of informed, diplomatic leg work which is not usually required in treating a family that presents with a depressed adolescent.

As a final reminder, it should be noted that in all of the above cases, both therapists and elder identified patients are fighting against the very same phenomenon: the very real possibility of giving up too soon and assuming that nothing will work, anyway.

BEHAVIORAL PROBLEMS AND CHRONIC PHYSICAL ILLNESS

If dementing illness were not enough for the family therapist to contend with, the immersion of the elder into the "medical model" for real physiologic disease creates even more opportunities for differences to emerge in treating families with elders. Most elders have at least two chronic physical ailments requiring the attention of a physician, (e.g., hypertension, arthritis, and/or the entire remaining organ recital). When a family comes to visit, the elder already is labeled as a "patient." Worse still, in a project providing family therapy for elders at the Mental Research Institute, almost half the elders reported in the first interview that they "had a problem," in that they not only identified themselves as having physical problems but psychological problems as well, a double-identified patient.

Compare the earlier interview of a family with an IP elder, with an initial interview of a family in which the IP is a 15-year-old boy having problems in high school. When the teenager is asked why he is in the office, predictably he will give a surly look to someone in the family, even the therapist, and say, "I don't know. I don't have any problem." From experience with families of all ages, the position of labeling oneself as the IP has the effect of making it more difficult for family members to become usefully involved. In families with elders, consequently, therapists have to work harder to engage family members to come to family sessions.

Another complication of physical illness associated with behavioral problems is that it often difficult to ascertain exactly who is in the family system. For example, if an elder is hospitalized in a nursing facility while recovering from a broken hip, members of the staff may be more instrumental in his or her life than visiting relatives. In these days of Prolixin-oriented-fast-food-community-mental-health-centers, family therapists working with younger IPs rarely work with families in which battle lines are drawn between who "owns" the IP; family or staff? This situation can be very different in working with elders where conflicts between family and staff actually may be producing behavioral problems in the elder. By way of example, the morale of caretakers in most long term care facilities and most skilled nursing facilities is almost universally low. The work is hard, the pay low, and status, particularly for RNs and LVNs, even lower. Often this leads to the staff feeling taken advantage of by owners and operators of the facility, and the objects of projected anger of family members of patients. This experience is often valid. As a result of their sense of guilt and helplessness, a family member may complain to a nursing staff member about "Dad's dirty fingernails" when the nurse had been working hard to provide bedsore-free care to an incontinent bedfast elder who refuses to cooperate with the staff's continued attempts at a bowel and bladder control training program. The personal pain and anguish of family members resulting from guilt and helplessness often manifests in infrequent visits or outright abandonment of elders. Often staff may then receive the projected anger of their patients.

It is not difficult to see how hostility between staff and families might adversely affect not only staff and visitors, but the elder as well. Certainly one or more meetings in a "neutral corner" is useful, where family, directly involved staff, and the elder, should be present. The purpose of the meeting is family therapy, including staff as members of "extended" family. As in all family therapy, it should be made clear at the onset of the first meeting, and reinforced in all additional sessions, that the therapist is not looking for victims and perpetrators, but how to work out problems in the here-and-now. Even in nonconflict situations between family and staff, having at least one meeting that includes the elder, essential members of the family, and essential members of the staff, with whom the family and elders will have to deal on a regular basis, is almost the only way to a viable, sensible, and successful psychotherapeutic treatment plan.

Family therapists who work with elders are more apt to find themselves in an institutional setting where the nagging question of who they work for is apt to come up. Just as it is easy to form a nontherapeutic alliance with a family member in a younger family, the same phenomenon can occur with elders when the "family member" may include the nursing home administrator. In such cases "a system is a system" regardless of how it is constructed. In such a situation, a good rule of thumb is that when a therapist working with a family and staff begins to see situations in which victims and perpetrators appear instead of a lot of hurting, stuck people, an outside consultant is needed on the case.

THE REASONABLE MIDDLE-AGED CHILD: MIRAGE AND MENACE

Anyone who has worked with families for very long soon comes to grasp fundamentally that what children, especially teenagers, and parents, especially parents of teenagers, say about one another usually has little relationship to what less-biased observers have to say about them.

In working with families of elders it is very important to remember that middle-aged children are as notoriously unreliable in describing problems with their parents as they are in describing the source of their problems with their teenagers. Even into advanced years, parents equally retain their notorious lack of reliability to impartially describe their middle-aged offspring.

The catch is that the middle-aged children can sound so remarkably convincing about the "true nature" of their parent's problem, that often the elders agree and label themselves the IP. Even in a case of disagreement and complaint, the elder's physical or behavioral problems tend to discount his or her credibility. After all, who would seem more reliable in the narration of a situtation—an articulate middle-aged child in the social and economic prime of life, or a frightened elder who may display at least one or two signs of a physical or cognitive impairment?

For those who perceive that, "middle-aged children are perpetrators; elders are victims," we have not been clear. We are not speaking to motives, nor to linear cause and effect, but, instead, to the fact that family members of all ages should be assumed to be involved in the problem, and equally unreliable and distorting. This points to a real need to see all family members together, not just individually, or worse still, not see the elder at all. The process of seeing and hearing for oneself is the same for treatment of both families with younger members and families with elders. It is just that, with families with elders, it is very easy to be misled by a sincere, but distorting, middle-aged child.

As an example of how remarkable this distortion can be, the authors were once requested to drop a case over the telephone by a very reasonable, concerned middle-aged successful businessman. He asked us not to honor his wife's wishes that we visit his mother-in-law, explaining that it would only get his wife's hopes up needlessly when it was clear that her mother was obviously senile. He sounded genuinely concerned and most sincere. Despite his request and because our client, his wife, had not fired us, we visited her mother. When we arrived at the board and care home, she was sitting in bed reading the novel *Centennial*. She was alert, witty, and quite sensitive and sensible about her current situation. When we expressed our confusion in seeing her so differently than her son-in-law had, she replied, "Oh, he's just a pain-in-the-ass paranoid schiz." Even the most reasonably well-meaning relative can lead a therapist down a very wrong path. All elders must be included in planning sessions, no matter how they are described by their caring family.

THE EXTENT OF THE FAMILY SYSTEM

The topic of who is really "family" was discussed briefly above in the context of working in a nursing home, but the problem goes far beyond this. The whole subject seems a bit incongruous: aren't we to be concerned about isolated elders rather than those who are "engulfed"? Being engulfed can be as pathogenic as being isolated. To be specific, the work of a family therapist can be sabotaged quite easily when the therapist does not know who is important in an elder's network of relationships.

Probably the most extreme example of this phenomenon is a case described by a colleague.

After several sessions with a three-generation family, where all members attended and worked with sincerity during the therapeutic session, nothing was changing in their lives outside the therapy hour. The therapist finally discovered the problem: it was not a three-generation family, but a four-generation family. After each session the family would go to great grandfather who would hold court in his room in the attic and discount the work that had gone on in therapy. When great grandfather finally was included in the sessions, the family finally began to make progress in the resolution of their individual and collective problems.

Physicians, attorneys, members of the clergy, and old friends and neighbors are the most obvious extension of the significant family system.

The well-meaning culprit often responsible for undoing the good done in family therapy is the out-of-town sibling (OOTS) of the local middle-aged child. The primary OOTS is usually in telephone contact with one or more of the following: the elder, secondary OOTS, other relatives, or the elder's physicians, attorney, or member of the clergy. Generally, actions taken are done out of great concern and involve considerable personal anguish on the part of the OOTS.

To combat the phenomenon of an unknown extended family system hindering therapy, there are some practices to handle differently than with younger families. First, take a very thorough history as to how the problem arose and came to be labeled, exactly how it was that each family member came to seek services, and with whom else they have discussed this problem. It is correct to prompt the family if no names of out-of-town relatives are volunteered. Second, ask each family member if there is someone else important to them that they would like to have at the session, even if it would be impossible for that person to attend. Third, thus armed, get releases to discuss the case with all professionals that are involved. Finally, follow up from session-to-session on what individuals might be missing, keeping open the possibility that those individuals might be invited to sit in on future sessions.

As to the matter of the ringing telephone, consider that it can be a device to calm as well as stir up problems. With the family's permission, frequently calling the OOTS to gain their perspective on issues and establish confidence in you, will work wonders in terms of taking pressure off local relatives.

HOUSE CALLS

Probably most family therapists who work with younger families have succumbed *once* to the temptation to make a "house call" because the identified patient refused to come in for therapy. A member of the family convinced the therapist that if only the IP could meet the therapist, the day would be saved. After having sipped from this poisoned well, most family therapists are not eager to take another drink. In the case of elders, the situation may be quite different.

First, there could be a real physical rason why the elder cannot travel to an office. Second, a site visit can be most useful to gain a measure of how an elder is dealing with activities of daily living. Finally, and most importantly for this discussion, initial reluctance to come to an office may represent a cohort reluctance rather than a personal resistance to treatment, failure to recognize a problem, or lack of motivation. Breaking the ice by visiting their turf seems to increase the likelihood of future visits to your office.

SUMMARY: SIMILARITIES AND DIFFERENCES

We have concentrated on the differences in practicing family therapy with elders to be, we hope, helpful. The differences are important but not insurmountable and, overall, there are far more similarities than differences. The greater danger is not that family therapy will be practiced imprecisely on families with elders, but that it will not be practiced enough, which would cause needless suffering among family members of all ages and no learning among therapists.

REFERENCES

Brody, E. The aging family. *Gerontologist,* 1966, *6,* 201–206.
Herr, J.J., & Weakland, J.H. *Counseling elders and their families.* New York: Springer, 1979a.
Herr, J.J., & Weakland, J.H. Communication within family systems: Growing older within and with the double bind. In P. Ragan (Ed.), *Aging parents.* Los Angeles: University of Southern California Press, 1979b.
Lear, Martha W. *Heartsounds.* New York: Simon & Schuster, 1980.

PART IV

Special Issues

9

MEMORY TRAINING FOR OLDER ADULTS*

Leonard W. Poon

Can elderly adults learn techniques to maintain and improve their memory abilities? Based on available evidence, the preliminary answer is an encouraging "yes." As we gain a better understanding of age-related changes in memory functions, we can begin to prescribe with more confidence memory techniques that can help individuals with specific memory problems. As yet, procedures for memory retraining for elders are at the formative stages. This chapter is intended to (1) explore some of the current difficulties in the diagnosis of memory problems; (2) examine laboratory findings on memory improvement with the older adult; and (3) examine six common questions about memory training with the aged.

DEFINITIONS OF TERMS

The main source of difficulty in diagnosing and treating memory problems lies in the multidimensionality of memory. In the last several decades, psychologists, neurologists, and neuropsychologists have attempted to establish models of memory and determine the relationship between memory and brain functions. While no model is completely satisfactory, it is now

* The preparation of this chapter is supported by the VA Medical Research Service.

GERIATRIC MENTAL HEALTH
ISBN 0-8089-1657-2

possible to identify some major characteristics of memory and factors that influence its functioning. Imagine memory as a multidimensional entity with interacting dimensions. One dimension of memory consists of dynamic processes related to the encoding, storage, and retrieval of information. Another dimension is the theoretical definition of different information storage capacities—*iconic* (sensory), *primary* (short-term), *secondary* (newly learned information), and *tertiary* (well-learned or very familiar) memory stores. A third dimension depends upon the modality-specific properties of the incoming information—verbal, spatial, visual, auditory, olfactory, etc. The functioning of any or all of these dimensions of memory is affected by differences in the characteristics of the total person—patterns of responses to environmental stresses, changing affective states, personality and cognitive styles, health, differences in intelligence, education, socioeconomic status, and both transient and stable neurological, hormonal, and physiological states. The many factors that can influence memory make it clear why the level of functional memory is fluid and subject to intra- and inter-personal variability.

Accordingly, any observed and subjectively perceived changes of memory may be attributed to changes in any one or combinations of the above dimensions. Differential diagnostic instruments for memory dysfunction would be incomplete if they only assessed the performance of specific types of memory without accounting for the impact of the environmental, physiological, and personal status of the individual assessed. Similarly, treatment of memory dysfunction must relate to individual differences in order to have lasting and effective results. This multidimensional model of memory should therefore be kept in mind for use as a guide in evaluating the adequacy of current practices in the diagnosis and treatment of memory problems.

ASSESSMENT AND REMEDIAL STRATEGIES

Among the factors found to influence memory, several investigators (Erickson, Poon, & Walsh-Sweeney, 1980; Gallagher, Thompson, & Levy, 1980) have recommended that careful analysis of relationships among memory complaints, memory performance, and depression could be helpful in assessing and planning treatment for individuals with memory problems. First, depression tends to exacerbate memory problems (Kahn & Miller, 1978; Miller, 1975), and the impact of extreme depression can be so devastating that the individual's cognitive abilities resemble those of patients with severe dementia. It has also been found that depression and memory complaints are positively related (Kahn, Zarit, Hilbert et al., 1975). Second, under some circumstances negative self-perception of one's memory abilities can have a significant impact on memory performance (Poon, Fozard, &

Table 9-1.

Possible Causes for Four Different Patterns of Memory Dysfunction

Pattern of Memory Dysfunction				
Complaints of Memory	Hi	Hi	Hi	Lo
Performance in Memory Testing	Normal	Normal	Lo	Lo
Level of Depression	Hi	Lo	Hi	Lo
Possible Causes				
	Depression	Environmental stresses	Serial testing is needed	Brain damage
		Minimal brain damage (mild stroke)	Depression	
			Brain damage	

Treat, 1978). And thirdly, different types of memory performance deteriorate with normal aging. Laboratory findings show that memory deterioration is primarily focused on the acquisition and retrieval of new information (episodic memory) while minimal decline is observed in the retrieval of familiar/personal/colloquial events (generic memory) (Smith & Fullerton, 1981). Episodic memory performance can be improved by memory training.

Table 9-1 displays several possible combinations of diagnostic outcomes based on three factors—performance, complaints, and depression—as well as possible etiologies. If a person who complains often of memory problems is shown to have normal memory performance but an elevated level of depression, the depression may be contributing to the self-perceived memory problem. As a first step, depression may be treated pharmacologically or by counseling and therapy. Memory training could be prescribed to demonstrate that the memory is normal and could be improved. If memory complaints are many, while memory performance is normal and there are no signs of depression, then some environmentally induced stresses or anxiety may be underlying the complaints. This symptom pattern also may be observed following an incident causing minimal brain damage, such as a mild stroke. In this situation preliminary clinical signs of neurologic damage may be negative and confirmation is sometimes made in follow-up examinations. Treatment may consist of therapy for situational stresses. Again, memory training could be prescribed to alleviate memory complaints as well as to bolster the confidence of individuals on their memory abilities.

Perhaps the most difficult situation to diagnose is that in which complaints are high, performance is low, and depression is high. In this situation, attention is needed to analyze the magnitude of dysfunction, and patterns of memory performance, as well as medical and affective assessment. Serial testing and treatment is indicated beginning with the depression. If memory problems still persist with the alleviation of depression then the possibility of brain damage increases. Treatment strategies could include therapy to alleviate depression and to minimize induced stresses, counseling with the family, and significant others to understand the situation and to help to create a supportive environment, as well as memory training to improve the memory.

Finally, when memory complaints, performance, and depression are all low there is a high likelihood of severe brain dysfunction. Given that treatable causes of brain dysfunction can be ruled out, counseling with the family and environmental modifications are helpful in minimizing adjustment problems.

MEMORY IMPROVEMENT

To remember something requires three steps: encoding, storage, and retrieval. Memory research on the acquisition of new information has shown that compared to young adults, the elderly adult is less efficient in encoding and retrieval, while storage does not seem to be affected by aging (Smith, 1980). It is noted, however, that encoding, storage, and retrieval processes are not independent and are difficult to untangle empirically; it is also difficult to draw simple conclusions about which one—or which combination of stages—is susceptible to aging. A quantitative analysis of the memory performance shows that elderly persons are indeed deficient in employing optimal organizational strategies during encoding.

Mnemonics, or memory aids, are techniques that first assist the learner to encode or organize information and then to retrieve that information on demand. Mnemonics are constructed on principles of learning and memory that attempt to (1) provide meaning to the material; (2) organize or file the information in a systematic, retrievable manner; (3) form meaningful associational networks; (4) take advantage of visualization; (5) concentrate on the material during encoding; and (6) provide feedback during the learning process.

The majority of the available mnemonics utilize the imagery mnemonic method. That is, the learner is taught to imagine or visualize the to-be-remembered information in some meaningful and organized manner. The following are brief descriptions of four popular mnemonic systems (for a more detailed description of these processes in layman's terms see Higbee, 1977; Lorayne & Lucas, 1974). First, the *link* or the *chain* system is used to remember a sequential list of events. As a first step, a visual image of each item in the list is formed. Then, meaningful associations are formed in a sequential manner between the first and second items, between the second and third items, etc.

The following is an example of a link system, chaining a list of ten words. This is the so-called "airplane list" employed by Crovitz (1979).

> The first word is airplane. Remember that however you like. The next word is giraffe, because the airplane is filled with giraffes sitting in the seats. The next word is bologna, because each of the giraffes is holding a bologna and taking bites out of it. The next word is moon, because the moon is really made out of bologna and not green cheese. The next word is elephant, because there is an elephant on the moon, not a man on the moon. The next word is ball, because the elephant is hitting a ball with his trunk. The next word is grass, because the ball is covered with grass, not leather. The next word is wall, because the grass is growing all the way to the Great Wall of China. The next word is cabinet, because the President's cabinet is having a meeting inside the wall. The last word is street, because the cabinet gets fired and goes off down the street looking for work.

Crovitz has demonstrated that most people could recall the ten words on the list in both forward and reverse sequences using this system.

One disadvantage of the link system is that, since the items are linked in a sequential manner, forgetting one item may affect the retrieval of subsequent items.

A second mnemonic system is the loci system, which does not seem to have some of the disadvantages of the link system. Loci, the pleural of locus, is derived from the Greek word *topo,* which means place or location. The system dates back to 500 B.C., and the origin is attributed to a story told by Cicero. A poet named Simonides was called outside from a banquet. During his absence the building collapsed, and he had to identify the bodies by the places the guests had been sitting—hence the method of loci.

The method first requires the learner to visualize a walk through familiar locations in some natural or logical order in which items to be remembered would be deposited. To retrieve these items, the learner would simply take a mental walk through the familiar locations. The loci system was used by Greek and Roman orators to remember long speeches without having to refer to notes.

Both the link and loci methods emphasize the acquisition and recall of sequential information. The *peg-word* or *book* system employs a similar approach except that it allows the retrieval of discrete information (say, the 12th item) without having to go through the sequence by utilizing the number sequence. If one associates the first item with the number 1, the second item with 2, and so on, then one can recall any item directly by its number. The main problem is that numbers are quite abstract and it is difficult to associate a number with an item.

To circumvent the problem of using numbers, a system that uses rhyming syllables and words to represent the numbers was introduced by the Englishman John Sambrook in 1879. His system uses nursery rhymes, for example: one two buckle my shoe/three four shut the door. Sambrook's peg-word system, using nouns that rhyme with numbers, so that numbers can be remembered more easily, is as follows:

One-bun	five-hive	eight-gate
two-shoe	six-sticks	nine-wine
three-tree	seven-heaven	ten-hen
four-door		

This system requires the learner to remember the peg words and then to associate the item to be remembered with the peg word.

Another more complicated mnemonic procedure employs the phonetic system to present numbers so that a mental filing system can be established. Briefly, each of the digits from 0 to 9 is represented by a consonant sound, which is then combined with vowels to code numbers into words. The words are then more meaningful and thus easier to remember. This procedure is quite complex and requires some time to master.

Two points should be emphasized about intentional remembering. One, it takes effort to systematically organize the to-be-remembered information; few people, regardless of age, can remember information effortlessly. Two, different individuals may prefer different mnemonics—a particular mnemonic may not be appropriate for all learners. It is therefore important for an individual to experiment with different mnemonics and employ one that is most suitable. It is possible that some healthy older persons who claim to have faulty memory may never have learned *how* to remember efficiently. The following is a review of experimental evidence on the use of mnemonics to improve learning and memory in brain-damaged patients and community-dwelling elderly individuals.

Brain-Damaged Patients

Studies have shown that some patients with organic disease of the nervous system, or with unilateral brain damage, could master mnemonic systems. An example of a demonstration was conducted by Patten (1972) who employed a peg-word method to teach the patient to remember lists of U.S. Presidents, grocery items, etc. Four patients with dominant hemispheric lesions and poor verbal memory were able to master the system and then improve their memory performances. Initial memory testing of these patients revealed:

1. A general pattern of disorientation for time and dates.
2. A forward digit span of about seven items and difficulty with backward digits.
3. Ineffective utilization of cues.
4. A fairly good memory for colloquial information, but poor recall of work-related information.
5. Poor recall of verbal information when a distraction task was interposed between presentation and retrieval.

After four weeks of memory therapy, patients showed improvement in their ability to remember a series of items. Some could master up to 100 items. Furthermore, they generalized and transferred the system to other everyday memory demands, such as appointments. In addition, improvement in other impaired abilities (e.g., in the ability to communicate verbally) and improvement in the patients' self-esteem were reported.

Three other patients with poor performances on memory tests did not improve significantly. One patient had Alzheimer's disease, one had a third-ventricular tumor, and the other had problems with recent memory after operative clipping of an aneurysm located in an anterior communicating artery. It was observed that these patients could not form vivid images. Furthermore, they were not aware of their memory deficits or interested in improving memory functioning.

Jones (1974) examined the facilitation effects of visual mnemonics with left- and right-temporal-lobectomy patients and patients with bilateral mesial temporal lobe lesions. Normal subjects matched on age and sex were used as controls.

Three lists of 10 paired associates were used for each group. The first list was used for baseline assessment. The second was used with imagery instructions and pictures depicting paired associates. The subjects generated their own images on the third list with no imagery instructions. Recall on all three lists was measured 2 hours after each task commenced.

As expected, the left-temporal-lobe group performed significantly worse than both the right-temporal-lobe and control groups on the paired associate tasks. Interestingly, the left-temporal-lobe group significantly improved and maintained their improved performance level after receiving imagery instructions. The performance of these patients with left-temporal-lobe damage indicates that imagery may facilitate recall of verbal information.

Because their spatial abilities were impaired, the right-temporal-lobe group was expected to perform significantly worse compared to normal controls with imagery instructions. However, the results showed that their performance was equal to or only slightly worse than that of the controls. Jones (1974) postulated that the paired-associate learning list might have been too easy for right-temporal-lobe subjects, with the result that a significant performance difference could not be obtained between patients and normals. It also is possible that these subjects used verbal mnemonics to compensate for lack of spatial and imagery abilities.

Although patients with bilateral mesial-temporal-lobe lesions understood the imagery instructions and could describe images, they were unable to improve their performances on immediate-recall tasks with imagery instructions. These patients could not retrieve any items in any lists for either immediate or delayed recall.

Baddeley and Warrington (1973) substantiated Jones's findings with bilateral-lesion patients in a list-learning study with adult amnesic patients who had no impairment other than memory dysfunction. The performance of these amnesic subjects was compared to that of control subjects with peripheral nerve lesions. Control and experimental subjects performed the following tasks: recall of lists clustered by categories and word sounds, recall of lists from different categories, and recall of an unrelated list of words using visual images.

The overall performance of amnesic subjects was significantly worse than that of control subjects. All subjects performed significantly better with the phonemically and taxonomically clustered lists. Two pertinent findings were specifically relevant to the amnesic subjects. First, although the amnesics could form visual images, they derived no benefit from imagery instruction in recall tasks. Second, these subjects could take advantage of phonemic and category cueing to improve their memory. Verbal mnemonics were shown to be beneficial for subjects, a finding consistent with those reported by Warrington and Weiskrantz (1971). In addition to the above studies, visual mnemonics have been demonstrated to be effective with other brain-damaged adult patients (Lewinsohn, Danaher, & Kikel, 1977) and educable mentally retarded (Lebrato & Ellis, 1974; Paris, Mahoney, & Buckhalt, 1974).

In conclusion, there is strong evidence that patients with initial signs of disorientation and some demonstrable brain damage could learn and efficiently employ a mnemonic (visual and/or verbal) system provided that patients are motivated, willing to practice the system, and that the staff is willing to work with the patient over a sustained period. Further, demonstration of an improved memory became a powerful reinforcer for the patients in their general outlook and self-esteem.

Community-Dwelling Elderly Populations

Most community-dwelling elders complain at one time or another of failing memory. However, experimental evidence shows that paired-associate and list learning can be improved when an appropriate mnemonic technique is provided for elderly persons.

Table 9-2 presents the results of a study comparing the effects of visual imagery, verbal elaboration, and no instruction on paired-associate learning (Hulicka & Grossman, 1967). Four groups of elderly and young subjects were employed. One group of subjects was instructed simply to learn 10

Table 9-2.

*Results from Age Group Comparisons for Use of Mediators in Paired-Associate Learning**

	% Correct			
	Young		Old	
	Baseline	Experimental	Baseline	Experimental
No instruction	72	70	28	35
Self image	72	81	28	53
Experimental image	72	78	30	45
Verbal instruction	71	71	28	47

* From Hulicka, I. M., & Grossman, J. L. Age group comparisons for the use of mediators in paired-associate learning. *Journal of Gerontology,* 1967, *22,* 46–51. With permission.

pairs of nonrelated words (no-instruction condition). When the first member of the pair was presented, the subject was required to retrieve the associate member. A second group of subjects was instructed to form images of the word pairs (self-image condition). A third group of subjects were given images to remember (experimenter-image condition). Finally, a last group was given the connecting words or phrase that was given to the experimenter-image group, but they were not instructed to form images. A baseline or no-instruction condition was administered to all subjects prior to the experimental condition.

The results in Table 9-2 demonstrate four points. One, there was a considerable age difference in the percentage of correct retrieval between old (28, 53 percent) and young (70, 81 percent) subjects. Two, there was limited improvement for the young subjects from the baseline to the experimental conditions. This lack of improvement was due to the high baseline performance—the young subjects could perform well without instructions. Three, for older groups there was a significant amount of improvement between the experimental and baseline conditions for the self-image (89 percent improvement), experimenter-image (50 percent), and the verbal-instruction (76 percent) groups in comparison to the no-instruction (25 percent) group. The study showed that older adults did not perform as well as young adults in the retrieval of newly learned information. When a mnemonic was provided, significant improvement was obtained by the older group, although performance did not reach the level of young adults.

If older adults have limited opportunity to practice the use of mnemonics for the acquisition of new information, would repeated practice of mnemonic techniques improve their learning skills? Treat, Poon, and Fozard (1981) examined the effects of practice on acquisition skills. Young and older adults participated in a paired-associate learning study in which lists of 10 paired-associates were presented. Some subjects were taught mnemonic techniques while controls were given no instructions. Subjects participated in three sessions and each session was two weeks apart. In each session the subjects learned two lists of paired associates. Trials to criterion, or the number of trials required for a subject to successfully learn all 10 paired associates, was employed to measure acquisition efficiency.

The results reported by Treat, et al (1981) replicated two general findings from the Hulicka and Grossman (1967) study: (1) there was a significant age effect, such that younger subjects were more efficient than older subjects; (2) for all subjects employment of mnemonics improved performance, and this improvement was significantly greater for older adults.

Three other aspects of the results provided insights into age differences in the acquisition of new information. First, the large magnitude of age differences observed in the first session was significantly reduced by the third session. The large age difference obtained in the first session may be inflated artificially because older adults were not familiar with the laboratory task and needed several sessions to adapt to the learning of unfamiliar information. Two, both the older mnemonics and no-instruction groups improved equally with practice. The no-instruction groups reported the use of self-improvement mnemonics to learn paired associates. Similarly, subjects who were asked to provide their own visual imageries performed better than subjects who were provided with specific imageries. Finally, transfer of learning skills pattern within and between sessions was different for young and older adults. The young adults performed efficiently after the first list, and there were no fluctuations in their performance across lists and sessions. Older adults performed significantly better on the second list, benefiting from practice derived from the first list. However, the benefit was not maintained in the next session, although there was a general improvement trend over the sessions.

Robertson-Tchabo, Hausman, and Arenberg (1976) reported the results of a study employing the method of loci to help older learners in serial recall. In this method, the learner takes a mental trip through his or her residence, stopping at 16 locations, which serve as clues to elicit appropriate responses. The method of loci capitalizes on the familiarity and natural order of the stopping places. Subjects were tested without instructions on the first and fifth day, and they were taught to use the method of loci on the second to fourth days.

The results of this study demonstrated three important points. First, there were large individual differences in retrieval performances among the elderly. Second, the use of the method of loci over three consecutive days for memorizing different lists did not produce interference for the elderly. And third, although the elderly successfully employed the method during the three training days, they did not use it spontaneously on the post-test, which was presented without specific instructions on how to use the method. In addition to the above two studies, two other studies (Treat & Reese, 1976; Treat, 1977) also have demonstrated that:

1. Young subjects spontaneously used efficient strategies.
2. Imagery instructions or practice served to enhance acquisition more for the elderly subjects.
3. Organizational techniques may be developed spontaneously by the elderly, given sufficient experience with a task.

The finding that the elderly, with practice, develop mediation strategies in paired-associate learning was corroborated in a dissertation by DeLeon (1974). He also found that based on subjects' reports of their use of mediation strategies, independent of treatment group, two groups of subjects were identified: those who used mediation and those who did not. Mediators performed significantly better than the nonmediators, corroborating the results of the facilitation effect of self-generated images reported by Treat (1977).

Successful application of the peg-word system with the elderly was also demonstrated by Hellebusch (1976). The study evaluated the effects of the standard peg-word system (e.g., one is a bun), sentence generation, and first-letter strategies on learning 10-item and 2-item self-paced lists and recalling them at both 3-minute and 2-week intervals after learning. The results showed that both peg-word and sentence-generation systems aided retrieval 3 minutes after presentation for both young and elderly adults. For the 2-week recall, however, the mnemonic strategies were found to benefit the young but not the old.

To evaluate whether or not subjects transferred the strategies learned earlier, the subjects were presented another self-paced list of 30 items to learn without specific instructions. By their own report, 83 percent of the young attempted to use mnemonic strategies, while only 44 percent of the elderly did so. Self-report data also indicated that 36 percent of the young subjects generalized their strategies from the unpaced tasks to a paced laboratory task. In contrast, only one older subject (out of the 48) generalized his mnemonic strategy.

Negative results on three mnemonic experiments with the elderly were reported from the laboratory of Smith and his associates (1981), based on a study of the effects of imagery on free recall and two studies on the use of the peg-word system. Mason and Smith, in experiment II (1977), reported no facilitative effects with younger and older subjects given instructions to form "a mental picture" with a list of 20 words, compared to subjects given standard free-recall instructions. The facilitative effect was found, however, with a group of middle-aged subjects.

Smith (1975) evaluated the effectiveness of the peg-word system in improving item recall with groups of young, middle-aged and elderly subjects. Experimental groups were taught a system very similar to that used by Patten (1972), reported earlier. The control groups were not taught the mnemonic system. The results showed no performance difference between the mnemonic and control middle-aged and elderly groups. However, a mnemonic facilitation effect was found for the young adults. The results essentially were replicated in Mason and Smith in experiment I (1977).

One important aspect of Smith's procedure may account for the negative results. Smith taught the mnemonic techniques to the elderly in a group setting, while the other studies taught the subjects individually. Given the complexity of the peg-word system and the importance of self-generated strategies, the elderly may need more time and individual attention to understand and master the technique.

DISCUSSION OF COMMON MEMORY QUESTIONS

A review of the literature shows convincingly that *most* community-dwelling adults *can* improve their memory performance, and that mnemonics—especially those that are individualized for a person—can provide dramatic memory improvement for most elderly persons. Following are six common questions regarding memory improvement for older adults.

1. *How long does it take an elderly person to master a mnemonic?*

Smith (1975) and Mason and Smith (1977) failed to produce a facilitating effect with the elderly using the peg-word method. However, it is possible that the peg-word system, which is fairly complicated and unfamiliar to most individuals, takes more time to master than was provided for in the design of their study. The learner must first master a list of novel pairs of peg-words then use this system to remember new information. Patten (1972) took up to four weeks to train successfully brain-damaged subjects to use the peg-word system. Hellebusch (1976) taught and tested his elderly subjects within the same session but was only able to obtain a minimal facilitation effect. Thus, evidence suggests that expectations of the time needed by the elderly to acquire and demonstrate proficiency with a mnemonic technique may need to be extended, particularly if the technique and stimuli are novel to the elderly learner.

2. *It has been demonstrated that the elderly* can *acquire specific mnemonic techniques, but* will *they use them for everyday remembering?*

In real-life situations an individual must employ a mnemonic spontaneously at the time of learning. Experimental findings show that elderly subjects tend not to use an acquired mnemonic when they are not reminded to do so. A question of practical importance is what types of training are needed by some elderly to enable them to employ the mnemonics spontaneously and to maintain the habit for long-term use.

3. *Would specific mnemonics be more applicable for specific memory situations, or could a mnemonic be generalized to different situations?*

Preliminary findings show that the elderly tend not to generalize the use of mnemonics from one situation to another. However, it remains to be demonstrated that generalization can be spontaneous or that some training would be needed to employ a mnemonic under different circumstances. While mnemonic techniques have been proposed for remembering different everyday information, e.g., names-faces, telephone numbers, etc. (Higbee, 1977; Lorayne & Lucas, 1974), these techniques await experimental verification on the degree of application with the elderly. It is important to note that the learner must experiment with different types of information. For some individuals general mnemonics may be useful for most information, while other individuals may prefer different mnemonics for different information.

4. *Does memory training reduce the magnitude of memory complaint for the elderly?*

Data from several memory training programs seem to show that memory complaints are reduced after training, but in a nonspecific way. Two successive studies employing 44 and 54 elderly participants in training sessions over a period of four weeks (Zarit, Cole, & Guider, 1981) replicated the finding that specific memory training tends to facilitate specific memory performance. However, they also found that subjective appraisals of memory were independent of treatment methods on a person's memory performance. Participation in a group discussing memory problems was sufficient to lower subjective complaints. This finding has been corroborated in other memory training programs with the aged (Perlmuter, Tenney, & Smith, 1980; Schaffer & Poon, 1982; Yesavage, 1981).

It is postulated that both specific and tangible as well as nonspecific and intangible benefits can be derived from a memory-training program. Actual memory improvement serves as a tangible reinforcer of the idea that one's memory is not as bad as first perceived and that it can be improved. The intangible benefit derives from overall improvement in self-esteem and self-confidence, and from the belief that one can improve one's memory, thereby an individual may have less concern about specific instances of forgetting (Zarit, Cole, & Guider, 1981).

5. *How much individual variability might one expect in a memory training program?*

Large individual variability is reported in the literature in both the acquisition rate of a mnemonic technique and in retrieval effectiveness during recall with elderly participants. The variability is illustrated in raw data reported by Robertson-Tchabo, Hausman, & Arenberg (1976) as well as in the work done in our laboratory (Poon & Walsh-Sweeney, 1981; Schaffer & Poon, 1982). Some elderly subjects performed as well as or better than the young adults. Some showed gradual and sustained improvement with repeated practice, while some showed no improvement or even deterioration with training (depending on their motivation to acquire a new learning system and to practice).

In one of our memory training studies (Schaffer & Poon, 1982) we have isolated two individual difference factors that could confound the training effects. One, there were individual differences in the rates of improvement *independent* of the treatment. Specifically, participants with initially low-baseline performance showed large improvements independent of the treatment or control conditions to which they were assigned, while participants with high-baseline performance generally had no room to improve or may even have shown some performance decline with training or practice. Two, high-verbal-IQ subjects tend to perform better in verbal-memory tasks independent of training given.

The implication of our findings on evaluation of memory group training is as follows. It is important that participants be distributed (yoked) equally on these two factors across the experimental and control groups in order to obtain a clear picture of treatment effectiveness. It may be fruitful to take a fresh look at existing memory training studies and pay particular attention to individual difference factors that could ultimately determine the success of the treatment effect.

6. *Since memory performance could be affected by neurologic, biochemical, and physiologic influences, can drug therapy improve memory performance for the elderly?*

While pharmacologic–cognitive intervention models are appealing, limited success in cognitive facilitation has been found in controlled studies with elderly adults, e.g., vasodilators, cholinergic drugs, neuropeptides, etc. (Marsh, 1980). Antidepressants might be appropriate to overcome some memory problems induced by depression. However, the magnitude of cognitive facilitation by pharmacologic means, if any, is within the range of practice effects (about 15 percent); mnemonic training—even with large individual variability—produces comparatively larger effects (about 50–100 percent).

Pharmacologic intervention with elders has so far had disappointing results (Hines & Fozard, 1980; Marsh, 1980). Ferris, Reisberg, & Gershon (1980) found predominantly negative results in their review of representative studies of neuropeptides (ACTH4–10 and ACTH4–9) in normal and cognitively impaired subjects. Some positive results have been reported in clinical studies with small samples, in which the effects of vasopressin on cognitive functions were observed (Ferris, Reisberg, & Gershon, 1980). Legros, Gilot, Seron et al. (1978) reported significant improvements in tests of memory and attention when vasopressin was administered to elderly inpatients. However, their results may have been contaminated by practice effects (Poon, 1978). Mohs, Davis, and Darley (1980) reported no substantial effect of choline chloride in a series of four memory studies with young and elderly adults.

CONCLUSION

Exciting future research awaits the collaboration of biomedical and cognitive researchers (1) to define a set of diagnostic and evaluative tools that examines the efficacy of treatment effects; and (2) to evaluate the effects of cognitive and pharmacologic intervention that improves memory and cognitive function for older adults.

In conclusion, memory can be objectively measured by the efficiency of the encoding and retrieval system. On one hand, its flexibility can be limited by neurologic, physiologic, and environmental factors. On the other hand, its efficiency can be maintained and improved by the reacquisition and conscious application of mnemonic techniques for most elderly adults. Memory is also subjective, experimental and selective. One's actual and self-perceived memory abilities can be affected by the "expectancy" of one's memory. Viable memory-training programs should address both mnemonic and attitudinal components.

The acquisition of mnemonic skills, like the acquisition of other skills, requires a commitment of effort and time. The development of memory skill is analogous in some ways to the acquisition of tennis-playing skills. Proper tennis techniques frequently feel awkward to students because the target behaviors are in conflict with playing habits that are inefficient. Similarly, mnemonic techniques initially may feel awkward to the learner. In both learning situations, the student may require many hours of instruction and practice until the target behaviors are integrated into the student's repertoire. The increased proficiency can then bolster the confidence and overall self-esteem of the older individual.

REFERENCES

Baddeley, A.D., & Warrington, E.K. Memory coding and amnesia. *Neuropsychologia,* 1973, *11,* 159–165.

Crovitz, H. Memory retraining in brain-damaged patients: The airplane list. *Cortex,* 1979, *15,* 131–134.

DeLeon, J.M. Effects of training in repetition and mediation on paired-associate learning and practical memory in the aged. Unpublished Ph.D. dissertation, University of Hawaii, 1974.

Erickson, R.C., Poon, L.W., & Walsh-Sweeney, L. Clinical memory testing of the elderly. In L.W. Poon, J.L. Fozard, L.S. Cermak et al. (Eds.), *New directions in memory and aging: Proceedings of the George A. Talland memorial conference*. Hillsdale, New Jersey: Lawrence Erlbaum Associates, 1980.

Ferris, S.H., Reisberg, B., & Gershon, S. Neuropeptide modulation of cognition and memory in humans. In L.W. Poon (Ed.), *Aging in the 1980s: Psychological issues*. Washington, D.C.: American Psychological Association, 1980.

Gallagher, D., Thompson, L.W., & Levy, S.M. Clinical psychological assessment of older adults. In L.W. Poon (Ed.), *Aging in the 1980s: Psychological issues*. Washington, D.C.: American Psychological Association, 1980.

Hellebusch, S.J. On improving learning and memory in the aged: The effects of mnemonics on strategy, transfer, and generalization. Dissertation Abstract (1459-B Order No. 76-19, 496), University of Notre Dame, 1976.

Higbee, K.L. *Your memory: How it works and how to improve it*. Englewood Cliffs, New Jersey: Prentice Hall, 1977.

Hines, T., & Fozard, J.L. Memory and aging: Relevance of recent developments for research and application. In *Annual review of gerontology and geriatrics* (Vol. 1). New York: Springer, 1980.

Hulicka, I.M., & Grossman, J.L. Age group comparisons for the use of mediators in paired-associate learning. *Journal of Gerontology*, 1967, *22*, 46–51.

Jones, M.K. Imagery as a mnemonic aid after left temporal lobectomy: Contrast between material-specific and generalized memory disorders. *Neuropsychologia*, 1974, *12*, 21–30.

Kahn, R., & Miller, N. Adaptational factors in memory impairment in the aged. *Experimental Aging Research*, 1978, *4*, 273–290.

Kahn, R.L., Zarit, S.H., Hilbert, N.M., & Niederehe, M.A. Memory complaint and impairment in the aged: The effect of depression and altered brain function. *Archives of General Psychiatry*, 1975, *32*, 1569–1573.

Lebrato, M.T., & Ellis, N.R. Imagery mediation in paired-associates learning by retarded and non-retarded subjects. *American Journal of Mental Deficiency*, 1974, *78*, 704–413.

Legros, J.J., Gilot, P., Seron, X. et al. Influences of vasopressin on learning and memory. *Lancet*, 1978, *i*, 41–42.

Lewinsohn, P.M., Danaher, B.G., & Kikel, S. Visual imagery as a mnemonic aid for brain-injured persons. *Journal of Consulting and Clinical Psychology*, 1977, *45*, 717–723.

Lorayne, H., & Lucas, J. *The memory book*. New York: Ballantine Books, 1974.

Marsh, G.R. Psychopharmacological issues. In L.W. Poon (Ed.), *Aging in the 1980s: Psychological issues*. Washington, D.C.: American Psychological Association, 1980.

Mason, S.E., & Smith, A.D. Imagery in the aged. *Experimental Aging Research*, 1977, *3*, 17–32.

Miller, W. Psychological deficit in depression. *Psychological Bulletin*, 1975, *82*, 238–260.

Mohs, R.C., Davis, K.L., & Darley, C. Cholinergic drug effects on memory and cognition in humans. In L.W. Poon (Ed.), *Aging in the 1980s: Psychological issues*. Washington, D.C.: American Psychological Association, 1980.

Paris, S.G., Mahoney, G.J., & Buckhalt, J. Facilitation of semantic integration in sentence memory of retarded children. *American Journal of Mental Deficiency,* 1974, *78,* 714–720.

Patten, B.M. The ancient art of memory-usefulness in treatment. *Archives of Neurology,* 1972, *26,* 25–31.

Perlmuter, L.C., Tenney, Y.J., & Smith, P.A. The evaluation and remediation of memory problems in the aged. Memory and Learning Center, Boston GRECC, Report #1, Sept. 1980.

Poon, L.W. Vasopressin and memory. *Lancet,* 1978, *i,* 557.

Poon, L.W., Fozard, J.L., & Treat, N.J. From clinical and research findings to intervention programs. *Experimental Aging Research,* 1978, *4,* 235–254.

Poon, L.W., & Walsh-Sweeney, L. Effects of bizarre and interacting imagery on learning and retrieval of the aged. *Experimental Aging Research,* 1981, *7,* 65–70.

Robertson-Tchabo, E.A., Hausman, C.P., & Arenberg, D. A classical mnemonic for older learners: A trip that works. *Educational Gerontology,* 1976, *1,* 215–226.

Schaffer, G., & Poon, L.W. Individual variability in memory training for the elderly. *Educational Gerontology,* 1982, *8,* 217–229.

Smith, A.D. Interaction between human aging and memory. Georgia Institute of Technology Progress Report #2, 1975.

Smith, A.D. Age differences in encoding, storage and retrieval. In L.W. Poon, J.L. Fozard, L.S. Cermak et al. (Eds.), *New directions in memory and aging: Proceedings of the George A. Talland memorial conference.* Hillsdale, New Jersey: Lawrence Erlbaum Associates, 1980.

Smith, A.D., & Fullerton, A.M. Age differences in episodic and semantic memory: Implications for language and cognition. In S. Beasley & L. Davis (Eds.), *Communication processes and disorders.* New York: Grune & Stratton, 1981.

Treat, N.J. Age imagery, focused attention, and egocentricism in paired-associate learning. Unpublished Ph.D. dissertation, University of West Virginia, 1977.

Treat, N.J., Poon, L.W., & Fozard, J.L. Age, imagery, and practice in paired-associate learning. *Experimental Aging Research,* 1981, *7,* 337–342.

Treat, N.J., & Reese, H.W. Age, pacing, and imagery in paired-associate learning. *Developmental Psychology,* 1976, *12,* 119–124.

Warrington, E.K., & Weiskrantz, L. Organizational aspects of memory in amnesic patients. *Neuropsychologia,* 1971, *9,* 67–73.

Yesavage, J.A. Personal communication, 1981.

Zarit, S.H., Cole, K.D., & Guider, R.L. Memory training strategies and subjective complaints of memory in the aged. The Gerontologist, 1981, 21, 158–164.

10

ALCOHOL USE AND ABUSE IN OLD AGE

Dennis S. Stern
Robert Kastenbaum

Bill is a cook for the Salvation Army. He has been preparing food for others for 37 years, but at the age of 62 he is finding it difficult to keep up. He walked off his last job when they asked him to work extra hours preparing a large Christmas dinner. His work record had been erratic over the past 10 years, ever since his wife died of cancer. He had never gotten over her death. Whenever he thought about it, Bill would become upset and reach for a bottle of vodka to console himself. He never drank much when his wife was alive, but after she died he would go on a binge and drink a fifth of vodka every day until someone found him and brought him into a detoxification center. Bill just completed his second alcohol treatment program and hopes it will be his last.

John is 64 years old. He worked as a salesman most of his adult life, and tended to drink too much while entertaining clients in bars. He has been treated for his drinking problem in over 10 detoxification and alcohol treatment programs. Among other things, his alcohol abuse has cost him two marriages and numerous jobs. He lives alone now and tries to earn a living as a caddy at a local golf course, but based on his past experiences, he expects that this job will fall victim to his drinking excesses as well.

Bill and John are two examples of a problem that is facing a growing number of older adults in this country—namely, alcohol abuse. Until recently, scientists and health care professionals seemed unaware of the extent

GERIATRIC MENTAL HEALTH
ISBN 0-8089-1657-2

to which ethanol abuse represented a serious health problem among the aged. After all, results from a number of investigations indicated that the rate of ethanol consumption in general *and* the rate of alcoholism in particular declined significantly with age (Cahalan, Cisin, & Crossley, 1969; Drew, 1968). In addition, older Americans represented a relatively small and politically noninfluential proportion of the total U.S. population. As their numbers and political sophistication have grown, so too has public interest in health-related problems facing the elderly.

This chapter will re-examine one health-related problem affecting a number of older Americans—namely, alcohol abuse. We will begin with a discussion of the prevalance of alcoholism among the elderly. Next, the various methods currently available for treatment of the older problem drinker and effectiveness of these methods will be reviewed, including a description of several innovative treatment approaches that show promise for improving the likelihood of long-term rehabilitation of older problem drinkers. The chapter will conclude with an examination of some of the beneficial effects of alcohol use in later life.

PREVALENCE OF ALCOHOL ABUSE AMONG OLDER ADULTS

Many more Americans over the age of 60 years drink alcohol with immunity than suffer from alcohol-related problems (Cahalan, Cisin, & Crossley, 1969). In fact, Mishara and Kastenbaum (1980) reviewed a number of studies suggesting that moderate use of alcohol by elderly men and women in a social setting actually may have beneficial effects in terms of psychosocial functioning. It is important to keep this in mind as we begin our discussion of problematic drinking in old age in order to guard against the type of moralistic over-reaction that culminated in the "great experiment" called Prohibition.

Estimates of the rate of alcoholism among older adults are generally comparable to those established for younger age groups. Anywhere from 2 to 10 percent of elderly men and 2 percent of elderly women are thought to experience severe problems related to their consumption of ethanol (Armor, Johnson, Polich, & Stambul, 1977; Schuckit, 1977; Schuckit & Miller, 1976). The rates are even higher among elderly widowers, residents of nursing homes, and patients in general and psychiatric hospitals (Bailey, Haberman, & Alkane, 1965; Barchha, Stewart, & Guze, 1968; Graux, 1969; Simon, Epstein, & Reynolds, 1968). For example, it is probable that one-third or more of those older patients admitted to a psychiatric facility would qualify as alcoholic (Daniel, 1972).

Although rates of alcoholism among elders are equal to those of younger groups, problem drinking in old age is a situation that should not be neglected. Health personnel often fail to identify the alcohol-related components of problems presented by clients in the geriatric range. Furthermore, there are clear indications that alcohol abuse among the elderly is increasing and will continue to do so. Jacob A. Brody, an official of the National Institute on Aging, described several of the factors involved in his background paper for the White House Conference on Aging. Brody (1981) reminds us that problem drinking among the elderly will increase at least in proportion to growing numbers of older people in our society, a well-documented trend that has not yet reached its peak. He identifies four factors that may promote increased alcohol abuse in this age group: (1) retirement, with its associated boredom, role status loss, and reduced income; (2) the death of significant others, with its pointed reminder of personal mortality; (3) health problems and physical limitations; and (4) loneliness, especially among elderly women.

The older person in our society, then, has multiple psychosocial susceptibilities to developing a drinking problem, and these susceptibilities are more likely to increase rather than decrease in the years ahead.

For a number of reasons the reputed rate of alcoholism among elders may actually underestimate the extent to which alcohol misuse creates serious problems. Inappropriate diagnostic criteria represent a major reason for what is, in all likelihood, an underestimation of problem drinking in older adults. The traditional diagnostic criteria for alcoholism typically include specific impairments in physical, psychological, and social/occupational functioning. Usually, however, these criteria fail to incorporate adjustments for the age of the patient even though it has been shown that significant differences in certain aspects of biological, psychological, and social functioning between younger and older adults exist (Bengston, 1973; Finch & Hayflick, 1977; Kimmel, 1974). For example, as a person ages, his or her tolerance to ethanol usually declines, due in part to the natural slowing down of the metabolic process (Wallgren & Barry, 1970), and partly to the increased ratio of body fat to body water (Vestal, McGuire, Tobin et al., 1977). Consequently, intoxication for the older drinker tends to occur at lower quantities of ethanol than would be the case for his or her younger counterpart. The health care provider who relies on a traditional quantity–frequency criterion for the diagnosis of alcoholism (e.g., National Council on Alcoholism, 1972) therefore often excludes a number of older people who drink excessively given the amount of alcohol their bodies can tolerate and who are in need of treatment for alcohol abuse. Reliance on traditional social/occupational impairment criterion may exclude other problem drinkers as well. The most obvious example would be "loss of job" due to alcohol abuse (American Psychiatric Association, 1980). Since many older citizens who drink are already retired, other criteria that reflect their social functioning are required to assess adequately the degree of impairment that exists in this area, and which might be a function of alcohol abuse.

In order to avoid some of the pitfalls inherent in the use of inappropriate criteria for the diagnosis of alcoholism in the aged, the terms, *problem drinking* and *alcohol abuse* will be employed in the remainder of this chapter. These are generic terms that are intended to encompass a host of physical, social, economic, and psychological difficulties associated with excessive consumption of alcohol. Within that approach, *alcoholism* would represent a specific type of problem drinking or alcohol abuse. A variety of drinking patterns and alcohol-related problems can be subsumed under the rubric of problem drinking or alcohol abuse. As a result, the use of these terms provides us with the opportunity to identify and study certain types of alcohol-related problems that may be unique to a given group of individuals, such as the elderly (or women, or blacks, etc.) and that may have gone unrecognized under the traditional diagnostic approach.

There are additional reasons why rates of alcohol abuse among the elderly have probably been underestimated. To begin with, the older problem drinker may never come to the attention of the health care provider since people will often avoid urging an elderly friend or relative to seek treatment because they fear embarrassment for themselves or for the elder with the problem (Droller, 1964). Even if the older drinker seeks professional consultation for reasons other than problematic drinking, the clinician may find it difficult to distinguish alcohol-related problems and those associated with old age in general, since a number of similarities between the two do in fact exist. For instance, brain damage, gastrointestinal disorders, and cardiovascular disease constitute clinical symptoms of alcoholism according to criteria established by the National Council on Alcoholism (1972). Yet, it has been shown that these same symptoms increase in frequency among nonalcoholic older adults as well (Timiras, 1972).

Alcohol is itself a drug, and even a relatively small intake can contribute to serious difficulties when interacting with some other drugs. Older people do take a lot of drugs—both through medical and self-prescription. As Lundin (1978), Moore (1978), and others have observed, elderly adults use more drugs more often than younger age groups. The specific combinations of alcohol and a drug that can lead to problems are too varied to encompass here. Nonetheless, a substance that of itself would not create difficulties interacting with alcohol may become an active menace when another drug is added to the picture. It is always advisable to consider the total configuration of substances the older person is using in connection with possible alcohol-related problems. Some older people are, furthermore, overdosing themselves on drugs alone, including over-the-counter as well as prescribed medications, thereby creating a dangerous situation that might be exacerbated by alcohol use. This represents a particular dilemma in the case of persons over 60 years of age, since elders consume more medication than any other age group (Goldberg & Roberts, 1976).

Once recognized, the older drinker may still go untreated due to a "natural reluctance" among health care providers "to separate the patient from his (or her) one remaining source of pleasure" (Rathbone-McCuan, 1975). The attitude that treatment of an aged individual, who has a limited life expectancy anyway, is not worth the time and effort of the clinician is, unfortunately, also widespread (Kastenbaum, 1978). For all of the above reasons, the older problem drinker may go unrecognized and, more importantly, untreated. In the health and mental health communities, this results in an under-representation of the magnitude of the problem and need for programs specifically designed for the treatment of the elderly problem drinker.

It seems clear that excessive consumption of ethanol represents a serious problem to a substantial number of older individuals. We can expect to see more older men and women with drinking problems in the future as the post-World War II baby-boom generation reaches late-adulthood, and the proportion of elderly people in the United States increases. In fact, shortly after the turn of the century, the elderly are expected to account for approximately 16 percent of the population, up from the current level of slightly more than 11 percent. Those individuals who will be reaching old age in the coming decades also will be less influenced by the prohibition morality that no doubt prevented many among the current generation from drinking alcohol. Thus, it seems timely to consider the effectiveness of our existing methods of alcohol rehabilitation for older problem drinkers in order to ensure that quality care is available to those who need it now and in the future.

TRADITIONAL METHODS OF ALCOHOL TREATMENT

The first time Bill was treated for problem drinking, he spent 30 days in a hospital on a special alcohol treatment ward. He was required to take antabuse and to attend daily classes in which the various consequences of ethanol abuse were discussed and illustrated through film. In addition, he received individual counseling to help him cope more effectively with the loss of his wife. Everyday, he participated in group therapy sessions and in the evenings went to Alcoholics Anonymous (AA) meetings. A social worker helped him locate a place to live, following the treatment program, and a vocational rehabilitation counselor directed Bill toward various job opportunities as a cook with employers who were sympathetic to graduates of an alcohol treatment program. When Bill was not in class or receiving some type of counseling, he was encouraged to take part in one of several types of recreational activities, such as arts and crafts or swimming. Although Bill found some aspects of the treatment program helpful, there were a number of required activities that he felt were of little or no use to him in curbing his problematic drinking.

John was a veteran of a number of different alcohol treatment programs

(ATP). Some ATP's were similar to the one Bill went through, but others were quite different. For example, in one ATP, John was given antabuse and encouraged to attend AA meetings. That was the extent of the treatment.

The experiences of Bill and John highlight the two major types of alcohol treatment programs currently available to adult problem drinkers, whether young or old. The so-called *broad-spectrum* approach is the term commonly used to describe the type of program Bill underwent. In this approach, individuals are exposed to multiple forms of treatment in order to maximize the possibility that some modality or combination of modalities will prove effective in stemming the abuse. John, on the other hand, was offered only a single treatment modality. In this case, it was antabuse, but in other cases it may be insight therapy or group therapy. If the person happens to "fit" the approach utilized in the alcohol treatment program, a positive outcome is likely. However, those individuals who do not fit the treatment are likely candidates for relapse.

Overall, both of these treatment approaches seem to be somewhat effective (Armor, Polich, & Stambul, 1978; Baekeland, 1977; Emrich, 1975). Approximately one-third of those individuals who receive alcohol treatment can be expected to remain abstinent over varying periods of time following discharge from the program. When treatment success is defined more broadly to include individuals who are able to use alcohol in a controlled fashion, in addition to those who abstain completely, roughly two-thirds maintain the effects of treatment, at least for some period of time. Of course, there are some individuals who are able to overcome their problematic drinking without ever receiving formal treatment. Possibly as many as 40–50 percent of problem drinkers fall into this category (Mandell, 1979). Nonetheless, formal treatment appears to improve overall success rates by about 18–22 percent over and above what would be expected from no treatment when success is broadly defined to include abstinence *and* controlled drinking. Unfortunately, there is no way to determine if these rates of remission apply equally to adults of all ages since most studies fail to differentiate treatment outcomes among older versus middle-aged or younger problem drinkers.

Relatively little information is available on the effectiveness of current treatment methods for elderly problem drinkers. Results from the studies that do exist in this area suggest that many older problem drinkers respond favorably to the social interactive aspects of treatment programs, such as group therapy and group recreational events (Blaney, Radford, & MacKenzie, 1975; Droller, 1964; Glatt, Rosin, & Jauhar, 1978). For example, over the past two decades, Glatt and his colleagues (1978) have treated nearly 2000 elderly male and female problem drinkers in England. Based upon clinical observations, they recommend a comprehensive approach to the treatment of aged alcohol abusers that emphasizes social interventions, such as a therapeutic community, group therapy, and social support. They do not stress individually oriented methods, such as personal psychotherapy, because the "common occurrence of neuroticism and deviant personality noted in particular among youthful alcoholics" (Rosin & Glatt, 1971) is less prominent in older alcoholics, at least in the aged drinkers observed in their clinical work.

Likewise, Zimberg (1969, 1971) found that alcohol abuse in older patients could be eliminated primarily by the use of group socialization, although antidepressant medication was used selectively as well. While the results from these, and previously referenced studies, cannot be considered conclusive due to methodological flaws of various kinds, it is nonetheless striking that these researchers agree on the special importance of social interventions in the treatment of many elderly problem drinkers.

Unfortunately, not all seniors who have a drinking problem are likely to benefit from alcohol programs that stress social interventions. The researchers in this area have identified two distinct types of older alcohol abusers—the early- and the late-onset types. The so-called early-onset individual began to abuse ethanol when he or she was young and has simply continued to drink excessively with age. John is an example of an early-onset older problem drinker. It is thought that this group of elderly alcohol abusers resembles younger problem drinkers in that these individuals tend to drink excessively due to basic personality defects (Rosin & Glatt, 1971; Zimberg, 1978). On the other hand, the late-onset abuser like Bill, who began to abuse ethanol relatively late in life, is said to consume alcohol not in response to personality factors, but rather in reaction to the external stresses of aging, such as the loss of a spouse, forced retirement, decreased income, and declining physical health (Zimberg, 1978).

The distinction between early- and late-onset individuals may have important implications for the treatment and long-term rehabilitation of the older problem drinker. For example, in a recent study conducted by Stern (1983), 30 men 55 years of age and older were interviewed at least 30 days after they had completed an alcohol treatment program (ATP). This group of older problem drinkers was selected because they had all relapsed following their treatment, that is, each man had experienced at least one episode of alcohol consumption since leaving an ATP. It was hoped that by understanding the nature of the relapse process in older problem drinkers, modifications could be implemented in existing treatment programs. These programs would reduce the likelihood of renewed drinking by providing these individuals with special methods for coping with situations that have a high risk for relapse.

As might be expected, the results from the study indicate that the factors leading to relapse in early-onset older problem drinkers (n = 13) were quite different than the factors reported by their late-onset counterparts (n = 17). For late-onset men, social or interpersonal factors, such as arguments with family or friends or social pressure to drink, were the most frequently cited reasons for resuming drinking. In Bill's case, even though he originally began to abuse alcohol in reaction to his wife's death, the reason he gave for his most recent relapse was an argument that took place between him and his boss at the Salvation Army. Because of his inability to cope with this type of interpersonal conflict, Bill sought comfort and relief by drinking a bottle of vodka.

In contrast, the early-onset older problem drinkers more frequently cited intrapersonal factors, such as coping with negative emotional states or enhancement of positive emotional states, as the major reason for their relapse. For example, John resumed drinking one morning when he became overwhelmed by feelings of fear, loneliness, boredom, and self-pity. He had felt this way on many occasions and his response was always the same—he would go to a bar and drink until he could no longer feel anything. To the extent that intrapersonal factors represent a heightened responsiveness to inner stress, and interpersonal factors reflect a heightened responsiveness to external demands, the pattern of relapse reported above corresponds to the earlier described notion that personality variables play a central role in explaining alcohol abuse in early-onset older individuals, while external stressors are more figural in understanding late-onset problem drinking in the elderly.

This is an important difference to consider when designing a treatment program for older problem drinkers. The effectiveness of existing alcohol treatment programs might well be enhanced by identifying the type and etiology of the older individual's drinking problem, and then assigning him or her to the treatment modality that is most appropriate. The late-onset patient is likely to be treated successfully and most expeditiously, both because the problem is less longstanding and less deeply rooted in his or her personality than is true for the early-onset alcohol abuser, and because social interventions can be provided with relative ease. Other former problem drinkers in the treatment program can serve to provide the alcohol abuser with ongoing monitoring of his or her sobriety, or controlled drinking, and to serve as the new support system that is crucial to maintaining the individual's emotional well-being. Similarly, because late-onset problem drinkers tend to have relatively intact personality structures, they usually possess the inner resources necessary to acquire new coping mechanisms, such as assertiveness, and to implement them in their daily lives quickly and effectively.

On the other hand, the early-onset problem drinker has, by definition, manifested a drinking problem much longer than his or her late-onset counterpart. It may be difficult to ascertain whether alcohol abuse has occurred in response to a deficient personality structure, or whether personality deficits have been exacerbated by the person's drinking over time. In either case, the problem drinking in such individuals is longstanding and often chronic, making it much more difficult to treat effectively. Early-onset problem drinkers may have undergone many alcohol treatment programs, and often they have achieved sobriety and then relapsed—for reasons described elsewhere in the literature (Stern, 1983). Such individuals often require more intensive and prolonged treatment than are offered by the social network and skills-building approaches, which have proven so effective for the more intact alcohol abusers whose drinking problems developed more recently. Individual psychotherapy, which is aimed at helping the patient modify the way she or he views the world, feels, and copes with problematic drinking, may be crucial to achieving permanent control for the elder who began abusing alcohol much earlier in life.

There are other characteristics that, because they are unique to older problem drinkers, should be given careful consideration when planning treatment programs for the elderly. To begin with, older alcohol abusers suffer from more health problems than do younger alcohol abusers. Advanced age, in combination with the deleterious effects of excessive drinking on the older person's health, make thorough physical examinations a vitally important part of the process of intake when the individual enters the alcohol treatment program. Ongoing medical care will also constitute an indispensable component of a quality ATP. Purveyors of such programs can anticipate that, while the health-care aspects the ATP's for the elderly are likely to be more complex and costly than those for younger people, the duration of treatment for this age group is likely to be shorter, particularly for the late-onset older problem drinker (Schuckit, 1977). When planning treatment interventions, it should also be borne in mind that elderly alcohol abusers are often characterized by a pattern of consumption in which they are more likely both to drink daily and to consume less alcohol per occasion than are their younger counterparts.

Finally, the program developers and professionals in charge of implementing the ATP must come to an understanding of the profound impact which loss and isolation have on the drinking behavior of many elderly alcohol abusers. Older problem drinkers are much more likely than their younger counterparts to be separated, divorced, or widowed, and to be living alone prior to entering an ATP (Schuckit, 1977; Schuckit & Miller, 1976; Schuckit & Pastor, 1978, 1979). Social rehabilitation of these individuals constitutes a key element in their treatment, by alleviating the painful isolation that may underly the cause and/or perpetuation of the drinking problem. As the elderly alcohol abuser is helped to develop a system of social supports to replace those which he or she has lost, and to understand the importance of such supports in maintaining both his or her emotional well-being and sobriety, the abuser becomes increasingly able to control his or her drinking behavior. Of course, efforts made toward social rehabilitation during treatment need to be continued as part of the aftercare program in order to maintain the beneficial effects of the alcohol treatment program.

As discussed in the next section, there are alcohol treatment programs currently in existence that have incorporated a number of special features designed to meet the needs of a large proportion of aging problem drinkers who seek rehabilitation.

ALCOHOL TREATMENT PROGRAMS FOR THE ELDERLY PROBLEM DRINKER

Hospitalization for detoxification and rehabilitation is a widely used approach to the treatment of alcohol abusers. An innovative adaptation of this approach to the needs of elderly alcohol abusers currently is being implemented at Long Beach, California's Memorial Hospital Medical Center (Glassock, 1979). Hospital staff have designed a 3-week inpatient program called the Alcoholism Treatment and Education Center (ATEC) that can accommodate the special requirements of the older problem drinker while providing treatment to younger alcoholics concurrently. For example, more time is allotted to the elderly patient for detoxification, and special attention is given to prescription drugs the patient may be taking that interact adversely with alcohol and exacerbate its effects. Discharge planning includes a thorough evaluation of the living arrangements and social support networks that await the elderly patient following discharge from the program. Special efforts are made to involve family, friends, and neighbors in discussions of long-term recovery. In addition to the traditional program features such as didactic lectures, films, orientation to Alcoholics Anonymous, and individual, group, and family counseling, older patients attend a special daily therapy group where problems or changes associated with the aging process are addressed. Elderly patients who have advanced to the later phases of treatment are encouraged to work with peers who have recently entered the ATEC.

Once discharged from the ATEC, the older problem drinker is encouraged to attend the twice-weekly meetings of Helping Hands, a free support group open to all elderly alcohol abusers. Helping Hands is designed to help maintain sobriety through mutual support, information sharing, and peer socialization. Members of Helping Hands and ATEC personnel have worked to establish ties with a number of social service agencies in the Long Beach area that can provide the recovering elderly problem drinker with additional community resources and support. For example, one community agency works closely with a local Helping Hands chapter to encourage the treated seniors to become active in such programs as Meals on Wheels and the Retired Senior Volunteer Program (RSVP). Participation in these types of programs helps the older alcohol abuser to engage in some type of meaningful activity and to develop new skills that will enhance his or her sense of competence and mastery. Contact with social service agencies also allows

ATEC staff and Helping Hands members to educate others in the community about the problems of alcohol abuse in late adulthood, and to offer help to older individuals whose misuse of alcohol has heretofore gone undetected or untreated. Although the effectiveness of the ATEC program has not yet been demonstrated empirically, it does represent a promising innovation in traditional inpatient approach to treatment of the elderly problem drinker.

Another innovative alcohol therapy program focuses on the grief-work process. With advancing age each new loss or threat of loss can rekindle earlier sorrows and deprivations. The number and variety of losses experienced by older people can lead to bereavement overload (Kastenbaum, 1969), a condition in which the individual's ability to function and to work through new losses has been overwhelmed by previous unresolved losses. When the individual personality is repressed to begin with and situational factors mitigate against open expression of loss, the problem intensifies. An instructive example of how this understanding can be applied to an alcohol therapy program is described by Turnquist and Christopherson (1981). Their program encompasses the Alcoholism Treatment Unit at Tuscon VAH and at West Center, the alcohol rehabilitation unit of Tuscon General Hospital. Both units are primarily inpatient facilities.

This therapy program for elderly alcoholics was based on a grief-work model with particular attention given to the individual's current phase of reaction. According to this model, shock is the first response to loss. "The mind and body take a temporary respite from the intensity of the immediate impact of the loss. This enables the person to build up resources and go through necessary everyday functions. A good physician does not give a person sleeping pills or tranquilizers at this stage unless absolutely necessary. Often, however, a person will medicate oneself through alcohol" (Turnquist & Christopherson, 1981). A depressive phase follows next that is especially dangerous for those who have turned to alcohol. Reliance on alcohol, or some other drugs, may influence the person to remain in this phase for an extended period of time, effectively arresting the normal progress through grief work.

When alcohol use interferes with recovery from loss there may be an additional "side-trip" as Turnquist and Christopherson put it, "a particular kind of guilt—the 'if only' type—through which the person will relive and review all the ways in which he or she might have prevented the loss or could have done something different. This squirrel cage mental state can be frozen through the use of chemicals" (Turnquist & Christopherson, 1981). Under normal conditions, shock and depressive phases are followed by *reconstruction,* an active state that includes emotional acceptance of the loss and seeking new relationships and activities that replace, but do not substitute, what has been lost.

The work of Turnquist, Christopherson, and their colleagues is devoted to helping elderly people with alcoholic problems move through the complication of chemical dependence and on to renewed life. Their instructive case histories are recommended for those interested in this apporach. The total therapeutic program includes didactic materials and procedures on the nature of addiction, self-evaluation procedures, group therapy, and one-to-one counseling. This combination of techniques is used flexibly according to individual needs, and the approach could be instituted at many treatment facilities.

A nontraditional method of treating the older problem drinker has been developed by the staff of the North of Market Senior Alcohol Program in San Francisco (NIAAA, 1982). Rather than hospitalizing an individual, the staff of the North of Market program attempts to treat the elderly alcohol abuser in his or her own home whenever possible. A five-person team consisting of a social worker, a nurse, a recovering alcoholic, a psychology student, and a Mennonite volunteer, visits each client at least once a week for 1–2 hours. In addition to regular home visits, activities are offered to the older problem drinker that will prove meaningful and valuable. For some clients, arts and crafts are sufficient; for others, volunteer work outside the home is effective in reducing relapse. Greater social interaction is also encouraged for senior clients by offering a neighborhood recreational drop-in facility where participants can play cards, go on field trips, attend AA meetings, or just sit around and talk with others. Unfortunately, as many as 70 percent of the seniors who are referred to the program refuse in-home treatment even though a majority of clients seem to improve. Nevertheless, in-home treatment of elderly problem drinkers represents a viable and economical alternative to hospitalization. Perhaps soliciting the help of family and friends will overcome the initial reluctance of many older alcohol abusers to participate in this type of treatment program.

Treatment of the older problem drinker is also taking place in a nursing-home setting. For example, in 1973 the Queen Nursing Home and Treatment Center in Minneapolis began to offer alcoholism treatment services in conjunction with standard nursing home care (NIAAA, 1982). The program imposes certain restrictions on the problem drinker that are designed to keep his or her money in the care of a staff member, and monitoring visits by family and friends to prevent the patient from accepting gifts containing alcohol. Each able-bodied patient is assigned a daily chore within the nursing home as well as some type of craft such as painting or sewing. As the program progresses, the individual's funds are returned gradually to him or her in the form of an allowance. Queen personnel have special training in substance abuse and other problems of the elderly so that the social, psychological, and physical problems associated with old age can be addressed along with the patient's abuse of ethanol. Since Queen staff members consider alienation as much a problem as alcohol abuse, each patient is encouraged to attend in-house AA meetings and the various other social events that regularly take place. In addition, the staff is taught to be responsive to the emotional as well as the physical needs of each patient. A special effort by staff to be open and giving is considered essential to help combat the "illness" of alienation in this elderly group.

The Alcoholism Treatment and Education Center at Memorial Hospital, the Tuscon VA and General Hospitals, the North of Market Senior Alcohol Program, and the Queen Nursing Home and Treatment Center illustrate how alcohol treatment programs designed to meet the specific needs of older problem drinkers can be implemented in a variety of settings. Wherever the treatment occurs, whether in hospital, nursing home, or the patient's own home, social involvement both during and following treatment is likely to be an important ingredient in the rehabilitation of many older problem drinkers. However, as our understanding of the processes of aging continue to grow, it will be necessary to study and explore other approaches to the rehabilitation of the elderly alcohol abuser that incorporate this expanding knowledge. It is through the reciprocal process of scientific inquiry and innovative clinical practice that improvements in the treatment of older individuals with alcohol-related problems are most likely to occur.

SOME BENEFICIAL EFFECTS OF ALCOHOL USE IN LATER LIFE

To conclude this chapter, the authors will shift from examining alcohol abuse to reviewing its potisive use in old age. There is a persistent historical tradition, starting from the earliest surviving documents from ancient civilizations and threading through all the intervening centuries, to the effect that moderate use of alcohol is a blessing, a boon for the elderly. Wine, for example, has at times been described as "the milk of old age."

The clinical research literature now confirms that *moderate* use of alcoholic beverages—especially beer and wine—can be beneficial to those older people who choose to use them. Studies conducted and reviewed by Mishara and Kastenbaum (1980) have demonstrated positive effects on morale, self-image, social interaction, and restful sleep with many populations of institutionalized elders. Furthermore, one series of studies with independent elders in the community indicates some positive effect on aspects of control of behavior, memory, and flexibility of thought.

These studies emphasize the importance of situational context: an environment in which alcohol use can become part of constructive social interactions. There also is emphasis on moderate use—typically, a single serving of beer or wine is all that the older person requires to obtain a beneficial effect. No adverse physiological effects have been reported in these studies, all of which have involved self-screening, and many of which have involved medical and nursing clearances as well. The individual's general health, including any current use of medication, should be considered before coming to a conclusion about the advisability of alcohol use. The differential effects of various types of alcoholic beverages also should be kept well in mind. Each beverage has its characteristic percentage of ethanol and a distinctive configuration of other components. A particular elderly person might find one beverage enjoyable but not another, or experience a sense of benefit from one but disagreeable sensations from another.

A general negative stereotype toward the use of alcoholic beverages by the elderly simply is not supported by clinical experiences and research, and must be considered a manifestation of veiled ageism. Many adults know how to integrate moderate alcohol intake into their life pattern, and some of these people are our parents and grandparents.

REFERENCES

American Psychiatric Association. *Diagnostic and statistical manual of mental disorders (3rd ed.)*. Washington, D.C.: APA., 1980.

Armor, D.J., Johnson, P., Polich, S., & Stambul, H. *Trends in U.S. adult drinking practices*. Summary report presented for National Institute on Alcohol Abuse and Alcoholism under Contract No. ADM 281-76-0020. Santa Monica: Rand Corp., February, 1977.

Armor, D.J., Polich, J.M., & Stambul, H.B. *Alcoholism and treatment*. New York: Wiley, 1978.

Baekeland, F. Evaluation of treatment methods in chronic alcoholism. In B. Kissin & H. Begleiter (Eds.), *The biology of alcoholism. Vol. 5: Treatment and rehabilitation of the chronic alcoholic*. New York: Plenum Press, 1977.

Bailey, M., Haberman, P., & Alkane, H. The epidemiology of alcoholism in an urban residential area. *Quarterly Journal of Studies on Alcohol,* 1965, *26,* 19–40.

Barchha, R., Stewart, M.A., & Guze, S.B. The prevalence of alcoholism among general hospital ward patients. *American Journal of Psychiatry,* 1968, *125,* 133–136.

Bengston, V.L. *The social psychology of aging*. New York: Bobbs-Merrill, 1973.

Blaney, R., Radford, I.S., & MacKenzie, G. A Belfast study of the prediction of outcome in the treatment of alcoholism. *British Journal of Addiction,* 1975, *70,* 41–50.

Botwinick, J. *Aging and behavior*. New York: Springer Publishing Co., 1978.

Brody, J.A. Alcohol and alcohol abuse. *White House Conference on Aging* background paper. Bethesda, Md.: National Institute on Aging, 1981.

Cahalan, D., Cisin, I.H., & Crossley, H.M. *American drinking practices: a national survey of drinking behavior and attitudes*. Monograph No. 6. New Brunswick, New Jersey: Rutgers Center of Alcohol Studies, 1969.

Daniel, R. A five year study of 693 psychogeriatric admissions in Queensland. *Geriatrics,* 1972, *27,* 132–155.

Drew, L.R.H. Alcoholism as a self-limiting disease. *Quarterly Journal of Studies on Alcohol,* 1968, *29,* 956–967.

Droller, H. Some aspects of alcoholism in the elderly. *The Lancet,* 1964, *2,* 137–139.

Eisdorfer, C. (Ed.), *Annual review of gerontology and geriatrics.* (Vol. 2). New York: Springer Publishing Co., 1981.

Emrick, C.D. A review of psychologically oriented treatment of alcoholism. II. The relative effectiveness of different treatment approaches and effectiveness of treatment versus no treatment. *Journal of Studies on Alcohol,* 1975, *36,* 88–108.

Finch, C.E., & Hayflick, L. (Eds.). *Handbook of the biology of aging.* New York: Van Nostrand Reinhold, 1977.

Glassock, J.A. Rehabilitating the older alcoholic. Aging, 1979, 19-24, 299–300.

Glatt, M.M. Experiences with elderly alcoholics in England. *Alcoholism: Clinical and Experimental Research,* 1978, *2,* 23–26.

Glatt, M.M., Rosin, A.J., & Jauhar, P. Alcoholic problems in the elderly. *Age and Ageing,* 1978, *7* (Suppl), 64–66.

Goldberg, P.B., & Roberts, J. Influence of age on the pharmacology and physiology of the cardiovascular system. In M.F. Elias, B.E. Eleftheriou, & P.K. Elias (Eds.), *Special review of experimental aging research: Progress in biology.* Bar Harbor, Maine: EAR, Inc., 1976.

Graux, P. Alcoholism of the elderly. *Review on Alcohol,* 1969, *15,* 61–63.

Kastembaum, R. Death and bereavement in later life. In A.H. Kutscher (Ed.), *Death and bereavement.* Springfield, Ill.: Charles C. Thomas, 1969.

Kastenbaum, R. Personality theory, therapeutic approaches, and the elderly client. In M. Storandt, I.C., Siegler, & M.F. Elias, (Eds.), *The clinical psychology of aging.* New York: Plenum Press, 1978.

Kimmel, D.C. *Adulthood and aging.* New York: Wiley, 1974.

Lundin, D. Medication taking behavior of the elderly. *Drug Intelligence and Clinical Pharmacy,* 1978, *12,* 518–521.

Mandell, W. A critical overview of evaluations of alcoholism treatment. *Alcoholism: Clinical and Experimental Research,* 1979, *3,* 315–323.

Mishara, B.L. & Kastenbaum, R. *Alcoholism and old age.* New York: Grune & Stratton, 1980.

Moore, S.R. Medication taking behavior of the elderly. *Drug Intelligence and Clinical Pharmacy,* 1978, *12,* 739–741.

National Council on Alcoholism. Criteria for the diagnosis of alcoholism. *American Journal of Psychiatry,* 1972, *129,* 127–133.

National Institute on Alcohol Abuse and Alcoholism (NIAAA). Alcohol and the elderly. Treatment approaches. *Information and Feature Service,* 1982, *103,* 2–4.

Rathbone-McCuan, E. A treatment typology for the elderly alcohol abuser. *Journal of the American Geriatrics Society,* 1975, *23,* 553–557.

Rosin, A.J., & Glatt, M.M. Alcohol excess in the elderly. *Quarterly Journal of Studies on Alcohol,* 1971, *32,* 53–59.

Schuckit, M.A. Geriatric alcoholism and drug abuse. *The Gerontologist,* 1977, *17,* 168–174.

Schuckit, M.A., & Miller, P.L. Alcoholism in elderly men: A survey of a general medical ward. *Annals of New York Academy of Sciences,* 1976, *273,* 558–571.

Schuckit, M.A., & Pastor, P.A. Alcohol-related psychopathology in the aged. In O.J. Kaplan (Ed.), *Psychopathology in the aging*. New York: Academic Press, 1979.

Schuckit, M.A., & Pastor, P.A. The elderly as a unique population: Alcoholism. *Alcoholism: Clinical and Experimental Research*. 1978, *2,* 31–38.

Simon, A., Epstein, L.J., & Reynolds, L. Alcoholism in the geriatric mentally ill. *Geriatrics,* 1968, *23,* 125–131.

Stern, D.S. Determinants of relapse in older male problem drinkers. Doctoral dissertation. Cincinnatti: University of Cincinnati, 1983.

Timiras, P.S. *Developmental physiology and aging*. New York: MacMillan, 1972.

Turnquist, M., & Christopherson, V.A. Grief work with older alcoholics in treatment. Tuscon: University of Arizona Agricultural Experiment Station Paper No. 3536, 1981.

Vestal, R.E., McGuire, E.A., Tobin, J.D., Andres, R., Norris, A.H., & Mezey, R. Aging and ethanol metabolism in man. *Clinical Pharmacology and Therapeutics,* 1977, *21,* 343–354.

Wallgren, H., & Barry, H. *Actions of alcohol* (Vols. 1 & 2). Amsterdam: Elsevier, 1970.

Zimberg, S. Outpatient geriatric psychiatry in an urban ghetto with nonprofessional workers. *American Journal of Psychiatry,* 1969, *125,* 1697–1702.

Zimberg, S. The psychiatrist and medical home care: Geriatric psychiatry in the Harlem community. *American Journal of Psychiatry,* 1971, *127,* 1062–1066.

Zimberg, S. Diagnosis and treatment of the elderly alcoholic. *Alcoholism: Clinical and Experimental Research,* 1978, *2,* 27–29.

11

SEXUALITY AND THE ELDERLY

Alex Comfort

Discussions of age effects still turn almost exclusively on male sexuality.Male anxiety about changes in sexual performance with age has been always more manifest—partly the result of the fact that male sexual performance depends on what the Bible calls the outward and visible sign of an inner and spiritual grace. But, in fact, the literature contains remarkably little about age effects on women. When it comes to discussing the question of pharmacological effects on sexual function, there has been considerably detailed documentation on males, but rarely any documentation on females. One of the assignments that this generation must undertake is documentation of these changes on a more impartial basis, so that it is possible to counsel elderly women as well as men. This is difficult at the present time due to lack of information.

Perhaps the most interesting feature of changes in human sexual physiology and age-induced performance, when compared with changes in the speed of memory encodement, is that, apart from one rather spectacular event, the programmed determination of fertility in menopause, changes are otherwise minimal. The folkloristic view of old age as being occupationally impotent, uninterested and nonfunctional in sexuality, tends to be the expression of a self-fulfulling prophecy.

GERIATRIC MENTAL HEALTH
ISBN 0-8089-1657-2

SEXUALITY IN ELDERLY MEN

The prime objective change in males is slight slowing of response and a reduction in intensity and regularity of the drive that lies behind sexual response. This trend, however, shows great individual variation. For some people sexuality is relatively unimportant, while others think of virtually nothing else. Between the two fall the majority. There is, cross-sectionally, a reduction in the drive underlying sexuality that may be partly physiological and partly due to social pressures not to be sexual that we bring to bear on the old.

There are also physiological changes. After the age of fifty, purely psychic erection,—erection produced by thinking about sex—becomes less frequent. Morning erection is maintained, and is still incorrectly said to be caused by a full bladder. In fact, morning erection is a carry-over from the terminal period of REM sleep. Whether the subject awakes with a morning erection depends on whether he awoke from REM sleep or from one of the other levels. REM sleep becomes a smaller proportion of the total sleep time in old age. The sexually-directed erection comes to depend increasingly on direct penile stimulation. It takes longer to induce than it does in younger males. A notice that is fixed to an aircraft cockpit panel, "Do not attempt landing until the undercarriage is fully locked in the down position," is a piece of advice that should be given to older males who are anxious about their performance.

There are, in addition, one or two minor physical changes: The angle of the erect penis to the abdominal wall becomes greater (that is, 90° as opposed to 45° in youth), and the inevitability of orgasm becomes less marked. There is a more gradual movement from tumescence to orgasm and a loss of the crescendo preorgasmic "inevitability" seen in younger males. With age, the retraction of the testes by the cremaster muscle during orgasm into the pod overlying Poupart's ligament ceases to occur.

A far more important change, and one that sometimes upsets male patients, is that orgasm ceases to occur at every act of intercourse, if intercourse is frequent. This is an important change, because—whereas in the Oriental tradition the avoidance of orgasm was recommended in order to prolong pleasure or for mystical reasons—in our tradition the orgasm is considered to be a certificate of success. For the male, erection is the equivalent of a valid credit card, and orgasm is the presumed equivalent of general solvency.

These changes are extremely variable in individuals. Some do not show them at all; others show them quite markedly. This is but another example of the fact that, with aging, nearly all physiological parameters tend to diverge and show a much greater scatter. The changes described as "age related" are commonly present by age 60. Like *benign senile forgetfulness* or changes in visual accomodation, the effects described tend to bottom out.

Neither sexual response nor visual accomodation gets worse after age 50. Time is reached when the oculist can give us what we might call our terminal spectacles, because we are not going to change very much after that, unless we have actual eye disease. In the same way, late-life male sexual response reaches a final level.

The chief importance of these objective changes is that sexually active and unanxious men, who are accustomed to prolonged sexual play and intercourse and are not bothered particularly by performance anxiety, simply see them as a case of getting more miles per gallon. But for the man whose stereotype of virility—and it is a very common one in our culture—depends on hasty performance followed by hurried orgasm may interpret change as a loss of function, and the consequent anxiety can in itself induce sexual failure.

It can be said with confidence that impotency is never the result of chronological age alone. Still it does increase with age and the increasing frequency is due to a variety of causes: (1) the prevalence of diabetes, which may be the presenting symptom of other forms of vascular autonomic insufficiency—from rare ones such as Leriche's Syndrome to more common ones such as general atherosclerosis; (2) the increasing prevalence of conditions like hypertension, which lead to medication, prostatic enlargement, and can lead to overenthusiastic surgery; (3) the fact that many elders are on either psychoactive drugs or on antihypertensives, all of which are capable of interfering with erection, ejaculation, or both; and (4) the social expectation of impotency in age. This last is reinforced by the loss, ill-health, or aging of the partner, obesity, increased sensitivity to alcohol—which, after performance anxiety, is the second most common cause of sexual failure in males of all ages. The increased incidence of undiagnosed depression, also can present as anhedonia, and is often, but not always, accompanied by a loss of sexual interest.

In spite of all these factors, objective loss of potency verified by penile plethysmography, which is the only good way of verifying it, is relatively rare, even in advanced age. What we see depends on the exacerbation of psychosexual problems with age. There are many sexually dysfunctional people in all age groups, from adolescence on. If we add the folklore of sexuality to the folklore of age, we have a double strike against the patient. Old people lose interest in sexual activity as a result of loss of competitive self-esteem, which society tends to enforce. We are increasingly familiar with the impotency that goes with job loss. Something similar is seen in the elderly. For others, loss of function is a welcome excuse to abandon an activity that they have always found rather embarrassing or guilt-inducing.

High-dominance individuals, whose sexual attitudes have always been positive normally, stay both potent and active throughout life, if they have the opportunity and avoid disabling disease. Androgen deficit rarely plays any part in this declining sexual function, nor are androgen supplements a good treatment for old-age potency problems. When they work, it appears they do so not by re-sexualizing the patient but by increasing physical strength and well-being, which in turn is expressed as a revival of sexual interest. Fertility may also persist in males up to the ninth decade.

Given the opportunity, neither sexual style nor sexual orientation changes with age. Preferences, and the position on the scale of human bisexuality, normally remain unaltered. At middle-age crisis we may, however, sometimes see a repressed option surfacing as part of a general reassessment of goals. Middle-age crisis is a time when people tend to review what they have done and consider what they had better do soon if they are ever to do it. That may be experienced sexually in what is sometimes called "sexual indiscretion", or in a change in orientation, where a repressed homosexual component surfaces in heterosexual people and vice-versa (the former is the more usual in our culture). As to the style or attitude of the patient, there are elders who received their sex education 60 or 70 years ago and who retain the mores they acquired then, and others who have updated their mores and are much more in keeping with those of the younger generation. Older people, for instance, may now cohabit without being married when they would not have done so in the society in which they were brought up.

The subjective experience of aging reflects the changed responses of the patient's contacts. This can lead to anxiety and rejection of sexuality, especially among those of either sex who have come to use sexuality as a way to manipulate other people. When they feel that they cease to be attractive they may resign from it completely, rather in the way that some people go to pieces when they retire from a job. How far sexuality will remain active and rewarding depends very much on the individual patient and a great deal more on basic attitudes then on physiology. It very often can be compromised severely, however, by the mistaken belief that there is something physically wrong. In the case of the elderly, the mistaken belief that major physical losses are inevitable with the passage of time can be accepted and acted-out by playing the role of counterphobic "oldness."

Medical students sometimes ask why we have so many drugs that interfere with erection, whereas we have no reliable aphrodisiac. The reason is the extreme complexity of the male erectile mechanism. At the effector level, there is overriding central control, and it is obvious that mood and situation and thinking about sex can produce arousal. On the other hand, the main cerebral effect over the lower spinal reflex is inhibitory—which is why hanging or decapitating leads to reflex erection. For erection to occur, blood has to be diverted into a complicated system. The corpora cavernosa, containing the hydraulics, have to be filled, and then the flow has to be regulated at a level that is sufficient to prevent thrombosis but not at a level that will empty the corpora. This is carried out by what the Germans call *bolters polstern* in the sides of the emissary veins of the corpora cavernosa. Moreover, for the system to operate, both the sympathetic and the parasympathetic systems have to be intact, because both adrenergic and cholinergic fibers are involved. We have recently learned that, at least in males, the neuroreceptors in the corpora, the glans, and the rest of the genitalia, when studied by immunoflourescence, are neither adrenergic, nor cholinergic. The agent to which they are sensitive is the vasoactive intestinal peptide (VIP). At the present time, we are in the process of finding out just what this VIP system means. It possibly accounts for loss of erectile capacity in diabetes, in which we know the VIP system is disorganized. It actually may give us a clue to therapeutic measures in cases where this occurs. Almost anything can disorganize so complex a system, but there is apparently no drug that can trigger all of it, hence the lack of an effective aphrodisiac. Moreover, the ejaculatory reflex and the engorgement of the glans are on a separate reflex apart from erection. The two normally occur one after the other, but they can also occur out of synchrony, which explains why with a drug like Mellaril some patients show no disorganization of sexual function, some show a lack of erection, and others show lack of ejaculation. One may, in fact, notice exactly the same subdivisions in sexual histories in normal males. There are some males who lose their erection when overtired, situationally stressed, under the influence of alcohol, or otherwise impaired; there are others who, under the same circumstances, retain their erection but fail to ejaculate. Large numbers of drugs have one or both effects, and they differ, probably according to the general susceptibility of the individual to these effects.

SEXUALITY IN ELDERLY WOMEN

Persistence of sexual function in women lamentably has been documented less well. But it seems to persist far more effectively than in men. Until lately, in our culture, women traditionally have been the passive objects of intercourse rather than active initiators of it. There is no evidence that the capacity for orgasm declines at any age in women. Women are known to have become orgasmic for the first time at ages in excess of 80. Coition can be impaired by vaginal atrophy, lack of lubrication, kraurosis, pelvic conditions such as cystocele, prolapse, and stress incontinence—but these are all conditions surgically remediable.

The most common reason for sexual inactivity in older women is social convention and lack of opportunity. The latter arises from the fact that there is a four-year differential between the average age of males and females in marriage, the male tending to be the older partner. The mortality of males is in general higher than that of females. The large number of what are termed "surplus" older women is partly due to a discouragement not imposed on the older males. The older male who loses a partner tends to raid a younger age-group for a mate, whereas the older woman is discouraged from doing so and is subject to mockery if she does. Older women who have no partners are not in general lacking either in inclination or ability to engage in sexual contacts, they are lacking in opportunity and trying to make the best of it.

STUDIES ON ELDERLY SEXUALITY

In reading statistical studies of sexual behaviors with age, it is necessary to recall that most of these cut cross-sections of populations that will include the unanxious and sexually active, those who were dysfunctional at younger ages, and those who never had intercourse—a complete mix. Very misleading results may be obtained. In spite of a high incidence of psychogenic dysfunction at all ages, it appears that older people always have been just as sexually active as any other group, but kept their own counsel about it, for obvious reasons. Perhaps the earliest study was that of Raymond Pearl in 1916, who recorded 4 percent of males aged 70–79 having intercourse every third day, and a further 9 percent having it weekly (Pearl, 1930). Kinsey's figures show a decline in coital frequency with age (Kinsey, Pomeroy, Martin et al. 1948, 1953). But these figures are cross-sectional, not longitudinal. Finkle, Moyers, Tobenkin et al. (1959), questioned 101 men aged 56–86, and he found 65 percent under age 69 and 34 percent over age 70 were still potent, on their own statement, with 2 out of 5 over 80 averaging at least 10 acts of intercourse a year. But on further inquiry it was found that a number of men in the sample had never had intercourse, and others, though they had been potent, disapproved of masturbation and had no partner. So, aside from REM sleep erections, they would have no way of judging their potency. In the over-70 group, the main reason given for inactivity was either "no desire" or "no partner." Of all men over 65, only three gave "no erection" as a reason. Newman and Nichols (1960) questioned patients of both sexes aged 60–93 in their sample. They got a 54 percent overall "still active" figure for that rather wide age range. They found that among those over 75, 25 percent were still active, but decline was chiefly the result of illness, either of self or spouse. "Those who rated sexual urges as strongest in youth rate them as moderate in age; those that described sexual feelings as weak or moderate in youth describe themselves as being without them in old age." They also found that early starters were late finishers (Newman & Nichols, 1960).

Pfeiffer, Verwoerdt and Wang (1968) at Duke studied 254 people of both sexes. The median age for stopping sexual intercourse was 68 in men and 60 in women, the difference being partly attributable to the age differential already mentioned. The figures for regular and frequent intercourse were 47 percent between 60 to 71 and 15 percent for age 78 and older.

This study was longitudinal. Over a 5–year period 16 percent of all ages noted a decline in sexual activity, but 14 percent reported an increase. These figures had no very close relationship of decline to the chronological age. Pfeiffer et al. strongly support the view, however, that this study reflects the experience of a mixture of high and low sexual-activity individuals. Those whose sexual set is low, either for physiological or for emotional reasons, tend to drop-out early, often with recourse to age as an excuse. Social pressures, ill health, medication, and lack of a socially acceptable partner tend to take some toll among others, but for those who are sexually positive and active, aging neither abolishes the need nor the capacity for intercourse. As a matter of fact, it is very much like riding a bicycle; people give it up either because they are too infirm to ride one, or somebody told them they looked silly or because they don't have a bicycle. There may be a difference with the current generation who may have higher sexual expectations when they reach old age, if they are, by then, correctly informed as to what they should and should not expect to occur.

TREATMENT FOR THE ELDERLY

What can we do to help the elderly? Sexual counseling and therapy depend upon permission-giving and correcting false impressions, and that is true for every age group. In the case of the old, we have to correct impressions both about sex and age. Apart from a much more strenuous exclusion of physical and iatrogenic causes of impotency, and of such factors as obesity and alcohol, counseling is identical in form at all ages. The therapy of impotency in older men is the same as in younger men: it depends on removal of performance anxiety and teaching of sexual attitudes that de-emphasize performance as a purely Olympic activity, instead of an enjoyable interpersonal experience involving the whole body.

Therapy also causes us to look rather carefully at our preconceptions. We have passed through periods in which an old man would not consult a physician on this subject lest it be thought indecent; then through periods when, if he had consulted a physician, he would have been given hormones or advised to consort with a younger prostitute; and, again, through a period when he would have been subjected possibly to psychoanalysis; and more recently still, a period when he would have been lectured about getting in touch with his body. We are now entering a period in which we realize that many of those women, who were not long ago lectured on their anorgasmia and on getting in touch with their bodies, had hyperprolactinemia. In the same way, in older males who display sudden and unexplained loss of sexual function—although it is true that performance anxiety is the commonest cause—undiagnosed Peyronie's disease is quite common. It is also more common in people who are on beta-blocking agents. Practolol, before it was withdrawn, was a well-documented cause of loss of sexual function, but there have been cases where it was associated even with propranolol.

There are also cases in which, although erection is obtained, the stability of the penis is reduced through stretching of the ligaments at its base. One sees this in Marfan's syndrome, but one also sees it in old people who do not have a specific collagenosis. These patients will complain of an inability to penetrate. Another often overlooked factor is that the older male requires more friction in order to achieve an erection. If his wife at the same time is on large amounts of estrogen for post-menopausal symptoms, her lubrication increases at a time when his friction should increase. He may say he "doesn't feel anything" and presents as impotent.

The physician must look at the mechanical situation i.e., penile erectile function. Fortunately, we no longer have to rely on anecdotal evidence. Penile plethysmography during sleep, or the much cheaper and simpler expedient of putting an adhesive piece taken from the edge of a sheet of U.S. stamps around the flaccid penis at bedtime to see if it is burst in the morning, will indicate adequately whether erection is occuring in sleep. If it is, then at any rate there is nothing fundamentally wrong with the hydraulics. By excluding physical causes and medication changes, one may finally be left with morale changes and false attitudes.

We probably require a warning against the excessive psychiatric interpretation of dysfunction. It pays to listen to what the patient says: he may tell you that he cannot have intercourse with one particular woman, but when investigated, you may find that the woman is too difficult to penetrate. There are women with whom it is possible to have intercourse without an erection, particularly in a rear-entry position, and there are others whose vaginas are so placed that it is rather difficult to penetrate without a very stiff erection. Variation in position will sometimes overcome this. Here we often face the problem, as with the disabled, that when elderly patients say that they cannot perform sexually, they mean they cannot perform sexually within the parameters imposed by their own concept of what is normal. A woman who "cannot have intercourse" with an arthritic hip may mean that she cannot have intercourse in the "missionary position," and has not been prepared to try any other. Some older women dislike the idea of touching male genitalia with the hand. Very often a discussion of attitude is required: there may be a lot of it to confront before getting to the counseling problem. On the other hand, there may be none, as not all old people are rigid or naive in such matters.

The keen, young physician does have to be careful not to get into the impertinent situation of trying to "turn old folks on." Enthusiastic youngsters sometimes do this. The physician has to have a reasonable degree of judgment in not disturbing those who wish to retain the privacy of their sexual experiences or are not particularly anxious to be turned on, and those who are actually very frustrated and upset by what they conceive as loss of a very important function that they have always enjoyed, but are too proud or too modest to talk about with the physician. Therefore, it is important that we afford the opportunity to every older patient to talk about it. One of the factors that many old people experience, even if they are not dysfunctional and have no problems with their present sexual situation, is great relief in the fact that it is now decent to discuss and ask about experiences that were not decent to discuss or ask about years ago. Many old people are quite relieved to be able to talk more frankly about sexuality than they could in youth.

One encounters other problems when pressures are placed on older people by sons and daughters who have a Freudian anxiety about sexuality of their elders. More cynically, some potential heirs very much dislike the idea of a parent getting remarried at an advanced age, when they almost have their hands on the stock portfolio. To those children, the old have to be encouraged to say, "Well, I did my job in bearing you or in begetting you. Get lost!" and "I've had the reproductive side of sex; I think I am now of an age to enjoy the recreational side of it." Sexuality is validating at all ages, especially so for the old as well as for the disabled. It militates against infantalizing the old so that they can retain the same privacy and sexual freedom of choice that they had when they were young adults. Any institution that denies that right is doing the old a disservice. There were times in the past when geriatric institutions divided old husbands and wives. It is rather important for the physician to realize that even terminal illness requires that room be left for sexual leave-taking.

The special geriatric problems we see are related both to changes in physiology and the circumstances of age. Masters uses the term "widower's impotence" to describe the condition of a man whose wife has been an invalid for a long while and who has been inactive sexually (Masters & Johnson, 1970; 1966). He may have even felt that it was slightly disloyal to her to masturbate while she was incapacitated. After her death, he wishes to marry again, and may find that the combination of disuse atrophy, mourning for his deceased wife, and guilt at his relief over her death, interfere quite seriously with function. Unfamiliarity with the new partner and performance anxiety, of course, are other contributors to dysfunction.

We find an excellent picture of performance anxiety in the old bridegroom in the story of the marriage of January and May in Chaucer's *Canterbury Tales*: The old man marries a young girl and doses himself the night before with every sort of medication. Next morning he is so delighted he could perform that he sings, and the "slacke skin about his neck gan shake." We can avert this kind of anxiety with some factual advice.

There are other reassurances we need to give. Women in particular need to be reassured about pelvic surgery and menopause. There are still women, though fewer now, who believe that menopause desexualizes them. In fact, menopause often leads to a sexual renaissance because women no longer have to bother about contraception. Pelvic surgery, if it is skillfully performed, does not interfere at all with sexual performance, but very few surgeons take the trouble to discuss these anxieties with women and make certain that they really understand what is being done and what will and will not result. There was, in fact, one older gynecological textbook stating that when a woman is over the age of seventy, the vagina can simply be sewn up, since it will not be needed. Insensitivity is, luckily, disappearing, like that of surgeons who imagine that you need not conserve function in aged males. We have managed to reduce the incidence of radical prostatectomies, particularly the transperineal variety, which interfere quite seriously with function. Generally speaking, a transurethral resection should not interfere with potency and when it does, one usually finds that there were considerable problems before the operation. So it behooves the surgeon both to take a sexual history before the operation and to explain its consequences.

> Special and more serious psychiatric problems sometimes arise. The story goes as follows: An old man with a sprightly, elderly wife became paranoid and came to the conclusion that she was involved with a neighbor, to whom she had been introduced by "two old yentas at the club." In the end, this gentleman bought a revolver to frighten her. He frightened himself, because his son-in-law had him committed to a hospital. Ten or fifteen years previously the patient had to have a prostatectomy. He did not want it and held if off for as long as he could, but his wife insisted he must. Just before the operation, the young surgeon sidled up to the wife and said, "You do realize, Mrs. X, that you won't be able to have any more children after this." As she was 68 at the time, Mrs. X thought this was self-evident. What the surgeon found himself unable to say was, "Does your husband realize that he won't ejaculate normally?" When the patient found he could not ejaculate, he was furious. He rapidly became impotent and blamed his wife for the whole procedure.

In this event, the paranoia turned out to be an offshoot of a senile dementia, Alzheimer's type, and was not entirely psychogenic. The case, however, does illustrate the evils of over-reticent and under-explicit communication.

One will encounter cases of established and organic impotency. This diagnosis can be made if, on proper nocturnal plethysmography, the patient is found not to have erections and there is clear-cut evidence that multiple sclerosis, diabetes, or some other irremediable cause of impotency exists, or if very extensive pelvic or perineal surgery has been performed. For those patients there is now a technique involving insertion of either a Small-Carrion prosthesis, which is a semi-rigid vinyl rod that provides a simulation of an erection, or a hinged device that can be locked up and down, and has a baseplate that is said to be more satisfactory. Many patients have claimed that a prosthesis is satisfactory, but it is remarkable how rarely the surgeon has consulted the partner.

One may find that the partners are "playing games:" the man is not getting great satisfaction out of intercourse, and the partner is putting up with it in order to sustain his ego. One has to ask the patient, "Do you really want this, or are you prepared to realize that there are other types of sexual activity that can be equally rewarding and can provide orgasm in both partners?" The physician may indicate it is time for a change. Unfortunately, the morale-boosting value of erection and intromission, buoyed up by some Freudian formulations on the subject, are so ingrained in our culture that there are those who would rather have an erection than have pleasure. To be successful, one must very carefully find out what the patient actually wants and what will be most reinforcing. I would certainly not withhold a surgical prosthesis in an elderly impotent subject if it was of any help to both of the partners. But it should be discussed jointly with the two of them, with due regard to possible postoperative complications. A prosthesis may be better avoided in younger people who have multiple sclerosis, because the impotency that occurs very often self-reverses. Similarly, it is a common finding in old men that there are periods in which they are not sexually active and periods when they "recover." In such cases success becomes chancier and more intermittent as age advances. Small events such as an attack of flu or being over-tired more easily disturb sexual activity in older men than they do in younger men.

As a general measure, androgen therapy is not usually of any value. However, even apart from the hypogonadic, there are cases where it seems to work. We would prefer to use something like mesterolone, which is not read by the body as testosterone, and does not therefore inhibit the androgenous supply. (Mesterolone is not an approved drug in the United States.)

Work on proclactin remains tentative. We know that women who are hyperprolactinemic are also dysorgasmic as a rule. This hyperprolactinemia can otherwise be relatively asymptomatic, although it may induce menstrual irregularity. Anorgasmia from this cause may respond to bromocryptine. A proportion of males who are impotent have microadenoma of the pituitary. They, too, respond to the administration of bromocryptine or one of the other antiprolactin drugs. On the other hand, in any case of impotency in which blood prolactin levels are normal, bromocryptine is no more effective than placebo. Androgen is ineffective in the presence of excess prolactin.

If one asks "In general what helps old people most with sexual problems?", the answer would be to identify the approach that helps disabled people in the same circumstances most, namely the opportunity of a well-led group discussion with other couples their own age. After getting over the initial reticence and "losing" those group members who really are too embarrassed to talk, patients will enlarge on the problems they have had, and by discussion will build each other's morale. There needs to be a trained leader on hand to answer questions, moderate the discussion, and protect individuals from prying by the group as a whole. Given this, the approach is very effective. When sexual group therapy with the disabled was proposed, it was objected, "You can't talk about that, you'll embarrass them." In fact, it was the staff who were embarassed, not the patients. It was necessary to say to the nursing director of a hospital for the disabled, "What do you imagine the patients talk about when you aren't there?" In fact, when offered the therapy, they beat a path to the door. One group consisting of either disabled couples or of couples where one was able and the other disabled, very soon got into a competition of comparing notes as to how to overcome particular disabilities, how to circumvent them, and how to maintain a rewarding sexual relationship in the presence of physical problems.

The elderly do not always have sexual problems. Even so, group discussion sometimes is very beneficial. One of the great curses of sexuality in our society is its privacy, and the fact that we have very little opportunity of comparing notes by discussion with other people and finding out how far our own experience is unique, which it very rarely is. For that reason, introducing discussions or lectures on the subject of sexuality into elderly communities, to older patients, or into senior citizen groups and organizations, often is appreciated very much. Those who find such occasions impertinent or distasteful will stay away.

REFERENCES

Finkle, A.L., Moyers, T.G., Tobenkin, M.I., & Karg, S.J. Sexual potency in aging males: Frequency of coitus among clinic patients. *Journal of the American Medical Association*, 1959, *170*, 1891–1993.

Kinsey, A.C., Pomeroy, W.B., & Martin, C.R. *Sexual behavior in the human male*. Philadelphia: Saunders, 1948.

Kinsey, A.C., Pomeroy, W.B., Martin, C.R., & Gebhard, P.H. *Sexual behavior in the human female*. Philadelphia: Saunders, 1953.

Masters, W.H., & Johnson, V.E. *Human sexual response*. Boston: Little, Brown, 1966.

Masters, W.H., & Johnson, V.E. *Human sexual inadequacy*. Boston: Little, Brown, 1970.

Newman, G., & Nichols, C.R. Sexual activities and attitudes in older persons. *Journal of the American Medical Association*, 1960, *173*, 33–35.

Pearl, R. *The biology of population growth*. New York: Knopf, 1930.

Pfeiffer, E., Verwoerdt, A., & Wang, H.S. Sexual behavior in aged men and women. *Archives of General Psychiatry*, 1968, *19*, 753–758.

SUGGESTED READINGS

Cameron, P., & Biber, H. Sexual thought throughout the lifespan. *Gerontologist*, 1973, *13*, 144–147.

Cooper, A.J., Ismail, A.A.A., Smith, G.C., & Lorraine, J.A. Androgen function in psychogenic and constitutional types of impotence. *British Medical Journal*, 1970, *3*, 17–20.

Finkle, A.L., & Prian, D.V. Sexual potency in elderly men before and after prostatectomy. *Journal of the American Medical Association*, 1966, *196*,139.

Polak, J.M., Mina, S., Gu, J. & Bloom, S.R. Vipergic nerves in the penis. *Lancet*, 1981, *ii*, 217–219.

Wagner, G., & Metz, P. Impotence (erectile dysfunction) due to vascular disorders—an overview. *Journal of Sex and Marital Therapy*, 1980, *6*, 223–233.

Wagner, G., Bro-Rassmussen, F., Willis, E.A., & Nielsen, M.H. New theory of erection involving hitherto undescribed vessels. *Lancet*, 1982, *i*, 116–118.

12

MINORITY ELDERLY IN MENTAL HEALTH SETTINGS: CLINICAL ISSUES

Barbara Solomon

It has been well documented that the elderly are underrepresented as consumers of mental health services (Butler & Lewis, 1973; Kramer, Taube, & Redick, 1973; Rosen, Anderson, & Bahn, 1967). There is equally compelling evidence that the so-called "oppressed minorities"— American Indian and Hispanic— are also underrepresented in the caseloads of mental health agencies (Kramer, Rosen, & Willie, 1973; Sue, McKinney, Allen et al., 1974; Thomas & Sillen, 1972). Numerous reasons for this underutilization by minorities have been posed including lack of minority service-providers, preference for informal help systems, and negative stereotyping by nonminority mental health professionals. Similarly diverse reasons have been given for underutilization of mental health services by the elderly such as mental health professionals' lack of knowledge about aging and negative stereotypes of the elderly. Although definitive data are not available as to the relative validity of reasons given, the experience of most mental health professionals would confirm the notion that minority elderly do not often receive help with their mental health problems either because of cultural barriers reflected in the elderly individual's attitude toward mental health services or in the attitude of service providers toward the elderly individual. This chapter will discuss some major issues

GERIATRIC MENTAL HEALTH
ISBN 0-8089-1657-2

that have relevance for ongoing efforts in the field of clinical gerontology to serve minority elderly effectively.

Preliminary to any discussion of clinical issues is the definition of relevant terms that have been used imprecisely in much of the social science as well as mental health practice literature. For example, *the elderly* have been most often defined in terms of normative age for mandatory retirement from the work force, which until recently was 65. Legislative changes now permit workers to stay on the job until age 70 without fear of termination because of age. However, the concept of retirement is problematical for many minority elderly who have never been afforded the luxury of retirement. They are often excluded from even the meager benefits of the Social Security system due to employment in uncovered jobs or erratic employment on temporary jobs (Stanford, 1978). A cross-cultural study of elderly in San Diego recently found that most minority group elderly considered aging to be determined not by retirement status but by extent of physical-mental impairment (Stanford, 1978). The implication is that those persons who are still working or who maintain active lives despite having retired from full-time employment would not be considered elderly by themselves or others of their racial/ethnic group.

If the determination of when one is elderly or not is difficult, the determination of whether one is a member of a racial or ethnic minority group would appear to be quite straight forward. However, membership in a particular racial or ethnic group by virtue of one's birth is rarely the issue in predicting an individual's attitudes or behavior. It is more often the extent to which that individual exhibits what has been referred to by anthropologists as *behavioral ethnicity* (Harwood, 1981; Stein & Hill, 1977). Behavioral ethnicity is indicated when members of an ethnic or racial group learn distinctive values, beliefs, behavioral norms, and languages or distinctive dialects during the process of socialization. Furthermore, these distinctive cultural artifacts govern interaction not only between and among members of the group but also in their interaction with others in mainstream social institutions. Behavioral ethnicity is different from ideological ethnicity, which is based on customs that are neither central to a person's social life nor necessarily learned from early socialization; it is fragmentary, situational, and voluntaristic. The anthropologist Schneider has referred to these customs as "Symbols" empty of elaborate social distinctions (Parsons, 1975).

It is behavioral ethnicity which has the most import for the mental health practitioner. Collectivities of behavioral ethnics (usually first and second generation immigrants or minorities with a history of exclusion from mainstream educational and political institutions, e.g., Blacks, Hispanics, Asian/Americans and American Indians) vary in rates of morbidity and mortality for different diseases (Alers, 1978; Bullough & Bullough, 1972; King, 1975; McDermott, Deuschle, Adair, et al. 1960; Shiloh & Shiloh, 1974). They also differ in their conceptions of illness and mental illness and how they should be treated, and in interactions with health professionals (Harrison & Harrison, 1971; Quesada & Heller, 1977).

Holzberg (1982) has described the qualitative dimensions of ethnicity as a sense of exclusiveness and awareness that one is a member of a distinct social group. Feelings of shared particularity may be reflected by membership in ethnic-specific social institutions and participation in ethnically segregated clubs or voluntary associations. She suggests, however, that ethnicity is relevant for all elderly, not just the traditional, oppressed minorities (Holzberg, 1982). Thus, any attempt to distinguish these latter groups in regard to values, traditions, communication style must take those same phenomena into account in the dominant group as well as in other minority groups such as white ethnics. However, it should be apparent that behavioral ethnicity is not an "either you have it or no you don't" proposition. Some members of the group have more behavioral ethnicity than others.

This conceptualization of ethnicity as an ordinal variable permits us to avoid the mistaken response in seeing only similarities with other groups rather than differences. For example, most subgroups in the American ethnosystem have significant extended family networks and strong religious orientation. Yet, despite the fact that these ethnic collectivities may share beliefs or behavior patterns, they may vary from each other in the particular manner in which they adhere to these same beliefs and behavior patterns.

Viewed from the perspective of mental health practitioners, having to predict variation in beliefs and behavior within ethnic groups, the data indicate that the more educated and affluent members of an ethnic group will tend to differ in their beliefs and behavior from less educated and less advantaged members of the same ethnic group. In other words, persons of lower socioeconomic status tend to demonstrate to a greater degree behavioral ethnicity in matters of health and mental health matters than do those of higher socioeconomic standing. The relationship between socioeconomic class and behavioral ethnicity may not hold in regard to future age cohorts since the deep economic recession in this country has meant that many persons who are middle class in orientation have been dropped precipitiously into a lower socioeconomic level. Whether their reference group will continue to be middle class or not is not clear at this time. Since the elderly in most groups tend to be closer to the unique historical experience of the ethnic group, it could be expected that they are more likely to reflect behavioral ethnicity than will younger persons of the same group.

THE CHARACTERIZATION OF MENTAL HEALTH PROBLEMS BY MINORITY ELDERLY

In the past two decades, despite the increased interest of the behavioral sciences on minority racial/ethnic populations, there have been only a few large scale studies that sought to provide accurate descriptions of minority elderly. Some studies have included data on the incidence and nature of minority mental health problems. It does appear that minority group elderly tend to somatize their emotional problems and are, therefore, more likely to seek help in primary health settings. When Ring and Schein (1970) sampled 388 households in a Black middle-class community in Philadelphia, they found that over 87 percent of the respondents said they would consult a physician for a mental or emotional problem, whereas only 19 percent indicated a psychiatrist. Of those who had experienced problems of obesity, severe headaches, dependence on medication, insomnia, excessive drinking, marked anxiety, depression, insecurity, or hostility during the previous 6 months, more than 84 percent had consulted a doctor.

After age 65, 79 percent of all persons have at least one chronic physical disorder. In a study conducted in England, Kidd (1962) found that 69 percent of those admitted on a geriatric medical service were also mentally ill, while 43 percent of those admitted to mental hospitals had significant physical illnesses.

Whereas black and Hispanic elderly are more likely to be seen in primary health settings rather than mental health settings, Asian-Americans are even less likely to be seen in mental health settings. In the case of the Chinese, those elderly with mental and emotional problems often somatize them and go for herbal treatments. Chinese medical theory encourages this practice by being deficient in psychological vocabulary and by analyzing and treating somatic and psychosomatic illnesses identically. Similary, among Puerto Ricans the dichotomy between somatic and psychological symptoms appears not to be drawn as rigidly as it is in the wider American culture. Indeed, Puerto Ricans are very likely to associate physical symptoms with psychosocial causes; e.g., suffering and worry are thought to damage the nerves, cause pains in the chest around the heart and throat, as well as difficulty in breathing (Murillo-Rhode, 1976; Padilla, 1958).

Whereas minority elderly are likely to somatize emotional problems, they are also likely to demonstrate a fatalistic acceptance of accompanying discomforts. Minorities experienced negative valuation and systematic exclusion from the opportunity system that often produces a generalized expectancy that any change in their situation will not be subject to their personal effort. Most studies seeking to discover significant differences in fatalism among ethnic groups and social classes have indicated that blacks and lower-class people are more fatalistic in their outlook than are whites and middle-class people (Lefcourt, 1976; Lessing, 1969; Scott & Phelan, 1969; Strickland, 1972). Varghese and Medinger (1979) have reviewed the extensive literature comparing prevalence of fatalism among ethnic minority groups and have concluded that significant levels of fatalism are found among American Indians. It is also more prevalent among certain groups of Italian-Americans and Chinese-Americans. They also point out, however, that research findings have supported the notion that when personal income is controlled for, blacks and Hispanics do not appear to be significantly more fatalistic than whites of the equivalent socioeconomic status.

Varghese and Medinger (1979) warn against generalizing the well-replicated association between fatalism and psychosocial adjustment when focusing on minority clients. Fatalism has adaptive consequences for people living under restraining conditions. Thus, for minority elders who have had to face severe environmental stressors without the environmental resources available to other groups, the development of a fatalistic orientation may have been a protective mechanism in helping the individual to cope with stress. The issue of fatalism does, however, have implications for the minority elderly's response to mental health problems. It seems most likely that those who experience such problems and have a more fatalistic orientation will not perceive the problems as amenable to change by their own personal efforts, but only by virtue of fate, chance, or religious intercession.

There is some evidence that some minority elderly may have advantages in later life that were not experienced earlier. For example, relative to their previous status and insecurity during youth and middle age, many of the black aged enjoy somewhat higher status and security. The reasons include a more stable income, strong intergenerational family ties, some progress toward racial equality, and the achievement of survival to old age (Palmore, 1976). Yet those who do become emotionally disturbed or socially dysfunctional have apparently failed to reap these substantial benefits or to perceive themselves as particularly advantaged.

Who are those minority elderly who, despite changing social conditions, have not been able to experience themselves as competent, well-functioning individuals? In some cases, they have experienced new losses— such as loss of job, health, or spouse— that have been so stressful that they have reached the proverbial breaking point. In this sense they are not unique. However, perhaps even more of these minority elderly are among a disproportionately high percentage of their group who have experienced the cumulative effects of economic instability, chaotic family life, and an oppressive social environment.

THEORETICAL FRAMEWORKS

The major theoretical approaches serving to explain disordered behavior and to generate principles of therapeutic intervention have all been utilized to some extent in the delivery of mental health services to elderly populations (Zarit, 1980). Psychodynamic approaches place emphasis on the elderly individual's intrapsychic functioning. Symptoms such as anxiety and depression are considered to reflect an underlying mental illness, and it is thus deemed necessary to treat the intrapsychic conflict expressed in symptoms. In contrast, behavioral theorists propose that maladaptive behaviors of elderly persons are governed by principles of learning. A behavioral approach would identify factors in the environment or in the person's prior learning that must be modified in order to change problem behavior. Another approach is based on humanistic psychology and stresses the natural tendency of all individuals regardless of age-stage to strive for growth and development or what has been termed *self-actualization*. Problem-solving in this context focuses on helping the individual to achieve optimal functioning through a supportive therapeutic relationship characterized by warmth, nonpossessive caring, and validation of personal worth and dignity. Each of the approaches carries some attendant risk when utilized with minority elderly.

A psychodynamic insight-oriented framework for mental health practice with minority elderly may be ineffective if it ignores environmental stressors that have contributed to the mental health problem. Jackson (1980) has conceptualized the unique environmental stressors that are experienced by minority elderly. The first set of stressors are defined as *institutionalized victimization,* which are intentional acts of discrimination against minority group persons. Thus, a now-retired black mechanic may have experienced innumerable incidents of discrimination both directed toward him personally (e.g., having to train whites, who are then promoted over him) and toward blacks in general (e.g., segregation of public facilities in the South). He may also have experienced another set of stressors that Jackson refers to as *systematic discrimination*. This is the application of criteria labeled as neutral but that in reality are discriminatory and produce unequal results. For example, the mechanic may have applied for a special government management training program but was denied it because he lacked supervisory experience. However, due to discriminatory policies on his job it was impossible for him to get the supervisory experience. Given these environmental stressors over a lifetime, the impact on self-esteem may be devastating and contribute to depression in later years. Thus, an exploration of one's early life experiences may only exacerbate the problem.

Zung's triadic approach to treatment of depression in the elderly emphasizes the potential effectiveness of simultaneous drug treatment, psychotherapy, and physical and occupational therapies to influence behavioral changes, changes in premorbid personality, and in the external milieu (Zung, 1980). It is this latter change goal— change in the external milieu— that is crucial when dealing with minority elderly. In the case of the mechanic described above, the likelihood is that his environment is still likely to reinforce his negative valuation and contribute to his low self-esteem rather than reduce it. It is therefore, likely that intervention may need to extend beyond the exploration of intrapsychic issues to bring about actual change in his environment.

It is sometimes assumed that behavioral or social learning theories of practice eliminate the stigmatizing effect of having to define behavior as deviant or pathological in order to prescribe a treatment. However, for persons with strong feelings of powerlessness, characteristic of those minority elderiy experiencing psychosocial problems, there is a heightened possibility that even successful modification of problems will be viewed as something that was done to or for them rather than something that was controlled by themselves. This may be better than the continuation of problematic behaviors (such as incontinence or poor personal hygiene), but far less than would be accomplished with some additional consideration of increasing positive response from others in the environment (such as enhancing opportunities for social participation). Otherwise, we may have a continent but deeply unhappy person. This is based on a hypothesis for which there is some documentation; that is, those persons who are able to change a negative response to themselves to a more positive response from the wider social system will demonstrate greater reduction of powerlessness than will those persons who are not able to effect such change.

The humanistic approaches focus on the self, particularly on how one feels about one's self and how one's goals can be optimally achieved. The value orientations of ethnic groups, which incidentally are held most strongly by elderly members, eschew the personal for the collective. Thus, this approach would appear to be unacceptably narcissistic. Futhermore, it has been well documented that the problems of many minority group members are tightly interwoven with environmental problems (such as income maintenance and/or deteriorating neighborhoods) so that the nonspecific, abstractly conceptualized goals of humanistic therapy may be considered irrelevant and inappropriate by minority elderly.

In fact, many people generally described as mentally ill may be perceived as persons deprived of adequate social solutions to the problem of individual growth and development (Ullman, 1969). For those experiencing negative valuation from the larger society to an intense degree, powerlessness is a more virulent stressor than anxiety or guilt. Consequently, empowering the client to take or maintain control over his life situation becomes a more immediate treatment goal than reduction of anxiety or guilt.

THE THERAPEUTIC ENCOUNTER

Although the mental health practitioner may be sensitive to the differential applicability of the several theoretical approaches to treating characteristic mental health problems of the elderly, there is still the problem of convincing the minority elderly of the relevance of psychosocial treatment of the problems. This will inevitably involve the establishment of a relationship with a helping professional who is most often from a different ethnic group. It also will demand that goals and content of the helping process be consistent with the values and lifestyle of the minority elderly client.

The Setting

As indicated earlier, minority elderly are underrepresented in mental health settings precisely because they do not interpret their mental health problems as derivatives of some inner psychological state but more often as a function of somatic difficulties, bad luck, or God's will. Thus, the physician, the minister, or even the fortune teller, may be seen as a more appropriate "helper" than the psychiatrist, psychologist, or social worker. Furthermore, the settings in which these latter professionals work — mental health centers, psychiatric out-patient clinics, mental hospitals — are not perceived as appropriate settings in which to find the more acceptable help sources. On the other hand, primary health-care facilities and churches may be much more likely places to encounter minority elderly persons with mental health problems. Rather than accepting the fact that minority elderly often do not go to traditional mental health agencies for service, it should be questioned as to whether it might be possible to provide such services in the settings where minority elderly *do* go for help.

While hospital utilization by the elderly increased considerably after the introduction of Medicare, a significantly larger proportion of all elderly utilize the physician's office, making it the center of the health care delivery system. Yet, it is in the hospital that potential access to mental health professionals is greatest for the minority elderly (Shanas & Maddox, 1976). Thus, the nature of the American health system continues to make mental health services less accessible to most elderly populations.

In a report of a recent conference sponsored by the National Institute of Mental Health on the integration of mental health services into general health settings, it was stated: "Mental health problems require the resources of many professional groups within the health field as well as in other social support agencies. . . . In our view, the inclusion of mental health services as an integral component of primary health care offers the only feasible means of substantially improving the distribution of mental health services for the population as a whole" (Coleman, 1979).

Whereas the primary health care setting appears to be an appropriate setting within which to offer mental health services to the elderly, there are some obstacles when the focus is on some ethnic elderly minority. For example, Chinese elderly often utilize traditional practitioners until symptoms become particularly severe. They will furthermore, avoid hospitalization, regarding it a place to die. It is reported that elderly Chinese men in rooming houses are sent most frequently to the hospital by fellow roomers who do not want them to die in the rooming house (Gould-Martin & Ngin, 1981). Similarly, the Hispanic elderly may also utilize folk medicine and not participate in mainstream primary care, thereby making it more difficult to provide access to mental health services through the general health care delivery system. The problem of access to general health services is most acute, however, for the American Indian elderly. They are the victims of inferior health status and inadequate health care throughout their lives, and health services currently available have been criticized for failure to contribute to either physical or emotional well-being (Block, 1979). The integration of physical and mental health services is less an issue to this group than availability of basic health care. Clearly, there would be little access to mental health professionals through a primary health resource, but traditional practitioners may provide an approximation of supportive or preventive health services.

The church is another setting in which mental health services are more likely to be accepted by minority elderly than in a traditional mental health agency setting. Although voluntary associations often have been perceived as a means of continuing the social integration of the elderly, the majority of persons do not belong to such groups, with the exception of the church. For example, church membership tends to be maintained well into the seventies (Lowenthal & Robinson, 1976).

It should be pointed out that the particular church affiliation differs interethnically; for example, Hispanics are more likely to belong to Catholic churches and the largest proportion of blacks belong to a Protestant denomination. At the same time, religion in the sense of a belief in a single faith and relative intolerance of other faiths, is alien to most Japanese-Americans. For example, many Japanese-Americans claim a Buddhist religious background but may attend an all-Japanese Christian church; many elderly Japanese attend both Buddhist and Christian churches in large numbers. The implications of this diversity of religious orientations among ethnic elderly indicates that it is not a simple matter of placing mental health services in the church context. Religious organizations differentially will be hospitable to the presence of mental health services offered by mental health professionals, depending upon the particular theology and how it defines emotional problems.

Establishing the Relationship

Although the setting may make it possible for the helping professional to have access to minority elderly who may be experiencing emotional problems, there is still a period of testing that occurs in any therapeutic encounter in which the client attempts to determine whether the helping professional does, in fact, have the expertise to deal with the problem. It may be important here to reflect on the basis that individuals will give others permission to be an influence in their lives. Most urban, middle-class individuals determine status on the basis of social position. Sociologists have referred to this as *gesellschaft orientation,* that is, how one relates to another is dependent upon that person's status relative to his own. The alternative or *gemeinschaft orientation* is more widely held by rural or lower-class people; this orientation is highly personalistic so that one's relationship to another is less dependent upon the particular social position held than by that person's personal attributes. In the former instance, one would expect that the professional's credentials, such as degrees earned and licenses held would be highly important. On the other hand, in the latter instance, one would expect that more weight would be given to the professional's personal characteristics, such as warmth and ability to communicate effectively.

There are behavioral norms associated with interpersonal transactions that occur across ethnic/racial, class, and age levels in this society. Thus, elders, particularly among ethnic subgroups, are to be given respect and deference. However, if the elder is a member of a minority ethnic group, he or she has most often *not* been given respect by members of the majority group. Similarly, lower class persons tend to defer to middle class authority figures. This is most likely to occur when the lower class person is a member of a racial/ethnic minority and the middle or upper class person is not. This complex interaction among race, age, and class is important to understand when attempting to establish a helping relationship with a minority elderly person. In some ethnic groups, such as Asian-Americans and Hispanics, it is extremely unlikely that an elderly male would find it easy to place himself in a relationship perceived as subordinate to a female mental health professional. In such instances, it is important to develop the relationship emphasizing a supplicant client and more powerful practitioner. In other instances, it may be just as difficult to convince elderly Asian-American or Hispanic women to engage in a peer collaborative effort with a male professional who is also a member of the Anglo majority. At such times, it would seem important for the professional to accept the authority without becoming authoritarian. This means that a more directive stance would be acceptable as long as the client is provided opportunities to become intensively involved in problem-solving efforts and encouraged to utilize these opportunities.

Language and style of communication are important, especially if an effective helping relationship is to be established. For those ethnic elderly who are not fluent in English, it may be of the greatest urgency to have a practitioner who is fluent in their primary language. For others, it is still important that their unique expressions and style of communication be understood and appreciated by the mental health professionals. The particular biases represented in our reactions to the speech of persons who are ethnically different need to be confronted. Studies have shown that the use of particular grammatical constructions and pronunciations may in fact trigger a wide range of negative characterizations towards the persons using them (Hertzler, 1965; Lambert, Hodgson, & Gardner, 1960). It is likely that this kind of stereotyping will influence the flow of communication and make the establishment of rapport and an effective helping relationship impossible.

It is important to understand the historical experience of the group to which the minority elderly client belongs, especially as it may influence expectations in cross-cultural encounters. For example, Mitchell-Kiernan has written:

> Black-Americans, for example, not infrequently report that they resent the use of their first names by service providers such as doctors and nurses and consider it a presumptuous practice. This may come as a surprise to a white nurse for whom the choice of first name is intended to create informality and friendliness. The resentment of Blacks toward this practice must be understood against a background of conventions that developed in the southern United States. Custom in that area called for the obligatory use of first names or kin titles such as Uncle or Aunty to all Blacks regardless of age or social status. In this system Afro-Americans were never accorded the respect of the title and last name. (1982, with permission)

There is similar residue lingering after the oppressive early years of many minority ethnic groups in this country so that mental health professionals working with members of a group should make every effort to learn its history and the implications of that history for cross-cultural encounters in the present.

Cultural Content

Members of minority ethnic groups simultaneously are like all other persons due to their common humanity, like some others who may have shared similar oppression in a society that disvalues cultural difference, and like no others in those areas where their unique history has shaped behavior, values, or attitudes. Thus, the challenge to the mental health professional is to be able to determine which set of determinants is operative in a specific problem situation.

All persons have some kind of social support system unless they are isolated totally, which occurs rarely even among the elderly. However, the nature of the support system reflects a great deal of variation, some of which is ethnically influenced. This is crucial in regard to the elderly and the delivery of services directed toward improvement of their physical and mental well-being.

The value of support networks is reflected in the fact that, although official statistics indicate that mental illness is not a major problem for Japanese-Americans, those who are afflicted are likely to be elderly, lower-class males who are isolated from family or peer group (Kitano, 1969). Common symptoms include hearing the voices of dead friends speaking in Japanese, emotional crying, heightened irritability, loss of toilet control, and withdrawal. The mental health professional who encounters such a disturbed person is not likely to be effective unless there is an effort made to create or replace the social support network. This requires consummate understanding of and access to the minority community, as well as skill in intervening in systems that extend beyond the "one-to-one" or even the family.

Although the importance of a kinship or peer group network in times of crisis has been recognized for many years in the helping professions, the systematic use of personal and social networks in mental health practice and the design of services is relatively new. During the seventies, the publication of several seminal works on natural helping networks marked increased attention to these resources. Social networks are considered to be a buffer to the individual against potentially overwhelming stresses from the external environment as well as a catalyst in promoting rehabilitation after of period of dysfunction (Caplan & Killilea, 1976; Collins & Pancoast, 1976). These social support systems are highly sensitive to subcultural variations and as such are influenced heavily by culture-specific skills that now must be acquired by the mental health practitioner, particularly if working with minority elderly clients. These include: (1) skill in identifying an existing support network and assessing its potential for assisting the elderly person with concrete services, emotional support, information and/or guidance; (2) skill in increasing the effectiveness of the support network in order to meet the needs of the elderly person; and (3) skill in developing alternative support networks when one does not exist. These skills can only be developed if there is a sound knowledge of the ethnic community, family relationships within it, characteristic informal helping structures, and intragroup attitudes toward both aging and emotional problems of living.

SUMMARY AND CONCLUSIONS

The mental health professional who is concerned with ameliorating the mental health problems of minority elderly cannot base effective intervention on sweeping generalizations expected to serve all ethnic elderly, regardless of the particular racial or ethnic group to which they belong. There is the need to recognize the special problems of the aged in our society who have not been served effectively in traditional mental health settings and who often do not perceive these settings as having any relevance to their problems. In addition, the problem is compounded when the elderly is also a member of a minority ethnic group that may have its own problematical relationship with the institutions of the dominant culture and that also may have its own ethnic-specific reservations about the efficacy of traditional approaches to mental health treatment of psychosocial problems.

There is a lack of information regarding the mental health problems of the minority elderly for a variety of reasons. The interrelationship of physical and mental health problems is so strong in this group that it is difficult to categorize problems as physical or mental. However, the minority elderly, as minorities in general, are more likely to view emotional difficulties as having physical origin and therefore to seek help in primary health care settings. Thus, mental health practitioners who are interested in working with the problems of this target population are more likely to encounter them in primary health care settings than in traditional mental health agencies or in the private practice of mental health practitioners. The church is another non-traditional setting that is likely to be perceived as an appropriate setting to bring mental health problems.

Regardless of the setting, it is crucial for the mental health practitioner to have considerable knowledge of the communication styles, lifestyles, value orientations, and history of the ethnic group in order to develop a satisfactory therapeutic relationship with a minority elderly client. Thus, when all of these things come together in the helping process, it should be possible to bring about significant changes in the lives of minority elderly to the same extent that it happens for those in the dominant population.

REFERENCES

Alers, J.O. *Puerto Ricans and health: findings from New York City* (Hispanic Research Monograph Series, No. 1). New York: Fordham University, 1978.

Block, M.R. Exiled americans: the plight of Indian aged in the United States. In D.E. Gelfand and A.J. Kutzik (Eds.), *Ethnicity and aging: Theory, research and policy*. New York: Springer, 1979, 184–192.

Bullough, C., & Bullough V.L. *Poverty, ethnic identity, and health care*. New York: Appleton-Century-Crofts, 1972.

Butler, R., & Lewis, M. *Aging and mental health: Positive psychosocial approaches*. St. Louis: C.V. Mosby, 1973.

Caplan, G., & Killilea, M. *Support systems and mutual help: multidisciplinary explorations*. New York: Grune and Stratton, 1976.

Coleman, J. Treatment of emotional problems by primary physicians. In D.L. Parron & F. Solomon (Eds.), *Mental health services in primary care settings: Report of a conference*. DHHS Publication No. (AD), April 2–3, 1979, 80–995. Superintendent of Documents, U.S. Government Printing Office, Washington, D.C., 1980.

Collins, A.H., & Pancoast, D.L. *Natural helping networks: A strategy for prevention*. Washington: NASW, 1976.

Gould-Martin, K. & Ngin, C. Chinese Amercians. In A. Harwood (Ed.), *Ethnicity and medical care*. Cambridge, Mass.: Harvard University Press, 1981, 30–171.

Harrison, I., & Harrison, D.S. The black family experience and health behavior. In C. Crawford (Ed.), *Health and the family*. New York: Macmillan, 1971.

Harwood, A. *Ethnicity and medical care*. Cambridge, Mass.: Harvard University Press, 1981.
Hertzler, J. *A sociology of language*. New York: Random House, 1965.
Holzberg, C. Ethnicity and aging: Anthropological perspectives on more than just the minority elderly. *Gerontologist*, 1982, *22*, 249–257.
Jackson, J.J. *Minorities and aging*. Belmont, Calif.: Wadsworth, 1980.
Kidd, C.B. Criteria for admission of the elderly to geriatric and psychiatric units. *Journal of Mental Science*, 1962, *108*, 68–74.
King, H. Selected epidemiological aspects of major diseases and causes of death among Chinese in the United States and Asia. In A. Kleinman et al. (Eds.), *Medicine in Chinese cultures: Comparative studies of health care in Chinese and other societies*. Washington, D.C.: U.S. Department of Health, Education and Welfare, DHEW Publication No. (NIH) 75–653, 1975.
Kitano, H.L. *Japanese Americans: The evolution of a subculture*. Englewood Cliffs, N.J.: Prentice-Hall, 1969.
Kramer, M., Taube, A., & Redick, R.W. Patterns of use of psychiatric facilities by the aged: Past, present and future. In C. Eisdorfer & M. Lawton, (Eds.), *The psychology of adult development and aging*. Washington, D.C.: American Psychological Association, 1973.
Kramer, M., Rosen, B., & Willie, E. Definitions and distributions of mental disorders in a racist society. In C.V. Willie, B. Kramer, & B. Brown (Eds.), *Racism and mental health*. Pittsburgh: University of Pittsburgh Press, 1973, 353–462.
Lambert, W.E., Hodgson, R., Gardner, R. et al. Evaluational reactions to spoken language. *Journal of Abnormal and Social Psychology*, 1960, *60*, 44–51.
Lefcourt, H. *Locus of control: Current trends in theory and research*. New York: John Wiley, 1976.
Lessing, E. Racial differences in indices of ego functioning relevant to academic achievement. *Journal of Genetic Psychology*, 1969, *115*, 153–167.
Lowenthal, M.F., & Robinson, B. Social networks and isolation. In R.H. Binstock & E. Shanas (Eds.), *Handbook of aging and the social sciences*. New York: Van Nostrand Reinhold, 1976, 432–487.
McDermott, W., Deuschle, K., Adair, J., Folmer, H., & Loughlin, B. Introducing modern medicine in a Navajo community. *Science*, 1960, *131*, 280–287.
Mitchell-Kiernan, C. Linguistic diversity in the service delivery setting: The case of Black English. In B. Bass, G. Wyatt, & G. Powell (Eds.), *The Afro-American family: Assessment, treatment and research issues*. New York: Grune and Stratton, 1982, 85–98.
Murillo-Rhode, I. Family life among mainland Puerto Ricans in New York City slums. *Perspectives in Psychiatric Care*, 1976, *14* (4), 174–179.
Padilla, E. *Up from Puerto Rico*. New York: Columbia University Press, 1958.
Palmore, E. Social and community concepts of aging. In L. Belak & T. Karasu (Eds.), *Geriatric psychiatry*. New York: Grune and Stratton, 1976, 227.
Parsons, T. Some theoretical considerations on the nature and trends of change of ethnicity. In N. Glazer & D.P. Moynihan (Eds.), *Ethnicity: Theory and experience*. Cambridge, Mass.: Harvard University Press, 1975, 65.
Quesada, G.M., & Heller, P.L. Sociocultural barriers to medical care among Mexican Americans in Texas. *Medical Care*, 1977, *15* (5), 93–101.

Ring, S.I., & Schein, L. Attitudes toward mental illness and the use of caretakers in a Black community. *American Journal of Orthopsychiatry,* 1970, *40,* 710–716.

Rosen, B.M., Anderson, T.E., & Bahn, A.K. Psychiatric patterns for the aged: A nationwide survey of patterns of utilization. *American Journal of Orthopsychiatry,* 1967, *37,* 223–224.

Scott, J., & Phelan, J. Expectancies of unemployable males regarding source of control of reinforcement. *Psychological Reports,* 1969, *25,* 911–912.

Shanas, E., & Maddox, G.L. Aging, health and the organization of health resources. In R.H. Binstock & E. Shanas (Eds.), *Handbook of aging and the social sciences.* New York: Van Nostrand Reinhold, 1976, 592–618.

Shiloh, A., & Shiloh, S. (Eds.). *Ethnic groups of America: Their morbidity, mortality and behavior disorders,* (Vol. II., The Blacks). Springfield, Ill.: Charles C. Thomas, 1974.

Stanford, E.P. *The elder Black.* San Diego: The Campanile Press, 1978.

Stein, H.F., & Hill, R.F. *The ethnic imperative: Examining the new white ethnic movement.* University Park: Pennsylvania State University Press, 1977.

Strickland, B. Delay of gratification as a function of race of the experimenter. *Journal of Personality and Social Psychology,* 1972, *22,* 108–112.

Sue, S., McKinney, H., Allen, D. et al. Delivery of community mental health services to black and white clients. *Journal of Consulting Clinical Psychology,* 1974, *42,* 794–801.

Thomas, A., & Sillen, S. *Racism and psychiatry.* New York: Brunner/Mazel, 1972.

Varghese, R., & Medinger, F. Fatalism in response to stress among the minority aged. In D.E. Gelfand & A.J. Kutzik (Eds.), *Ethnicity and aging: Theory, research and policy.* New York: Springer, 1979, 96–116.

Ullman, M. A unifying concept linking therapeutic and community process. In W. Gray, F. Duhl, & N. Rizzo (Eds.), *General systems theory and psychiatry.* Boston: Little, Brown, 1969, 253–266.

Zarit, S.H. *Aging and mental disorders: Psychological approaches to assessment and treatment.* New York: The Free Press, 1980.

Zung, W. Affective disorders. In E. Busse & D. Blazer (Eds.), *Handbook of geriatric psychiatry.* New York: Van Nostrand, 1980, 358.

PART V

Social Policy, Ethics, and Planning

13

PROVIDING CLINICAL GEROPSYCHOLOGY SERVICES IN COMMUNITY SETTINGS

Peter R. LeBray

Tremendous challenge and opportunity exist for those concerned with mental health care of older adults in community settings. Trends to shorten hospital stay, bolster ambulatory outpatient care, and develop a competitive mix of home health care promgrams favor new, innovative geriatric health care services.

This chapter will discuss role and functions, principles, applications, and special concerns in providing clinical geropsychology services in nursing homes and other community settings. It emphasizes the clinician's attitude, knowledge base, applied techniques, and service settings.

Clinical gerontology is an interdisciplinary field involving specialists in medicine, mental health, social services, administration, and allied health fields. The generic term used here is mental health provider (MHP). The role proposed for the MHP is that of *clinician–consultant*. This individual would be trained in a basic discipline (e.g., medicine, psychology, social work, nursing, or allied health) with special training in gerontology, geriatrics, and consultation. Also, the MHP would have expertise in a variety of consultation formats (e.g., client, agency, or program centered) and experience in a collaborative team approach to geriatric care (Butler & Lewis, 1982).

Over three decades of research have produced important data regarding psychological aspects of aging including cognitive, behavioral, conative, and

GERIATRIC MENTAL HEALTH
ISBN 0-8089-1657-2

personal adjustment in later life. Application of these findings is termed *clinical geropsychology,* an emergent specialty analogous to pediatric psychology. Clinical geropsychology compresses that body of knowledge involving application of clinical psychology methods to older adults. In effect, clinical geropsychology emphasizes *what is different* in mental health practice with elders (Birren, 1968; Burnside, 1978; Eisdorfer & Stotsky, 1977; Herr & Weakland, 1979; Hussian, 1981; LeBray, 1979; Raskin & Jarvik, 1979; Zarit, 1980).

Concern exists that advocating a clinical geropsychology may discriminate negatively toward elders, perhaps isolating them from the developmental mainstream (Gatz, Smyer, & Lawton, 1980; Smyer & Gatz, 1979). In response, there is no data in support of such a view. In fact, a focus on important differences in geropsychology application is *not* incompatible with a theoretical, developmental view (Erickson, 1959; Havighurst, 1963). It is well known that developmental roles and tasks differ in late life and that selected individual differences over the life course result in greater intra- than intergroup variability. Thus, the MHP must have working knowledge of these differences and sensitivity in terms of aging attitudes.

ATTITUDE

As one elderly patient recently lamented to this author, "You know, it's darned hard to grow old gracefully in this country today." Both MHP and geriatric patients are influenced by social values, customs, and attitudes toward aging and elders. Awareness of *attitude* is crucial in the provision of geriatric mental health services. If elders are stereotyped as frail, dependent, senile, and of low social utility, the MHP likely will be imbued with fatalism, cynicism, and frustration in attempts to serve elders and their families. Such negative attitudes represent ageism or stereotyping based on chronological age (Butler, 1963; Butler & Lewis, 1982).

Cohen (1977) has identified a number concerns that influence a therapist's interest and willingness to work with older patients. The elderly may stimulate the practitioner's unresolved conflicts about relationships to parental figures and arouse fears about the therapist's own aging. Another area of concern is the practitioner's belief that his or her skills and time will be wasted on elderly patients because they are not likely to benefit from treatment. Therapists may feel that the elderly are not capable of behavior change or that all psychopathology in later life is organic in nature.

Clinicians may be reluctant to work with the elderly because of the possibility of being overwhelmed by the complex and diverse problems an older person might present. Also, the patient might die while in treatment, thus challenging the therapist's sense of importance and power.

The myths and stereotypes about aging and the aged can interfere with a clinician's ability to correctly diagnose the mental health problems of the elderly. The practitioner's misinformation could even preclude a decision to provide treatment. This is compounded by a cultural insensitivity which has slowed societal and professional responsiveness to the problems of the aging.

The important issue of attitude is complex and difficult to analyze in an age-stratified society (Atchley, 1980; Riley, 1971), and complicated by attitudes of elders themselves (McTavish, 1971). Perhaps it is well for the MHP to analyze carefully attitudes toward his or her *own* aging also. Attitudes form the bases for major psychosocial theories that are important in defining policies and programs for elders. The "model" of the elder client held by the MHP significantly influences practice as denoted in the following theories.

DISENGAGEMENT THEORY. This theory postulates that in later life, it is inevitable, irrevocable and mutually agreeable that we begin to have less interactions with others and engage less frequently in social roles. This is mutually agreeable with society and results in the eventual disengagement of individuals and the social system (Cumming & Henry, 1961; Atchley, 1980).

ACTIVITY THEORY. The activity theory postulates that it is important to continue the role and activities of the middle years well into later life. Thus, opportunities for being active and engaging in leisure and other pursuits remains paramount, as exemplified in senior centers (Havighurst, 1963).

PATHOLOGY THEORY. The pathological viewpoint looks at social deviancy among elders and their departure from usual social norms and values. Behavior and social activities are considered on a normal–abnormal continuum. This theory often is applied in medical and health settings (Decker, 1980; Posner, 1974).

CONTINUITY THEORY. This theory suggests that personality in earlier years has a strong influence on one's adjustment during later years. In fact, we become more like ourselves in the period of later life (Atchley, 1971; Neugarten, 1968).

HETEROGENEITY THEORY. This theory results from recognition of individual differences and increased variability in the period of later life based on life-span developmental psychology (Goulet & Baltes, 1970; Nessleroade & Reese, 1973). This theory holds that there is increased variability during later life and increased *within-group* differences with respect to chronological age (Bengston, Kasschau, & Ragan, 1977).

KNOWLEDGE

Major Principles

In addition to attitude, the MHP clinician–consultant needs a solid knowledge base derived from gerontological research and familiarity with elders in various community settings. The following principles apply:

Lifecourse Changes

An important outcome of gerontological research is that individual differences appear to *increase* over the lifecourse (Baltes & Schaie, 1973; Goulet & Baltes, 1970). Using the cross-sequential design, researchers have demonstrated greater intra-group than inter-group differences based on age for a variety of cognitive, performance, and personality variables. Practical implications are that there is no single theory applicable to the aged. Rather, highly individualized assessment and treatment approaches are required (Datan & Ginsberg, 1975).

Further, there are serious limitations in applying cross-sectional (age differential) data in clinical practice (Schaie, 1977). The MHP needs to function in an "interventive research" fashion (Baltes & Willis, 1977), acknowledging the unique, multiple antecedants and determinants with each geriatric patient.

Holistic Approach

The multiple, interactive problems of the elder demand sensitivity in terms of the patient as a whole person. Functional and organic problems in the elder are likely to coexist, resulting in a "spiral of senility." For example, a socioeconomic factor such as fixed, limited income may affect physical health in terms of available funds to purchase needed medication. In turn, the elder becomes depressed and less active exacerbating the physical condition (e.g., congestive heart failure).

The holistic approach is person-centered and conceptualized as physical, psychological, social and philosophic overlapping spheres with interactive effects in the context of environment. The Whole Person Model can be very useful in individual assessment and therapy, agency and resource planning and community resource coordination (cf. Palmore, 1970; 1974). For example, the MHP involved in assessing elders can use the model as an interview guide with items pertaining to each area (health, cognition, social relations, outlook on life, living setting).

Community Resources

The geriatric clinician-consultant must be aware of community resources available to elders and have a working knowledge of such programs. Consonant with a holistic approach, geriatric care requires a team approach with the MHP serving as collaborator and coordinator. Family members, physicians, home health staff, clergy, volunteers and others may be involved in a patient care plan. Although not generally traditional, interdisciplinary programs appear both viable and beneficial for providing mental health services to older adults (Glasscoate, Gudeman & Miles, 1977).

Basic Discipline

As conceptualized here, the MHP clinician-consultant must have substantative training in a basic health care field. Further specialized training in gerontology and geriatrics is required with emphasis on what is unique in later life, interventions, application and evaluation. As Friedman and Steinheber (1977) noted, "Age should never be a barrier to appropriate investigation and treatment of any significant symptoms." A constructive attitude coupled with training in a basic health care discipline allows the MHP to serve and *learn from* elders. Specialized training in gerontology is increasing and more available through university centers, Veterans Admininstration health facilities, federal, state and local programs on aging, as well as professional organizations such as the Western Gerontological Society, Gerontological Society of America, and American Geriatrics Society.

Special Knowledge

To enhance effectiveness, the MHP must have special knowledge of important differences in the application of mental health services to elders. Table 13-1 illustrates elder client characteristics and correlates in terms of MHP roles and functions. Other salient differences are outlined as follows.

INTERVIEWING. Special techniques and approaches to interviewing confused, disoriented, demented elders (Burnside, 1980, 1981), or elders presenting a variety of illnesses (Schmidt, 1975), are noted in the literature. Attention to pacing, repetition, nonthreatening manner, multiple sessions, or observations, as well as corroboration are crucial (LeBray, 1980).

ASSESSMENT. Multidimensional formats (Pfeiffer, 1975; Robinson, 1980), brief and valid screening instruments (Goldfarb, 1974; Kahn, 1971; Kane & Kane, 1981), adaptations of psychometric tests (Oberleder, 1967), and special geriatric projective instruments (Bellak & Bellak, 1973; LeBray, 1982) are useful with elder clients. Since elders often present with both psychogenic and organic symptoms, careful attention to health history, practices, and functional observations represent significant clinical data (Caird & Judge, 1977; Mezey, Rauckhorst, & Stokes, 1980). While the MHP may not be expert in all aspects of holistic assessment, his or her observations can be constructively reported and discussed with team members who are (e.g., internist, psychologist, others).

Table 13-1.

Elder and MHP Characteristics

Elder Characteristic	MHP Characteristic
Long past, shorter future	Increase time with History taking
Multiple, interactive problems	Complete medical evaluation, team approach
Sensory and physical changes	Compensatory methods
Change in learning	Focus, repeat, pace, familiar
Reliability as a historian	Collaborate, case management
Reasons for services	Grief, depressions, Dementias, competency, behavior and family problems
Personal (ego) strength	Analysis vs. short-term intervention
Diminished financial resources	Sliding scale, public and Voluntary programs
Multiple needs	Home visitation, Community advocate
Advanced age	Role reversal
Chronic conditions	Optimal management vs. care

GROUP WORK. As an efficient use of limited time and staff, group work with elders differs significantly in content, process, and leader functions than with younger clients (Burnside, 1978). Based largely on elder inpatients, the following approaches are reviewed in current literature: resocialization, remotivation, reality orientation, reminiscing, rehabilitation, and retraining (Barnes, Sack, & Shore, 1973; Brintnell & Mitchell, 1981; Eisdorfer & Stotsky, 1977). Elder groups can be educational (e.g., retirement preparation), psychotherapeutic (Zarit, 1980), or social (e.g., resocialization), and serve affiliative (AARP), self-help (Alzheimer's Foundation), or a variety of psychosocial needs.

PSYCHOTHERAPY. Reviews of psychotherapy range from general discussions (Brink, 1979; Rechtschaffer, 1959), elders and families (Herr & Weakland, 1979), behavioral approaches (Hussian, 1981; Eisdorfer, Cohen,

& Preston, 1981; Richards & Thorpe, 1978), psychoanalysis (Blum & Tross, 1980; Verwoerdt, 1976), psychotherapy with demented elders (Verwoerdt, 1981), and special assessment methods (Raskin & Jarvik, 1979). Therapeutic goals of patient management, educating family and staff, using ancillary resources (e.g., protective services or volunteer visitors), and life review are features mentioned frequently (Storandt, Seigler, & Elias, 1978).

SERVICE DELIVERY. Traditional approaches for providing mental health services to elders simply are not effective (Kahn, 1971; NIMH, 1972, Cohen, 1977). As with *what* is done in terms of intervention, so are there important differences in *how* such services are organized. As Gatz et al. (1980) note, "Psychologists should infiltrate such settings as senior centers, congregate housing and apartment buildings with large numbers of older adult residents." Creative options are needed, and ten innovative institutional and community health programs serving elders are reviewed elsewhere in detail (Glasscoate, Gudeman, & Miles, 1977).

MAJOR SETTINGS

At present, there are at least a dozen major settings in which the MHP can provide geriatric mental health services, training, program development, and consultation (Table 13-2). The need is great since one estimate, based on epidemiologic data, indicated that some 81 percent of community-residing

Table 13-2.

Elder Group Settings
Long-term care facilities
Homes for the aged
Congregate, residential settings
Senior centers
Community mental health centers
Psychiatric hospitals
Voluntary organizations
Community service centers
Rehabilitation facilities
Home health agencies
Private mental health settings

elders who might benefit from mental health services are not receiving them (Kramer, Taube, & Redick, 1973). These programs would appear to be equally viable for younger, disabled adult populations (e.g., head injuries, neurologically impaired, developmentally disabled).

Congregate Care

In congregate settings such as nursing homes, retirement centers, and group residential facilities (e.g., homes for the aged, foster homes, domiciliaries), elders reside with supervision and assistance since they ostensibly are unable to manage living independently. The reasons they cannot live in independence may vary among the following: chronic or disabling conditions, lack of family or social supports, limited or inadequate finances, shortsighted public policies (e.g., public assistance may reimburse a nursing home but not a foster care setting), environmental factors (Lawton, 1977), or perhaps lifelong maladaptive patterns (Garetz & Peth, 1974). This author's observation is that many elders are institutionalized on a long-term basis not for specific medical or nursing care, but due to economic, social, or environmental factors. A social policy of "custodalism" (Kahn, 1971) appears to promote a high incidence of psychiatric disorders among inappropriately institutionalized elders.

Today in this country there are 50 percent more long-term beds in nursing homes than general hospital beds. While this accounts for only 5 percent of the aged population, this "20-billion dollar nursing home industry is a major challenge to the United States health care system" (Libow, 1982), particularly given the fact that the number of mentally ill elders in nursing homes well exceeds those in mental hospitals (Kramer, Taube, & Redick, 1973).

The range and types of problems in congregate and long-term care settings are very appropriate for geropsychology services, including: depressions, dementias, paranoid delusions, noisiness, restlessness or wandering, combativeness, inappropriate dependency on staff, persistent talk of a wish to die, incontinence, and family concerns with the resident and facility (Group for the Advancement of Psychiatry, 1971). Indeed, there are reports of highly successful programs in congregate settings (Eisdorfer & Stotsky, 1977; Hefferin, 1968; Glasscoate, Gudeman, & Miles, 1977; Hussian, 1981; Peth and Garetz, 1974, Stotsky, 1970; Libow, 1982). Individual psychotherapy, small group approaches (e.g., reminiscing, reality orientation, life review), in-service education programs, staff development, family programs, and community education represent some of the key services with institutional support the MHP can offer. The MHP with commitment and expertise will be challenged to develop innovative, constructive geropsychology services in long-term care facilities (LeBray, 1979).

Hospitals

General hospitals, psychiatric inpatient facilities, and both public and private rehabilitation centers, have a major role and responsibility in establishing and providing the highest quality health and mental health services to elder patients (Butler, 1975; Brocklehurst, 1973; Rossman, 1979; Tobias, 1976).

With expertise and commitment, the MHP can render valuable assistance in developing geriatric care programs (e.g., health screening, consultation, staff training) in hospital settings. It is both curious and disconcerting that every major hospital does not have a visible, viable geriatric health program addressing community residing elders' unmet needs. Libow (1982) discussed the important, useful relationship between teaching hospitals and nursing homes that "emphasize the goals and approaches of geriatrics, which are usually quite different from those of acute medicine." LeBray (in press) recently described a geriatric health clinic in a large urban medical center that uses a team format (physician, nurse, psychologist, social worker) to assess and treat elder patients.

What is needed, it seems, is collaboration among a few health care providers and hospital administrators to establish a geriatric team in both general and psychiatric hospitals. This team can be responsive to institutional, community, and staff needs in providing direct services, case consultation, staff training, and program development (e.g., day treatment, community education, professional continuing education programs). To do less is to ignore needs and challenges.

Community Mental Health Programs

The amended Community Mental Health Centers (CMHC) Act of 1974, for the first time, specified that elders are a subgroup of the population designated for specialized inpatient, outpatient, crisis, liaison and referral services. Implementation and evaluation of this charge seems limited given inadequate funds, resources, and expertise. Traditionally, federal, state, and local CMHC programs have provided few, if any, mental health services to elders. In fact, the report of the American Psychiatric Association Task Force on the 1981 White House Conference on Aging noted, "only 4 percent of community mental health center patients are elderly. Private practitioners and clinics provide but 2 percent of their services for the elderly. In fact, less than 1.5 percent of patient care expenditures for mental illness is provided for older people residing in the community" (APA, 1980). These data contrast sharply with the fact that up to 20 percent of community residing elders and one-half to three-fourths of institutionalized elders have significant mental health needs (Kramer, Taube, & Redick, 1973; APA, 1980)

The MHP has enormous opportunity and challenge in the CMHC

arena. As with hospitals, specialized programs addressing geriatric needs are required, including expert staff and adequate resources to develop a multidisciplinary, multipurpose geriatric team serving elders, families, general hospitals, nursing homes, and other health programs in the service area. Surveys and descriptions of a number of CMHC, nursing, and congregate care programs emphasizing geriatric mental health are available elsewhere (Glasscoate, Gudeman, & Miles, 1977).

Community Programs

Senior centers, home health agencies, voluntary organizations, and the private sector may all represent important consultation, treatment, and referral resources for the MHP with clinical geropsychology expertise. Specific examples of nontraditional mental health services depend on the initiative and creativity of the service provider. Considering the fact that individual differences increase in late life, geropsychology services that are innovative and variable might emphasize key areas such as prevention, consumer education, and community workshops on exercise, nutrition, family relationships, and transitions. Such activities as patient–family education, case finding, outreach, health screening, social skills training, preventive care or self-help groups can be established in senior high-rise buildings, adult day care, meal sites, community centers, clinics, or hospitals.

The key to starting such important psychosocial programs is to begin where it is possible to start. The MHP can survey the community, including contacts with agency staff, health care programs, churches, and voluntary groups (e.g., AARP, Rotary, Elks, and others). Needs and program plans that include objectives, staff, and budget, can be established and implemented. Examples of several nontraditional approaches include the following:

CHURCHES. Often, within a congregation, there are opportunities for volunteer supportive visitation of elders who may be home-bound. The MHP can instruct and supervise volunteers providing such services.

SENIOR CENTERS. Educational or small group approaches to important psychosocial topics as widowhood, life review, social skills training, or consumer issues can provide support to center participants. The MHP can confer with center staff and members in determining specific interests and needs.

DAY TREATMENT. The MHP can provide staff and client support depending on the type of program (e.g., respite, neurologically impaired, social, or medical model). Individual client assessment, including formal psychological testing, family conferences, small group interventions, behavioral treatment programs, and cognitive retraining, including memory enhancement and improved problem-solving, are examples of important, needed services.

SUPPORT GROUPS. Self-help or support groups can be vital to elders and families as sources of support, social activity, and community change. Examples include Stroke Clubs, Alzheimer's Disease Associations, Parkinsonian Societies, to name a few. The MHP, with rational help and local commitment of hospital, agency, and community groups, can assist in establishing, training, and supporting these important programs.

SPECIAL CONCERNS

The future holds promise for further development and application of clinical geropsychology (Welford, 1980) with increased recognition of the "special qualities about the nature of mental problems in old age that demand special attention and training" (Butler, 1975). Ideally, it will be professionals *and* elders (Pegels, 1981) exerting political pressure to cause health and social changes. The fragmented, acute care, illness-oriented emphasis that exists in much of health care today simply fails to do the job for older adults (Brody, 1973; Hendricks & Hendricks, 1977).

The problem of developing geriatric mental health services that are sensitive and responsive to the varying needs of elders is indeed multifaceted and complex. A significant aspect of the issue is whether elders are a viable political force in this country (Atchley, 1971; Binstock, 1972; Rule, 1977). It seems the missing ingredient to date in three White House Conferences on Aging is moving beyond recommendations to implementation. Although Medicare provides for important geriatric health care needs, it remains woefully inadequate in providing for mental health services to elders (APA, 1980).

It is advised that the MHP, in addition to the important role of clinician–consultant, also is obliged to function as an agent of advocacy and change (Butler, 1975). As reviewed in the final chapter, the *barriers* to change are multiple, including: political, economic, attitudinal, need of manpower, and lack of training.

Community and population barriers (Kahn & Tobin, 1981), such as elders' resistance to mental health care, require the MHP to know and interact with various sectors concerned with mental health care in the target or designated area of service. Special attention must be paid to the existing social milieu or network (Brody, 1981). In a sense, the principle for beginning a geriatric mental health service is basic; i.e., start where you can and with whom you can. Certainly there may be risks in establishing nontraditional programs, but the rewards can be attained (Glasscoate, Gudeman, & Miles, 1977).

From where will the MHP proposed here emanate? Manpower and training issues are crucial in addressing unmet health care needs of elders (Verwoerdt, 1981). Professional school training, continuing education, and criteria for certification in multidisciplinary, gerontological curricula are absolutely necessary to address future manpower needs in geriatrics. Gerontological researchers, academicians, and clinicians must interact, reciprocate, and educate cooperatively for a constructive future. In brief, much remains to be done.

CONCLUSIONS

On the basis that clinical geropsychology exists as a specialty field, emphasizing application of empiric differences that obtain in later life, this chapter has surveyed the roles and functions of the mental health practitioner. Principles and issues pertaining to attitude, knowledge base, application, and special concerns were reviewed, supported by the literature and author's clinical practice.

The future is ours to potentially experience and determine. The dynamic field of clinical gerontology and its subspecialty, clinical geropsychology, hold both enormous challenges and rewards for many lifetimes. If the reader is provoked and stimulated, then this review has added in small measure to a more positive approach to mental health care of the elderly.

REFERENCES

American Psychiatric Association. *The report of the American Psychiatric Association Task Force on the 1981 White House Conference on aging,* Nov. 1980.

Atchley, R.C. *The social forces in later life*. Belmont, California: Wadsworth, 1980.

Atchley, R.C. Retirement and leisure participation: Continuity or crisis. *The Gerontologist,* 1971, *11,* 29–32.

Barnes, E.K., Sack, A., & Shore, H. Guidelines to treatment approaches. *The Gerontologist,* 1973, *13,* 513–527.

Baltes, P.B., & Willis, S.L. Toward psychological theories of aging and development. In J.E. Birren & K.W. Schaie (Eds.), *Handbook of the psychology of aging*. New York: Van Nostrand Reinhold, 1977.

Baltes, P.B., & Schaie, K.W. *Life-span developmental psychology: Personality and socialization*. New York: Academic Press, 1973.

Bellak, L., & Bellak, S.S. *Senior apperception test*. Larchmont, New York: CPS, Inc., 1973.

Bengston, V.L., Kasschau, P.L., & Ragan, P.K. The impact of social structure on aging individuals. In J.E. Birren & K.W. Schaie (Eds.), *The handbook of psychology of aging*. New York: Van Nostrand Reinhold, 1977.

Binstock, R.H. Interest group liberalism and the politics of aging. *The Gerontologist,* 1972, *12,* 265–281.

Birren, J.E. *The psychology of aging*. Englewood Cliffs, New Jersey: Prentice Hall, 1968.

Blum, J.E., & Tross, S. Psychodynamic treatment of the elderly: A review of issues in theory and practice. In C. Eisdorfer (Ed.), *Annual review of gerontology and geriatrics* (Vol. 1). New York: Springer, 1980, 204–234.

Brink, T.L. *Geriatric psychotherapy*. New York: Human Sciences Press, 1979.

Brintnell, J.C., & Mitchell, K.E. Inpatient group psychotherapy for the elderly. *Journal of Psychosocial Nursing and Mental Health Services,* 1981, *19* (May), 19–24.

Brocklehurst, J.C. Geriatric services and the day hospital. In J.C. Brocklehurst (Ed.), *Textbook of geriatric medicine and gerontology*. London: Churchill Livingston, 1973, 673–691.

Brody, E. The formal support network: Congregate treatment settings for residents with senescent brain dysfunction. In N. Miller & G.D. Cohen (Eds.), *Clinical aspects of Alzheimer's disease and senile dementia*. New York: Raven Press, 1981, 301–332.

Brody, S.J. Comprehensive health care for the elderly: The continuum of medical, health and social services for the aged. *The Gerontologist,* 1973, *13,* 412–418.

Burnside, I.M. Interviewing the aged. In I.M. Burnside (Ed.), *Psychosocial nursing care of the aged*. New York: McGraw-Hill, 1980.

Burnside, I.M. One-to-one relationship therapy with the aged. In I.M. Burnside (Ed.), *Nursing and the aged*. New York: McGraw-Hill, 1981.

Burnside, I.M. *Working with the elderly: Group processes and techniques*. North Scitvate, Massachusetts: Duxbury Press, 1978.

Butler, R.N. Age-ism: another form of bigotry, *The Gerontologist,* 1963, *9,* 243–246.

Butler, R.N. *Why survive? Being old in America*. New York: Harper & Row, 1975, 174–259.

Butler, R.N., & Lewis, M.I. *Aging and mental health: Positive psychosocial approaches*. St. Louis: C.V. Mosby, 1982.

Caird, F.I., & Judge, T.G. *Assessment of the elderly patient*. California: Pitman Publishing Corp., 1977.

Cohen, G.D. Approach to the geriatric patient. In A. Reading & T.N. Wise (Eds.), *The Medical Clinics of North America, 1977,* 61 (July), 855–866.

Cumming, E., & Henry, W.E. *Growing old: The process of disengagement*. New York: Basic Books, 1961.

Datan, N., & Ginsberg, L.G. *Life-span developmental psychology: Narrative life crises*. New York: Academic Press, 1975.

Decker, D.L. *Social gerontology: An introduction to the dynamics of aging*. Boston: Little, Brown & Co., 1980.

Eisdorfer, C., Cohen, D.R., & Preston, C. Behavioral and psychological therapies for the older patient with cognitive impairment. In N. Miller & G.D. Cohen (Eds.), *Clinical aspects of Alzheimer's disease and senile dementia*. New York: Raven Press, 1981, 209–226.

Eisdorfer, C., & Stotsky, B.A. Intervention, treatment and rehabilitation of psychiatric disorders. In J.E. Birren and K.W. Schaie (Eds.), *Handbook of the psychology of aging*. New York: Van Nostrand Reinhold, 1977, 724–750.

Erickson, E.H. *Identity and the life cycle*. New York: International Universities Press, 1959.

Friedman, S.A., & Steinheber, F.V. *The medical clinics of North America symposium on geriatric medicine*. Philadelphia: W.C. Sanders Co., 1977.

Garetz, F. & Peth, P.R. An outreach program of medical care for aged senior high-rise residents. *Gerontologist,* 1974, *14,* 404–408.

Gatz, M., Smyer, M.A., & Lawton, M.P. The mental health system and the older adult. In J.W. Poon (Ed.), *Aging in the 1980s.* Washington, D.C.: American Psychological Association, 1980.

Glasscoate, R., Gudeman, J.E., & Miles, D. *Creative mental health services for the elderly.* New York: American Psychiatric Association, 1977.

Goldfarb, A.I. *Aging and the organic brain syndrome.* Washington, Pennsylvania: McNeil Laboratories, 1974.

Goulet, L.R. & Baltes, P.B. *Life-span developmental psychology: Research and theory.* New York: Academic Press, 1970.

Group for the Advancement of Psychiatry. *The aged and community mental health: A guide to program development.* New York: Group for Advancement of Psychiatry, 1971.

Havighurst, R.J. Successful aging. In R.H. Williams, C. Tibbitts, & W. Donahue (Eds.), *Processes of aging.* New York: Atherton Press, 1963.

Hefferin, E.A. Rehabilitation in nursing home situations: A survey of the literature. *Journal of the American Geriatrics Society,* 1968, *16,* 296–313.

Hendricks, J., & Hendricks, C.D. *Aging in mass society: Myths and realities.* Cambridge, Massachusetts: Winthrop Publishers, 1977.

Herr, J.J., & Weakland, J.H. *Counseling elders and their families.* New York: Springer, 1979.

Hussian, R.A. *Geriatric psychology: a behavioral perspective.* New York: Van Nostrand Reinhold, 1981.

Kahn, R.L. The mental health system and the future aged. In I. Rossman (Ed.), *Clinical geriatrics.* Philadelphia: Lippencott, 1971.

Kahn, R.H., & Tobin, S.S. Community treatment for aged persons with altered brain function. In N. Miller & G.D. Cohen (Eds.), *Clinical aspects of Alzheimer's disease and senile dementia.* New York: Raven Press, 1981, 253–276.

Kane, R.A., & Kane, R.L. *Assessing the elderly: A practical guide to measurement.* Lexington, Massachusetts: Lexington Books, 1981.

Kramer, M., Taube, C.A., & Redick, R.W. Patterns of use in psychiatric facilities by the aged: Present, past and future. In C. Eisdorfer & M.P. Lawton (Eds.), *The psychology of adult development and aging.* Washington, D.C.: American Psychological Association, 1973.

Lawton, M.P. The impact of the environment on aging and behavior. In J.E. Birren & K.W. Schaie (Eds.), *Handbook of psychology and aging.* New York: Van Nostrand Reinhold, 1977, 276–301.

LeBray, P.R. Geropsychology in long-term care settings. *Professional Psychology,* 1979, *10,* 475–484.

LeBray, P.R. *Interviewing the elderly.* Videotape, Audio Visual Department, Good Samaritan Hospital, Portland, Oregon 97210, 1980.

LeBray, P.R. *Geriatric sentence completion form.* Psychological Assessment Resources, Inc., P.O. Box 98, Odessa, FL 33556, 1982.

LeBray, P.R. Selected characteristics of geriatric clinic patients. *Hospital Staff* (in press).

Libow, L. Geriatric medicine and the nursing home: A mechanism for mutual excellence. *The Gerontologist,* 1982, *22,* 134–141.

McTavish, D.G. Perceptions of old people: A review of research methodologies and findings. *The Gerontologist* (Third Report), 1971–72, 90–101.

Mezey, M.D., Rauckhorst, L.H., & Stokes, S.A. *Health assessment of the older individual.* New York: Springer, 1980.

National Institute of Mental Health, Biometry Branch. *Distribution of patient care episodes in mental health facilities, 1969* (No. 58). Washington, D.C.: U.S. Government Printing Office, 1972.

Nesselroade, J.R., & Reese, H.W. *Life-span developmental psychology: Methodological issues.* New York: Academic Press, 1973.

Neugarten, B.L. *Middle age and aging.* Chicago: University of Chicago Press, 1968.

Oberleder, M. Adapting current psychological techniques for use in testing the aging. *The Gerontologist,* 1967, *7,* 188–191.

Pegels, C.C. *Health care and the elderly.* Rockville, Maryland: Aspen Publications, 1981.

Pfeiffer, E. A short portable mental status questionnaire for the assessment of organic brain deficit in elderly patients. *Journal of the American Geriatrics Society,* 1975, *23,* 433–441.

Posner, J. Notes on the negative implications of being competent in a home for the aged. *International Journal of Aging and Human Development,* 1974, *5,* 357–364.

Raskin, A., & Jarvik, L. (Eds.) *Psychiatric symptoms and cognitive loss in the elderly.* New York: Hemisphere Publishing Corp., 1979.

Rechtschaffer, A. Psychotherapy with geriatric patients: A review of the literature. *Journal of Gerontology,* 1959, *14,* 73–84.

Richards, W.S., & Thorpe, G.L. Behavioral approaches to the problems of later life. In M. Storandt, I.C. Siegler, & M.F. Elias (Eds.), *The clinical psychology of aging.* New York: Plenum Press, 1978, 253–276.

Riley, M.W. Social gerontology and the age stratification of society. *The Gerontologist,* 1971, *11,* 79–87.

Robinson, B.J. Assessment of the frail elderly. In I.M. Burnside (Ed.), *Nursing and the aged.* New York: McGraw-Hill, 1980.

Rossman, I. Environments of geriatric care. In I. Rossman (Ed.), *Clinical geriatrics.* Philadelphia: Lippencott, 1979, 668–680.

Rule, W.I.B. Political alienation and voting attitudes among the elderly generation. *The Gerontologist,* 1977, *17,* 400–404.

Schaie, K.W. Quasi-experimental research designs in the psychology of aging. In J.E. Birren & K.W. Schaie (Eds.), *Handbook of the psychology of aging.* New York: Van Nostrand Reinhold, 1977.

Schmidt, M.G. Interviewing the ill old. *The Gerontologist,* 1975, *15,* 544–547.

Smyer, M.A. & Gatz, M. Aging and mental health: Business as usual? *American Psychologist,* 1979, *34* (3), 240–246.

Storandt, M., Seigler, I.C., & Elias, M.F. *The clinical psychology of aging.* New York: Plenum Press, 1978.

Stotsky, B. *The nursing home and the aged psychiatric patient.* New York: Appleton-Century-Crofts, 1970.

Tobias, J.S. The special rehabilitation needs of the elderly. *Geriatrics,* 1976, *31,* 51–103.

Verwoerdt, A. *Clinical geropsychiatry.* Baltimore: Williams & Williams, 1976.

Verwoerdt, A. Individual psychotherapy in senile dementia. In N. Miller & G.D. Cohen (Eds.), *Clinical aspects of Alzheimer's disease and senile dementia*. New York: Raven Press, 1981, 187–208.

Welford, A.T. Where do we go from here? In L. Poon (Ed.), *Aging in the 1980s*. Washington, D.C.: American Psychological Association, 1980, 615–621.

Zarit, S.H. *Aging and mental disorders*. New York: Free Press, 1980.

14

MODELS OF MENTAL HEALTH CARE FOR THE ELDERLY

Carl Eisdorfer

The aging of our world population is the great, bittersweet success of our century. The data documenting lengthened life span and the increasing number and proportion of older persons in our population have compelling implications. The range of societal responsibilities that include the mental health needs of this population are staggering, but to date the consequences of these age changes in demography have been addressed poorly (Eisdorfer & Cohen, 1982; Neugarten, 1982). To recognize current problems stemming from this population shift is to appreciate only a part of what may be considered to be the emerging phase of another age of demographic change. It has taken us eight decades to move our population aged 65 or older (Brotman, 1981), from 3.5 percent to 11 percent. We now face an increase in the proportion of elders from approximately 10 percent of the population in the early 1970s to a projected near-20 percent over the next 40 years. This doubling in proportion will significantly strain our ability to deliver a range of human services (Eisdorfer, 1981). However, the crux of the problem is even more serious. The fastest growing subgroup of the population are those aged 75 years and older and, given the changing morbidity patterns of late-life diseases, longevity among the oldest portion of our population is expected to increase, even beyond current projections. The Census Bureau conservatively estimated that there will be 3.7 million persons over age 85 by the year 2000, but a recent

GERIATRIC MENTAL HEALTH
ISBN 0-8089-1657-2

report from the National Center on Health Statistics projects twice that number: 6.7 million men and women by 2000 (Kovar & Drury, 1980).

The process of aging brings with it an increased risk for problems and conditions requiring care of one sort or another, including mental health care. However, the aging of the most aged has resulted in a greater relative increase in those groups at risk for conditions needing care, and is leading to a serious, world-wide increase in the prevalence of mental disorders and chronic diseases (Kramer, 1980). This rising pandemic has important implications for health policy and financing, planning and delivery of mental health services, research, manpower, and training. Developing new approaches to the mental health care of the aging is not only timely, but overdue.

It would seem, at least on the surface, that having identified the size of the aging population as well as their problems, it should be an easy task to organize and deliver the care necessary to resolve their problems. Unfortunately, this task is not simple. Meeting the challenge of dealing with the mental health needs of an aging population requires a thoughtful analysis of the many conceptual approaches to systems of mental health care, which is the focus of this chapter. Our current health delivery system reflects the interplay between interactive systems—economic, societal, national, professional, and personal. These various conceptual systems and their interactions with each other determine how care is delivered.

Caring involves a transaction between deliverers and receivers within the societal or environmental context. Furthermore, the perceptions and beliefs of the deliverer and receiver, as well as others in the environment, mediate the nature of the transaction. These perceptions are, in turn, a function of the conceptual models of the individuals involved. If we accept the hypothesis that the conceptual models of the caregivers influence the course of an individual's treatment, it is clear that there are multiple models at play, some of which are competing, some conflicting, and some reinforcing each other. The difficulty for the professional is to identify all belief systems operating at a specific point in time and deal with them appropriately.

A DEVELOPMENTAL SOCIAL AND ECONOMIC MODEL

Perhaps the first model to consider is one that does not primarily relate to mental health or its related professional disciplines, but rather to that of the cultural context, which includes social and economic beliefs concerning the aged. Even at the risk of being simplistic, it is heuristic to conceptualize human development as spanning four economic categories. The first category is youth, those growing individuals not yet able to function independently without support. Society invests emotional, economic and supportive resources in this group in many forms, such as education, in the anticipation that such investment will yield future benefits that will contribute to the survival of the society. The second group are those who are in the productive part of their life; i.e., individuals who generate goods and services for the broader population. Third are the post-work group that the French refer to as *le troisieme age,* people who are reasonably healthy but have passed their 65th birthday, or some functional equivalent thereof, and are retired from paid employment. Finally, we have the fourth group, those aged, dependent individuals who cannot function independently and require home-based or institutional care.

From a societal point of view, this conceptualization of aging and human development has clear implications for the provision of help from the caring disciplines. For the first group, the young, we invest a full range of resources: education, health, nutrition, and any assistance necessary to bring people into the world and launch them into a trajectory so that they can reach a productive phase within our society. Whether we "invest" enough is a chronic debate, but the concept that youth are "entitled" to such investment is rarely challenged. The second group, those being productive, may on occasion need assistance to maintain their productivity. We may need to tide them over rough periods with such assistance as unemployment compensation or supplementary training. We also need to provide appropriate health benefits for periods of illness and disability. In some instances we provide tax incentives for specific factors such as employment-related educational programs. For the third group, which may be conceptualized as a *nonproductive* segment of society, we act as if they have no future productivity. They get little recognition for a range of interpersonal, family, and social services. Therefore, what they receive falls into one of two categories based on what they have earned, (i.e., deferred compensation, or what is derived from the humanitarian aspects of society, charity). The fourth age is a period where the dependent person progressively is more reliant on the beliefs of the broader society for the preservation of human life.

In our approach to mental health care of the aged, we should be careful that our thinking is not overly influenced by such models. Therefore, an examination of our beliefs concerning the role of elders is necessary. Are the aged indeed "over the hill" and a predictable burden on our charitable resources? Is it true that we cannot "teach old dogs new tricks" or do we adopt the view that elders should continue working until the end and die at their desk or lathe? Are there alternative roles for elders? Can we think of them as having special needs and special talents that emerge in later life, or is old age merely the downward slide of the productive years? The old may be seen as the cause of the burden on Social Security (i.e., they take more benefits out than they put in), as a burden on their families, or as the respected elders helping to teach values essential to society.

Politics, economics, and social structure thus have a significant impact on how we think about the aged (Estes, 1979) and determine how we allocate resources (Eisdorfer & Cohen, 1981). Indeed, the very quality of life in old age depends upon our socioeconomic structure and the way we choose to allocate societal resources.

NATIONAL MODELS: A COMPARISON BETWEEN THE UNITED STATES AND CHINA

National models are based upon national belief systems, and they predetermine the way care is provided. A comparison between China and the United States helps illustrate how national models influence the organization, style, and effectiveness of health care delivery. Two elementally distinctive approaches to health-care delivery characterize these two countries.

Health care is socialized in China. It is more important for people to be healthy on behalf of the society-at-large than it is for any single person to feel better. The ethos of a productive Chinese society diminishes individual well-being, stressing the best interests of the nation, which is clearly in sharp contrast to the United States where health care focuses on the individual and family. The Chinese stress a public health approach with control of health service delivery at the community level. Thus, health care is a national priority of the new Chinese society with a strong emphasis on the social components of care.

The United States has evolved a powerful technological orientation to health care emphasizing biomedical advances in the diagnosis and treatment of disease, whereas in China, social and environmental services are the important considerations related to health and disease. Caring services are organized and reside at the community level, and it is at the community level that decisions are made. For example, community groups determine to what extent a "sick" person will be allowed to work.

The implications of different conceptual models for health service delivery in China and the United States are clear. In China health care is universally available, there is a single standard of quality (at least this is the claim), and cost is not a barrier to care. A series of health-care services are coordinated within the community to provide both a regionalized, as well as a decentralized, system of health care. Although health care clearly is regionalized throughout the country, a hierarchical organization also is operational. The individual may seek treatment for complex health problems utilizing a full range of services from the barefoot doctor through the tertiary medical center.

The Chinese report that they have achieved fusion of both preventive and curative medicine which ensure of professional accountability and patient acceptability. A combination of folk practices and scientific methods are integrated into the practice of a form of medicine that is embedded within the very matrix of the culture. Many folk practices are well accepted and strengthen the cultural ties of the individual. Acceptability of new technological advances is mediated by how embedded they are in the culture.

The United States' health care system is dominated by a set of beliefs reflecting our private, entrepreneurial culture. National policy and models clearly can influence the economic viability of various health systems. For example, a salient issue in this country is the relative equilibrium between private versus nonprofit health care. There is no national control of education, placement of physicians, or the organization of specialty services or technology, except on a free enterprise basis.

These models clearly reflect the economic and health policy decisions imbedded in belief systems that shape the nature and quality of a country's health-care program. In the United States, Medicare is an economic system where transfer of payment is made to older persons, or their providers, for certain kinds of health care. Unfortunately, Medicare is inadequate to deal with most of the health care needs of the aged because the very nature of the reimbursement emphasizes acute episodic care, and these needs are characteristic of a younger-adult population rather than the aged (Lee, Estes, LeRoy, & Newcomer, 1982). Medicare was originally intended to reduce the cost of health care to the elder and the family. It was not designed on the basis of an analysis of the real needs of older people with chronic health problems in the United States, any more than socialized Chinese medicine was based on the needs of the Chinese people. Instead, both are based upon belief systems as reflected in the political setting of the country. Unfortunately, in the case of Medicare, cost considerations have become paramount in the provision of health care in the United States today. Attempts to improve Medicare, and consequently the coverage of older persons, which includes long term care, have been rejected by society in a bipartisan fashion, i.e., both unions and management have backed away because of their concerns about cost (Eisdorfer & Cohen, 1982; Somers, 1982).

Medicaid is another economic health program in the United States, designed to cover specific health-care costs for individuals who meet specific economic criteria. Medicaid is based on a welfare model in which limitations on care, especially long term care, are determined by certain provisions for an adequate standard of living rather than therapeutic need. Clearly any attempt to alter or improve health-care delivery nationally will have to deal not only with the factually-determined needs but with the prevailing beliefs about health care.

MODELS OF MEDICINE

Traditional models of medical care with all of their limitations (Eisdorfer, 1981; Engel, 1980) have dominated mental health care for the aged. Within the boundaries of the medical approach, we view the older person as someone at increased risk for illness, more likely to be frail, and more likely to have marginally functioning vital organs that complicate treatment. Perhaps more than any other single factor, the expectation that to be old is to be poor, sick, senile, and incompetent, and therefore a burden on society, has undermined efforts to improve mental health care for the aged.

In order to understand this tradition more clearly, the various conceptual models of medicine and their history need to be reviewed. While medicine has several conceptual models (Eisdorfer, 1981), there are three to review briefly—the anatomic, humoral, and behavioral.

The anatomic model derives from sticks and stones and broken bones, and cuts and bruises. Initially oriented toward dealing with the effects of trauma on organs of the body (e.g., closing wounds, setting bones, amputating limbs), this part of medical activity has improved our understanding of anatomy and has advanced techniques in surgery, including transplantation and microsurgery. These have led to daily miracles in our major medical centers and a level of societal prestige reflected in the legitimation of relatively high income for the practitioners of surgical disciplines.

The humoral approach was based initially on diagnosis and treatment of illnesses by balancing the four basic humors. This primitive conceptualization led, of course, to the fields of physiology, biochemistry, physical chemistry, and pharmacology as approaches to patient diagnosis and treatment by internists, pediatricians, and others. This strategy assures that the explanation for disease states is related to alterations in body chemistry (e.g., enzymes, electrolytes, hormones), and that treatment and cures involve changes in body chemistry (e.g., medications, diet).

Of great significance to mental health, the behavioral approach was first associated with a belief in spirits and a dynamic balance between angelic and demonic possession of the individual. With scientific refinement, however, we witnessed a splitting of the behavioral model into two subcategories: the organ-free and organ-involved. Two organ-free approaches exist. In the psychoanalytic psychodynamic model the psyche is embedded in a rather complex set of processes which are conceptualized as causal factors. Alternatively, the learning model holds that the person may as well be a "black box" into which stimuli are introduced and from which behaviors emerge by predictable formulae. Given certain knowledge of deprivation schedules, patterns of reinforcement, etc., we can control desirable and undesirable behaviors accordingly. While both of these submodels assume an intact organ of cognition (i.e., the brain), in neither model does the brain play a clearly defined role.

In contrast to the organ-free models, in the organ-involved approach to behavior the brain was identified as the target organ and mediation of the brain's structure or humors explain behavior. Thus, pharmacologic or other biologically involved changes in brain chemistry are basic to the treatment of disease in this model.

These narrowly defined conceptual approaches are not merely of academic consequence. They lead to pathways of training and transmission of beliefs about evaluation, diagnosis, management, and treatment. Thus, it would be fair to predict that a moderately depressed person brought to a behavioral specialist, who does not believe in the organic basis for behavioral problems (i.e., somatic or humoral), would be less likely to receive pharmacologic intervention and more likely to receive a purely behavioral intervention. This may very well be reflected not only in professional training, but also in licensure and/or certification of the individual.

Narrow conceptual issues rather profoundly influence our clinical techniques, and even the vocabulary of care is a function of the models we adopt. Terms such as *diagnosis* are used in contrast to the terms *assessment* or *evaluation* and, indeed, have differing implications. Treatment is distinguished from management; *patient* is contrasted with the term *client*. Each label reflects a rather narrow position that is understood by those who have been initiated appropriately to a particular conceptual model, each with its unique perception of the individual in need of help. An immediate set of concerns emerge from this analysis. Are clinicians or scientists too narrowly trained to recognize and deal with a given orientation to pathology? Can we switch to alternative strategies? Do we believe in the sanctity of the model we employ and do we have trouble crossing models?

Medical models traditionally view the aged in terms of diseases and the need for medical care. Not surprisingly, for every $30 we invest in medical aspects of health care, we are investing only $1 in the social and community services designed to improve the lives of older persons, prevent illnesses, or improve adaptation in the face of long-term illness (Brody & Spivak, 1981). Is the model of coping with diseases, frailty, and maladaptation a health, or mental health, model or would it be better served by alternative social models (e.g., educational or biopsychosocial models)?

CONCEPTUAL MODELS OF PSYCHOPATHOLOGY

In mental health care we are no less the victims of our conceptual models (Eisdorfer, Cohen, Kleinman et al., 1981). Our approach to diagnosis and management varies enormously, depending upon whether we accept the existence of a complex behavioral entity called mental illness, or whether we hold the view that there is no mental illness, but rather poor adaptation to an environment that may stimulate and exacerbate aberrant behavior. At one level of abstraction, it matters little whether the models are embedded in a biologic substrate, with the disease caused by a gene, virus, or a structural change, secondary to some other event (e.g., high fever). There are various permutations and combinations of beliefs. We even have psychological models embedded in biologic models. Thus, Jungian and Freudian instinctual conceptualizations are seen as embedded in the genetic structure of the species. Pathology models may range from the purely academic (i.e., inherited chemical deficit), to the purely psychological (i.e., aberrant behaviors may be learned). The learning may result from early preverbal interaction with individuals and objects during the development of the individual and/or result from subsequent experiences across the life span.

In contrast, if we assume that there is no such thing as mental illness or psychopathology, aberrant behavior may be seen as part of an adaptive continuum either because it is reactive to an aberrant situation, and consequently attention-getting, or it may be an expression of unresolvable conflict. Deviant behavior thus may be conceptualized as a learned reaction to a crazy society or behavior stemming from dealing with a parent who places the child in a crazy situation (e.g., "a double bind"). Socially we may note that antisocial behavior is a by-product of ageism, racism, sexism, social Darwinism, or some combination thereof.

There are, of course, other hypothetical models relating to deviant behavior. These include the labelling model in which certain groups or persons are identified as having special patterns that may normalize the abnormal. The elder with loss of memory may be recognized as having problems but not require help because "all old people become senile." Once a label is applied (as with a diagnosis), we deal with the label, ignoring the particular needs of the individual or even the reality of presumptions associated with the label. Thus, labels such as aged, senile, crazy, and depressed carry with them certain social and professional consequences that do not help the process of understanding and caring, but rather elicit and promote professional stereotypic behavior which further serves to reinforce the label.

TOWARD NEW MODELS OF MENTAL HEALTH CARE

We could enumerate a number of either broadly or narrowly conceptualized economic, social, and political models that may help us understand the mental health care of the aged. We have addressed only a few. Conceptual models are heuristic approaches that can help us understand and predict the behavior of the individual within the framework of the model. Each model is embedded in a hypothetical structure that should be testable by observation or prediction and, in turn, may help us elaborate an analytic and management strategy.

This seems fairly straightforward. Why, then, are there problems? The difficulty becomes manifested in the autonomy of approaches and in the nature of the beliefs of the individuals who decide which model or models are to be applied in a given instance. In a dyadic system where there is a professional and a patient, what happens if the professional adheres to only one conceptual model for all patients? It is not rare to find a patient relating to a professional who is focused narrowly on one model and trained to believe in one treatment. In effect, the professional fits the patient to the model and its concomitant pattern of evaluation and management. Is the patient's problem conceptualized as an insufficient blood level of a particular drug or an insufficient cortical level of a particular psychotherapeutic approach? If the patient fails to fit the therapy, do we not risk reconceptionalizing the patient as "resisting" the therapy or having a "crazy reaction" that is resisting the medication. In effect, we develop a moral judgment concerning patients who fail to respond to our ministration.

As Carl Sandburg said, "Nothing happens unless first a dream." Given the relative paucity of the data base in clinical psychopathology and the multiple models that may be brought to bear on a given individual, many models may be appropriate. We must evolve strategies of caring that go beyond our existent narrow models. It is incumbent upon us to deal effectively with the needs of the individual older patient. We are not likely to discover the potential of the aged unless we broaden our conceptual models and develop a notion of clinical care that transcends narrow approaches and the images they convey. Otherwise, we will be destructive to the person in the patient. Is the patient "'old," "mature", or "senile"? To what extent is age per se relevant to the treatment? Is the professional performing purely as a technician to provide care, with little or no understanding of the individual needs of the patient, or is he or she ready enough to learn more about individual patients, their problems, needs, desires, and resources, and then to interact with them to deal with the management issues? Can we use models as heuristic devices to stimulate research and study and to provide more insights without being controlled by the model? Does the model designed to broaden the cognitive network of the professional actually lead to the loss of individuality both to the professional and the patient/victim?

We need to begin with a reconceptualization of our model of the aged. The aged are now captives—the victims of a belief system that has most people over 65 identified with the small proportion of needy, dependent, and helpless individuals. Gerontologist Herb Shore once stated that older people could be conceptualized in three different ways: the no-go group, the slow-go group, and, of course, the go-go group. Are we so attached to no-go and slow-go images that those who can and do go lose their options?

Our beliefs concerning the role of elders in our society risk victimizing the aged. The models of the aged as deteriorated physical beings, bundles of diminished cells, depleted enzymes, low energy, decreased ability, and an increased burden on society, lead to operational consequences. It is no surprise that a substantial portion of our aged population, now numbering well over a million, reside in warehousing arrangements spending their last days in poorly-run, poorly-equipped, chronic-care facilities that are really mini-state hospitals. Since older people are already perceived to be at the margin of life and society, it seems clear why treatment for mental illness is not fully reimbursable and why medication is a substitute for personal interaction.

We must reconceptualize the roles of older people in our society. No longer should they be perceived as people with chronic, organic, and, therefore, untreatable problems, but rather as valued individuals who are functioning well in society, albeit with an increased risk for display of a host of difficulties ranging from alcohol and substance abuse to psychiatric illnesses, which include depression, paranoia, and dementia.

Narrow conceptual turfs reflect the educational background of most mental health professionals. Too often our description of a patient or client's problem and care are couched in terms that fit individual professional needs to provide or not provide care. In most instances, it emerges as a way of deprecating the potential contributions of others. We are told that medications are bad because they have side effects; psychotherapy fails to work or it does not address real-life issues; behavior modification is of little help since no insight is derived. Alternatively, conceptualizations and treatment strategies should be examined in terms of how they are effective, where they are best applied, and what the risks and benefits are to the patient and family, who have a right to play a role in clinical decisions.

Clinical programs must be undertaken to integrate medical and psychological care so that medical or behavioral manifestations of a disorder do not blind us to the possible underlying basis for disturbances that may be outside of our personal professional experience. Families or other social settings should be considered in evaluation and treatment of all types (Eisdorfer & Cohen, 1981). Second opinions should be solicited in mental health care. The role of the gerontologically trained mental health practitioner should be expanded. Fundamentally, however, research, broadly based education training across models, and sensitivity to the prejudicial issues involved are absolute requirements.

This is the great challenge in working with the aged. Just as we have seen that no single societal model applies to the elderly, we must also see that no single mental health conceptualization can apply to all the problems of the elderly. Furthermore, we must avoid such close identity with any particular model that we become wedded to it, or worse still, own it, or are disastrously owned by it. For the best approach to the care of those in need, we must sharpen our perceptions and be fully prepared for other insights and integration of the broadest range of ideas.

REFERENCES

Brody, S., & Spivak, S. Long term health care planning: The state of the practice. In C. Eisdorfer, (Ed.), *Annual review of gerontology and geriatrics* (Vol. 2). New York: Springer, 1981.

Brotman, H.B. Every ninth American. In United States Senate Special Committee on Aging, 97th Congress. *Developments in aging, 1980*. Washington, D.C.: United States Government Printing Office, 1981.

Eisdorfer, C. Care of the aged: The barriers of tradition. *Annals of Internal Medicine*, 1981, *94*, 256–260.

Eisdorfer, C., & Cohen, D. *Mental health care of the aging*. New York: Springer, 1982.

Eisdorfer, C., & Cohen, D. Management of the patient and family coping with dementing illness. *Journal of Family Practice*, 1981, *12*, 813–837.

Eisdorfer, C., Cohen, D., Kleinman, A., & Maxim, P. *Models for clinical psychopathology*. New York: Spectrum, 1981.

Engel, G.L. The clinical application of the biopsychosocial model. *American Journal of Psychiatry*, 1980, *137*, 535–544.

Estes, C. *The aging enterprise*. San Francisco: Josey-Bass, 1979.

Kovar, M.G., & Drury, T.F. Elderly people: The population age 65 and over. Tables prepared for the Annual Meeting of the American Public Health Association, Detroit: October, 1980.

Kramer, M. The rising pandemic of mental disorders and associated chronic diseases and disabilities. *Acta Psychiatria Scandinavia Supplement*, 1980, *62* (285), 382–397.

Lee, P.R., Estes, C.L., LeRoy, L., & Newcomer, R. Health policy and the aged. In C. Eisdorfer (Ed.), *Annual review of gerontology and geriatrics* (Vol. 3). New York: Springer, 1982.

Neugarten, B. Older Americans: a profile of social and health characteristics. In M.T. Kulczycki and M. Peisert (Eds.), *The hospital's role in caring for the elderly: leadership issues*. Chicago: Health Research and Educational Trust, June, 1982.

Somers, A. Long term care for the elderly and disabled: A new health project. *New England Journal of Medicine*, 1982, *307*, 221–225.

15

ETHICAL ISSUES IN MENTAL HEALTH CARE OF THE ELDERLY

Christine Cassel

In discussing issues of ethics with clinicians and investigators it is almost always better to begin with a case to be grounded in the concrete realities of day-to-day experience and use whatever abstract wisdom or philosophical methods will help us find our way through our daily confrontation with value conflicts. Bertold Brecht said, "The truth is concrete,"—a statement that may seem a self-evident truism or perhaps glib anti-intellectualism, but which holds a great deal of power and unexpected subtlety in questions of medical ethics.

Initially, however, one must indulge in a brief discussion of principles—broad premises of ethical action that often are basic to dilemmas in clinical medicine and mental health practice. In our pluralistic society one cannot assume that one's values are necessarily shared by others, or even that similar words encompass a similar scope of values. Therefore, a brief definition of terms is in order. It is of the utmost importance for productive and meaningful discussions of ethical issues that participants speak the same language.

One objection frequently encountered when trying to apply philosophical methodologies to clinical problems is the claim of "righteous pluralism." I have my ethics and you have yours and what's the point of discussing it any further (Equating ethics with personal values is an example of not using the same language.)? Pluralism, however, is a fact of life. In terms of the Brechtian criterion of truth, the inescapable fact of differing

GERIATRIC MENTAL HEALTH
ISBN 0-8089-1657-2

value systems is about as concrete a sociological observation as can be made. This diversity is, in fact, the source of much confusion about ethical issues, and it lies at the center of many ethical dilemmas. Nevertheless, it is rarely or ever the case that people in our culture hold values that are entirely mutually exclusive. Moral principles from diverse traditions tend to have great areas of overlap and commonality. One does not have to be a Jungian scholar to suspect a shared moral universe from which our sense of right and wrong flow, our images of good and evil are formed, and from which our expectations of praise and blame ensue. Thus, elucidating basic principles is a method for establishing a common basis from which to explore problems involving values.

Two of these basic principles are: (1) beneficence, or doing good, and (2) respect for persons and their autonomy. On the face of it, there are few who would (in public at least) deny the validity of these as moral principles. No doubt areas of disagreement as to what constitutes respect or goodness will occur. As happens in many situations that are referred to as ethical dilemmas, one sometimes is faced with deciding between several courses of action, each of which represents one of those principles, and must go against one of them in order to act consistently with another. In colloquial terms, this is what is known as being between a rock and a hard place. This is an all too familiar place for professionals working in the area of geriatric mental health care. To make the "most right" decision, and to feel satisfied with the process of that decision, one can be greatly helped by methods and ideas of philosophical ethics. Ethical analysis is not likely to present us with an answer that is conclusive in the sense that the solution to a mathematical problem is conclusive. But of course, these are problems of life, not of mathematics, and one must resolve to deal constantly in areas of ambiguity. However, ambiguity does not preclude clarity, and clarity of thought is an appropriate goal.

BENEFICENCE

The first principle to consider is usually referred to as beneficence, meaning simply "doing good." This is probably the oldest and most consistent principle of medical ethics. Most health professionals would agree that some such ideal underlies the motivations of all those involved in the care of the sick, and if it does not, it should. Its origin is in the corpus of Hippocratic works. "As to diseases," wrote the author of *The Epidemics,* "make a habit of two things—to help, or at least to do no harm (Reiser, Curran, & Dych, 1977)." The works attributed to Hippocrates contain many other exhortations to virtues more arcane, pagan, or just plain unacceptable, but this central notion has had a remarkable transcultural persistence. The physician should be committed to producing good for the patient and to protecting that patient from harm.

Clearly, this principle is not as simple as it might appear on face value. The growing literature on risk-benefit analysis is ample testimony to our uncertainty as to what balance of goods and harms exists in any given course of action. Some philosophers (Veatch, 1981) have used this objection to disvalue the Hippocratic tradition as a valid basis for a medical ethic, claiming that it places too much and unwarranted decision-making power in the role of the physician. Others object that it is oriented only towards the individual physician–patient relationship, taking no account of the public health role or social responsibility of the healer. It is not that these criticisms embody an expectation that Hippocrates should have anticipated the complex world of twentieth-century medicine. Rather a valid concern exists that the medical profession has concentrated its ethical sense too much on this paternalistic and individualistic model, and its limitations have made it difficult to effectively deal with the dilemmas of modern medicine.

AUTONOMY

The second principle is "respect for persons," or more precisely, respect for personal autonomy. It is on this principle that the whole idea and process of informed consent is based. Certain kinds of entitlements we call patients' rights are also related to the principle of respect for autonomy: for example, the right to refuse treatment, the right to a second opinion, and the right to death with dignity. It is much more recent in our culture than the Hippocratic principle, and finds its most articulate origin in the works of John Stuart Mill, social philosopher of the 18th century. In *On Liberty,* Mill argues that "social and political control over individual actions is legitimate only if necessary to prevent harm to other individuals affected by those actions. (Mill, 1926)." Notice that he does *not* say ". . . and to prevent harm to the individual himself." Mill was not one to claim spiritual revelation as the source of his principles, but rather had a careful utilitarian analysis in which it seemed to him that a principle of maximum and equal autonomy and liberty for everyone (except in situations where someone else's liberty was thereby reduced) would encourage the kind of diversity that would finally produce a most productive and creative society.

This principle is invoked often in the context of court cases. Society generally supports the rights of competent adults to whatever course of action they choose as long as it does not impinge on the rights of another. Unfortunately, in health care contexts the mention of patients' rights often has meant the declaration of an adversary relationship between physician and patient. Embracing the principle of respect for personal autonomy is sometimes difficult to reconcile with beneficence, as we shall see, and thus conflict can develop. The simplest, most eloquent and most relevant formulation of this principle came from a court case in 1914 in which Justice Benjamin Carozo stated, "Every human being of adult years and sound mind has a right to determine what shall be done with his or her own body (Schloendorff, 1914)."

In mental health care in general, and especially with the elderly, the principles of beneficence and autonomy often appear to be in conflict. The predilection to "help," to make life easier or better for someone in need, may threaten to invade the sacrosanct respect for self-determination of an elder who does not want to accept help. If such a refusal is seen as derived from the person's pride and sense of self-reliance, then it may be touching or even tragic, but it would be accepted by most people that the principle of autonomy prevailed over that of beneficence. On the other hand, if the elders were confused, or carried a psychiatric diagnosis of any sort, they may be seen as "incompetent" to decide for themselves, and paternalistic intervention would be a moral obligation, i.e., to respect such a person's refusal of care would be tantamount to abandonment. Here is the area where concrete issues must be weighed, such as in the following case study.

Case Study

Mrs. Smith, a 79-year-old, 87-pound female was admitted to the hospital with the chief complaint of "I'm feeling bad because of the trouble I've caused." She lived in a rural town with her 84-year-old husband, had very little formal education, and could not read or write. They had seven children, one or another of whom was able to look in on them frequently. She had lost 80 pounds over the past 2 to 3 years, and over that same period increasingly had become withdrawn and disinterested in social contact with her relatives. During the few months prior to admission, she reported feeling sad, losing her appetite, having difficulty falling asleep, and staying asleep. Three weeks prior to her first admission, she began to complain that she could not get the idea out of her head that she had committed an unforgivable sin and was going to die. On examination there was evidence of short-term memory impairment, periods of confusion, and inability to concentrate. An additional medical problem was a ten-year history of chronic congestive heart failure and atrial fibrillation treated with Digoxin.

Initial evaluation showed no exacerbation of her cardiac condition, and normal lab values including acceptable Digoxin levels. Electroencephalogram showed a grade II dysrhythmia with excess amount of theta waves and generalized slow background rhythm. CAT scan showed generalized atrophy without other abnormalities. Neurological diagnosis was senile dementia, probably Alzheimer's type.

Psychiatric consultants agreed with this but felt there was also evidence for a depressive component of her illness that might be reversible. A course of tricyclic antidepressants produced urinary retention and severe postural hypotension so that she became totally bedridden and afraid to walk. At lower doses these symptoms decreased somewhat, and she began to eat and move around a bit, although objectively her mood was not improved. Her family wanted to take her home at this point, and did so. The tricyclics were not continued because of what were felt to be unacceptable side effects.

Eight weeks later she was readmitted because, in addition to the persistence of her previous complaints, she had developed an incapacitating conviction that there were demons within her. She stated, "I am a wicked and evil person and the devil has been after me all my life and now is overpowering me." She reported hearing the demons' voices, said that if she were stronger she would kill herself to be rid of these demons, and implored those around her to leave her alone to die. In addition she insisted that family members taste her food before she ate it, and accused her physicians of wanting to blow her up and throw her off the roof.

At this time her heart failure had markedly worsened, but improved after two weeks of adjusted therapy and bedrest. She still insisted that she be left alone to die, and refused adequate nourishment.

These remarks were interpreted as further evidence of involutional depression, and electroconvulsive therapy (ECT) was recommended. With her unstable cardiac condition it was an intervention of quite significant risk, as was related to her family, but her physicians felt that her depression posed an even greater and more immediate life-threatening risk, and that, without treatment, she would surely die within a matter of weeks.

The patient initially had refused ECT, and her family recoiled at the idea of it, but after much discussion, her husband finally convinced his wife to consent to the treatment. She received nine electroconvulsive treatments, and responded with improved appetite, better self care, and increased positive interaction with hospital and staff. She was discharged to home and scheduled for outpatient follow-up. She was doing well on the subsequent two-monthly visits and then was not seen for seven weeks, at which time she required readmission for recurrence of severe depression. Her cardiac condition at this time was also decompensated, and she required ICU care. During this time she suffered a massive stroke and died within a few days (Weitzel & Puitilo, 1979).

Although this story is packed with ethical quandaries, it is not an unusual one. Rather it is probably a typical and even common sort of situation faced by mental health professionals who deal with aged patients. One central issue it raises, that will be discussed in detail, is that of mental competence and informed consent in persons with emotional disorders or impaired cognitive abilities. This is especially problematic when one must consider what constitutes "heroic" or extraordinary intervention in the elderly, and when such intervention is not indicated.

MENTAL COMPETENCE AND INFORMED CONSENT

The question of mental competence is highlighted because we accept the requirement for free and informed consent, in both treatment and research. This is a very recent addition to the rituals of medical care, and stems from increased emphasis on respect for personal autonomy of the patient. Even though psychiatric illness may threaten the very "personhood" on which the principle of respect for personal autonomy is based, current opinions lean towards seeing the psychiatric patient as an autonomous agent to the greatest degree possible. This includes the condition of informed consent as a prerequisite for treatment. There are three essential components to valid consent:

1. The patient must be competent.
2. The patient must have been informed of the risks and benefits of treatment, alternatives to the proposed treatment, and risks of nontreatment.
3. Patient consent must be voluntary, i.e., noncoerced.

Except in emergency situations, caring for patients is based on an implicit contract: the patient comes or is brought to the doctor seeking help; the doctor offers X and Y therapies; the patient agrees to accept one or both or something else, or, of course, may decide to accept neither—in which case the relationship is re-negotiated or the contract dissolved. A third possible outcome is that the patient's competency will be questioned. In most clinical practice situations this contract is never made explicit nor does it need to be. In certain situations, those that are likely to be of greater risk to the patient, or involving significant or invasive procedures, modern medicine has ritualized the contract by the process of informed consent.

The process of informed consent includes adequate disclosure of information, comprehension of that information, acceptance by the patient that the information is correct, and utilization of this information in deciding to give or withhold consent. Finally, the patient must be able to communicate his or her decision. There are obviously many places in this process where mental impairment calls into question validity of consent, but not all those problems can be equated with incompetence. Aphasia, for example, may limit understanding and communication, but, with special efforts, adequate communication can be established. Likewise, mental impairment in mild or moderate dementia is not incompatible with a level of understanding that makes it possible to evaluate basic risks and available options. However, attention and time must be given to the communication process with these patients.

The legal context in the United States regarding informed consent is often more confusing than helpful. There has been a lively and contentious debate about measures to protect patients' rights to make their own, well-informed decisions about their medical care and implications about the responsibilities of doctors and nurses to ensure that those rights are respected. The legal conundrum for physicians, as regards patients with questionable competence, involves the following dilemmas. The consent of an incompetent person does not legally or ethically give valid authorization to a physician to perform medical treatment. Unconsented medical treatment can be viewed by the law as "battery." On the other hand, the physician who withholds needed treatment from an incompetent patient because of the patient's refusal can be held legally, and ethically, negligent if no steps are taken to establish some other valid authorization. The above case of Mrs. Smith poses two challenges to the determination of competence: depression and dementia.

DEPRESSION

Depression has presented one of the classic "Catch 22's" of the competence conundrum, especially in the situation of refusal of life-saving therapy. The classic case is the patient with multiple organ-system failure in an intensive care unit who conveys a message that he wants to die and wants life support systems terminated. The aggressive heroic physicians counter with a diagnosis of depression, that medicalizes the patient's despair, revokes his autonomy, renders him incompetent, and his decision invalid.This is not to find fault with the psychiatric diagnosis of depression. One surely has an important responsibility to intervene promptly and effectively with patients in whom depression may be a life-threatening illness, and to listen for and attend to suicidal ideation. But, there are many psychological characteristics of persons in the dying process that are similar, if not identical, to those of clinical depression. When is it right to treat aggressively, and when, instead, to offer spiritual guidance and caring attention while allowing someone mercifully to die? This is the fine line that must be tread particularly in the care of the elderly. For the ICU patient one easily might inquire, who wouldn't be depressed in such a situation? Is this a normal response? Should the patient's wishes be honored as perhaps the only shred of personal autonomy he has left? Or should doxepin be added to the already long list of medications he is receiving, and efforts be redoubled to pull him out of this?

It is possible to view the symptoms of Mrs. Smith in a cultural context in which the diagnosis of psychotic depression becomes irrelevant or meaningless. Perhaps she had begun to tire of the strains of her life and her chronic illness, and had begun to look forward to death as a release. In some religious contexts, this is a normal part of the aging process. For this lady, there may have been unresolved guilt about some past events which she symbolized as "evil demons" within her. The sadness then was not that she had decided that her time had come, but rather that she did not see it as a joyous release leading to heavenly rewards. She was anxious and fearful of meeting her maker, and perhaps the treatment of choice in such a case would be a religious one. She may have needed spiritual counseling more than she needed ECT. Her paranoia may have grown out of this anxiety. Fear of doctors is common, and it is important not to see this as totally delusional.

It is crucial to attend to the disabling condition of depression in the elderly and not to write them off simply because of their age. But there is clearly more than simply changes in biogenic amines to explain the epidemic of depression in this age group. If chronic disease were not enough, there is economic strangulation, social abnegation, and loneliness. These things cannot be cured by tricyclics or even by ECT. Depression may be an appropriate response to the situation many elderly people find themselves in, and it may be that in some cases more good is done for patients and perhaps, indirectly, for the quality of society by respecting the perceptions and reactions of people as autonomous agents in their final days. Clinicians must probe deeper into the actual *meaning* of "psychiatric symptoms." Often there is a reality underlying these symptoms, the importance of which overwhelms the ability of medical treatment to ameliorate symptoms.

For patients whose prognosis is obviously hopeless, e.g., the person with widely metastatic cancer, the physicians would be more likely to "respect the patient's wishes," and let him or her "die with dignity." In fact, this really may not be respecting the wishes of another, but rather only be coincidental that both physician and patient have the same assessment of the situation. The real test of respect for autonomy of another person comes when one disagrees with the choices of another person or the values on which they are based (e.g., Mrs. Smith's doctors intuitively felt it was wrong to simply let her die). This test is strenuous, especially in a profession which draws its ethical tradition from two-and-a-half centuries of admonitions to do what *you* think is right. Before examining this tradition in more detail, the parallel problem as it relates to dementia will be examined.

DEMENTIA

In questioning the mental competence of a depressed person, one is concerned that the pathological mood disturbance will influence the person to make decisions that really are not in his or her best interest. An example of such a case was described to this author by Roth (1981). A patient who was severely depressed was asked to consent to ECT. When told that a very small percentage of patients had actually died from complications of the therapy, she responded, "Oh, good. I hope I'm one of them." Should this be considered a competent consent? It is clear that the patient *understands* what she has been told, but we question her *judgment*. On the other hand, in patients who have cognitive loss (i.e., dementia), the concern is their ability to understand the information given to them and to make use of it in the process of judgment.

The issue of competence in the demented patient strikes directly at the tension between the desire to do what is best for the patient, and its pejorative extreme, *paternalism,* and the desire to respect the rights and autonomy of that person, which has its pejorative extreme in something like "abandonment." The advances of modern medicine have not contributed to the solution of this tension either. Even though our ability to treat disease or symptoms has increased, the *risks* of therapy—and of some diagnostic procedures as well—has increased apace. One's ability to make accurate predictions of outcomes has not comparably improved, however. In fact, at best one usually can give a patient statistical probabilities to weigh the risks of disease against the risks of treatment, knowing how often even those statistics are reinterpreted or revised. In addition, often a cure cannot be offered, but rather some degree of symptomatic improvement in a disorder that may be progressive. Prolongation of life can be offered, but with persisting disability of some degrees. This is the reality of chronic disease with which may geriatricians are very familiar. Choosing therapies in this context is indeed a *value judgment.*

This means that "medical" decisions sometimes actually rest on value judgments that patients can best make for themselves. The normal (competent) patient may make a decision that the physician would not make for himself or herself, but in most cases there is little question that the patient has a right to decide in the context of his or her own value system. There may be a very fine line between considering a patient's decision "rational" and declaring him or her "incompetent." The legal criteria most commonly used to establish or test competence are the following:

1. Can the person make choices concerning his life?
2. Are the outcomes of these choices "reasonable"?
3. Are these choices based on "rational" reasons?

De jure competence rulings made by courts are generally in the context of setting up guardianship or conservatorship arrangements. They always consider specific aspects of competence (i.e., competence to handle finances, make a will, stand trial, etc.). In the *de facto* judgments that physicians, and often psychiatrists, are called on to make in the context of medical care, the specific issue is whether the person is competent to make decisions concerning his or her own medical care. A decision of incompetence in one of these areas is in most jurisdictions not relevant to other areas. One may not assume incompetence in reference to informed consent simply because the patient has a court-appointed guardian, for example.

It would seem that this is as it should be. The nature of these decisions is quite different. One may not be able to balance a checkbook, but still know quite well whether one wants to live or be allowed to die. But the degree of intellectual ability necessary for an ethically valid consent has not been established in either medical or legal terms. Most physicians will use some kind of notion of "rationality" in assessing competence, but it is often a more limited notion than that established in court cases.

The emphasis on rationality as a criterion for competence has a couple of significant limitations. Competence is a specific function; one is competent to make a will but not to perform neurosurgery. Thus, in considering problems of informed consent, the concern is about the competence of demented patients in relation to their ability to make decisions about their own medical care. It is interesting that many physicians seem less concerned if patients understand anything about medical facts, but rather base their judgments of competence on general cognitive ability, memory and judgment (i.e., performance on a standard mental status examination). The reason for this is twofold: first, demented elderly persons may bring out a paternalist reaction, and thus, are not expected to understand. Things are not explained to them as they might be with younger or normal-ability persons. Second, and most interesting, there is really only one way to judge the rationality, or reasonableness, of a patient's decision—and that is to compare it with one's own assessment of the situation. This is the primary criterion used by the courts in adjudicating competence in issues of medical decision making. The obvious limitation in this is that the physician or judge is weighing the decision in light of his or her own value system. Is it not possible for someone (e.g., Mrs. Smith) to make an irrational but valid decision, or a decision based on irrational thinking, which is consistent with a personal value system?

It has been pointed out in the psychiatric literature, that the question of competence only arises if the patient makes a decision that conflicts with the recommendation of the physician (Roth, Meisel & Lidz, 1977). A well known court case in Tennessee involving a woman named Mary Northern illustrates this dilemma. She was a 75-year old single woman with mild cognitive impairment who lived alone in a very poorly-kept apartment that she could not afford to heat adequately. She developed frostbite on both feet and subsequently gangrene with superinfection. When she was brought to the hospital, the physicians felt that bilateral, below-the-knee amputation was indicated. She refused, even though they emphasized that she had less than a 10 percent chance of survival without the operation. The surgeons then took recourse to the courts to have her declared incompetent on the basis of her "irrational" decision. Had she consented, the question of her mental competence to give informed consent would not have been raised (Supreme Court of the United States, 1977).

It may in fact be appropriate that a disagreement or cognitive dissonance is the threshold that triggers a questioning of patient competence. After all, health professionals are concerned as to what is best for the patient, usually are better informed than the patient, make their therapeutic recommendations in good faith, and therefore ought to be somewhat disturbed when the patient's decision seems irrational or even self-destructive. But that very same threshold ought also to signal the likelihood of a values dissonance, instead of, or in addition to, cognitive shortcomings.

Recent studies by Barbara McNeil and her group in Boston have shown that patients vary enormously in their attitudes towards risk-taking (McNeil, Weichselbaum, & Parker, 1978, 1981). More important, they differ as a group from the attitudes of physicians as a group. The cancer patients she studied generally opted for quality of life over the short term, rather than accept a riskier therapy with a chance for longer survival. While these studies were not done specifically with elderly persons, one might imagine that this trend would hold true or perhaps be even stronger. And yet if that elderly person has a mild cognitive deficit, her decision is more likely to be viewed as irrational and therefore incompetent. In fact, the law under which Mary Northern's case came to court was only valid for people over 60 years old—which is to say, if she had been 59 and had no obvious psychiatric disorders, her "irrational" decision could not legally have been considered evidence of incompetence.

Most writers in this field place a heavy emphasis on the criterion of rationality, but acknowledge that other aspects of personhood may be equally relevant. They do not discuss these simply because it is a more difficult job. Few measures have been developed for noncognitive function, and the whole area of personal values is a vague and imprecise one. This issue is important enough to take on some of that vagueness and imprecision in an attempt to at least begin to develop a fuller and more humane notion of competence in the elderly psychiatric patient.

Emotion, and other limbic phenomena, are in some way crucially linked to the formation and the meaning of individual values. Likewise, personality—that vague and yet distinct entity—is a crucial aspect of personhood, and certainly contributes to a person's attitude about life and death decisions concerning his or her own fate. True, these are not measured easily by a ten-point mental status exam, but the science of neuropsychology has progressed towards defining and clarifying some noncognitive functions of the brain. Work in behavioral neurology suggests there are some significant affective aspects to character that may be more relevant to certain areas of competence than strictly cognitive function (Hardy, 1981).

It may not be possible to ever quantitate these functions, but an awareness of and familiarity with the noncognitive aspects of brain function may help clinicians deal more humanely with the tension of evaluating competence in elderly demented patients.

Returning to the case of Mrs. Smith, it is difficult to determine if her decision to accept the ECT was a competent one. Usually a patient's competence is questioned when a recommended course of treatment is refused. But after her initial refusal, her husband finallly convinced her to consent. Not knowing more of the details, it is impossible to pass judgment on the meaning of that event—but it does point to a few important ways in which families and friends of patients can be helpful in clarifying confusing competence questions. For example, important information about the person's value context can be gleaned from discussions with family and friends. While it is possible that people develop new values or change their minds as they age, we generally expect that basic value orientations are consistent over time. If the family described Mrs. Smith as a fighter who never wanted to give up and die in her old age, and persevered in the face of great difficulties, there might have been grounds to assume that her pathological depression was making her suicidal and her initial refusal of treatment was a manifestation of her disease—and therefore an indication of her incompetence. The case as described suggests a level of anxiety that would not be consistent with a sanguine decision to allow death with dignity. The spiritual content of her distress should have been more extensively explored. One can certainly err by going too far to respect autonomy, and the mentally frail elderly is the most significant example of that.

While infantilizing elders should not be encouraged, it may be that, for many people of this age-group, a caring paternalism on the part of caregivers is long overdue and may be the antidote to the terrible neglect they have suffered in the past. Thomas Halper asked, ". . . of what value is liberty to one who is buffetted by the violent winds of the mind (Halper, 1980)?" In society and the medical system, aged persons with mild or moderate dementia may need, and even possibly deserve, some special protection against exploitation and neglect.

In retrospect, it may be easier to criticize "heroic" efforts to treat Mrs. Smith's depression because they were, in fact, finally futile. She died of heart failure. The interplay between her mental condition and her cardiac condition is something on which one can only speculate. But if the ECT had given her months or even a few years of meaningful life, would this not be worth struggling for, even at the cost of overriding her expressed wishes by declaring her incompetent? With a "positive" outcome, most health professionals would probably agree.

On the other hand, some gerontologists and advocates for rights of the elderly maintain that the most caring thing we can do for our patients is to respect their autonomy. George Alexander, for example, has argued eloquently, "It is important to recognize that however benevolent that intention of those who would seek to substitute other decision makers for the aged, persons deprived of the right to decide for themselves will have lost the most basic attribute of citizenship (Alexander & Levin, 1972)." Losing those rights, he seems to suggest, is a small step away from losing one's identity as a person. A few added months of life may not be worth the price of relinquishing one's autonomy.

Once a judgment of incompetence has been made, it is not easy to have it reversed. It takes a competent and aggressive legal advocate, and financial wherewithal to obtain that support. Once the label of incompetence has been used on a medical chart, its presence will continue to influence the attitudes of all health professionals who have access to it. It can deal a devastating blow to the level of respect a patient receives during contact with the health care system. Since confusional states in the elderly are often reversible, and levels of mental competence are more likely to fluctuate than not, it is clear that one ought to consider very carefully before placing such a far-reaching epithet in a permanent medical document.

Old people embody the mystery of their future as well as the history of their past. Trying to make decisions based on likely outcomes of disease and treatment is a lot like shadow boxing. The outlines are visible, but the reality is ephemeral. It is uncertain if research will ever enable us to know more accurately who will benefit from aggressive treatment and who will not, but for the time being the risk-benefit analysis can only be meaningful if it includes the manifold meanings of the treatment, the disease, and continued existence itself . . . to the patient.

REFERENCES

Alexander, G.J., & Levin, T.H.D. *The aged and the need for surrogate management.* Syracuse, New York: Syracuse University Press, 1972, p. 4.

Halper, T. The double-edged sword: Paternalism as a policy in the problems of aging. *Milbank Memorial Fund Quarterly,* 1980, *58,* 487.

Hardy, P. Personal communication. Department of Behavioral Neurology, Tufts New England Medical Center, 1981.

McNeil, B.J., Weichselbaum, R., & Parker, S.G. Fallacy of the five year survival in lung cancer. *New England Journal of Medicine,* 1978, *299,* 1397–1401.

McNeil, B.J., Weichselbaum, R., & Parker, S.G. Speech and survival: Tradeoffs between quality and quantity of life in laryngeal cancer. *New England Journal of Medicine,* 1981, *305,* 982–987.

Mill, J.S. *On liberty and other essays.* New York: MacMillan, 1926, p. 90.

Reiser, S, Curran, W., & Dych, A., *Ethics in medicine.* Cambridge, Mass.: MIT Press, 1977, pp. 5–9.

Roth, L.H. Personal communication, 1981.

Roth, L.H., Meisel, A., & Lidz, C.W. Test of competency to consent to treatment. *American Journal of Psychiatry,* 1977, *134,* 281.

Schloendorff, V. New York Hospital 211. *New York:* 125, 127, 129; 105 N.W., 92, 93, 1914.

Supreme Court of the United States. *Application for stay of mandate of Tennessee Court of Appeals, Middle Section at Nashville in re Mary Northern.* October Term, 1977.

Veatch, R.M. *A theory of medical ethics.* New York: Basic Books, Inc., 1981.

Weitzel, W.D., & Puitilo, R. Aggressive treatment of geriatric depression: What limits on intervention? *Psychiatrics Opinion,* May 1979, *16* (5), 9–14.

16

THE IMPACT OF SOCIAL POLICY AND PLANNING ISSUES ON GERIATRIC MENTAL HEALTH CARE

Valerie Crooks

The tasks of the mental health professional serving elderly patients and their families are sufficiently time and talent-consuming without the added frustration of dealing with disparate, confusing, and sometimes hostile social policies. Yet, the importance of social policy to daily clinical practice with the elderly cannot be easily ignored. Similarly, clinical practice ultimately has a profound influence on social policy. The current contradictions and ambiguities of mental health policies for the elderly are the result of conflicting professional values and technologies of practitioners as well as fragmented and uncoordinated health and social service networks. Consequently, understanding social planning and policy and their implications for practice is essential in providing comprehensive mental health services to the elderly.

This chapter will present an overview of mental health care of the elderly by examining prevalence, major policies and systemic factors, evaluating current and future trends, and finally by making legislative and program recommendations to policy makers, planners and clinicians.

GERIATRIC MENTAL HEALTH
ISBN 0-8089-1657-2

PREVALENCE AND UTILIZATION FACTORS IN GERIATRIC MENTAL HEALTH

In 1973, the World Health Organization estimated that the degree of psychopathology was more prevalent among the elderly (236.1 per 100,000) than any other age group (Butler, 1975). Numerous studies have estimated that from 18 to 25 percent of the elderly have significant mental health problems (Pardes, 1981). The most prevalent types of clinically diagnosed mental disorders among the aged are depression (10 percent) and dementia (5 percent) (Federal Council on Aging, 1981). Rate of utilization of psychiatric services is another useful indicator of the prevalence of mental disorders in the elderly. In 1975, there were 3.4 million admissions for psychiatric services and approximately 5 percent were patients 65 years of age and older (Redick & Taube, 1980).

In spite of the need for psychiatric services for the elderly, availability in recent years has been limited. The National Institute of Mental Health (NIMH) had estimated that in 1980 approximately 80 percent of the elderly who needed mental health care services did not receive them (National Retired Teacher's Association (NRTA) & American Association of Retired Persons (AARP), 1982). The percentage of elderly in institutional and community-based mental health settings over a period of 15 years is illustrated in Table 16-1. Compiled data strongly suggests a shift from public mental hospital care to more community-based care. Yet, with the exception of the nursing home, utilization rates for community care are far lower than the estimated need.

Table 16-1.

*Estimated Percent of Persons 65 and Over with Mental Disorders in Various Institutional/Community Settings**

	1964	1979
Public mental hospitals	51–70	30
Private mental hospitals	1–5	<1–2.9
General hospitals	13–17	11.7
Psychiatric units of		1.2
Nursing homes	43–75	16–61
Out-patient psychiatric clinics	8	6
Community Mental Health		4
Private		2

* Estimates derived from Birren & Renner, 1975; Cohen, 1980; Federal Council on Aging, 1981; Pardes, 1981; Rosen, Anderson, & Bahn, 1967; Sherwood, 1980.

POLICIES AFFECTING GERIATRIC MENTAL HEALTH

Since the sixties, three major legislative policies have had impact on mental health care of the elderly. First, in 1963, the Community Mental Health Centers Act was introduced and greatly facilitated the increasing shift from public institutional care to community-based care. The act was set up to provide five essential services that included 24-hour in-patient services, out-patient care, partial hospitalization, consultation, and education. Since large numbers of elderly were being discharged from state hospitals, it was expected that these community-based services would serve them along with all age groups. Second, in 1965, Medicare and Medicaid were established to provide for the health care needs of the elderly. These programs included provisions for in-patient and out-patient psychiatric services. Third, in 1980, the Mental Health Systems Act was passed and was designed to make funding available for broader and more coordinated mental health services to the needy elderly and to link community nursing homes to services. Nominally, each of these three efforts supports a reasonable community-based mental health care system for the elderly. In reality, however, a statement made 13 years ago still applies: "Public policy in mental health care of the elderly is confused, riddled with contradictions, and shortsighted limitations and in need of intensive scrutiny geared to immediate and long-term action" (U.S. Senate Special Committee on Aging, 1971).

LIMITATIONS IN ACCESS AND BUDGET

Accessibility to the variety of mental health care settings has been particularly influenced by federal health legislation and budgets. The 640 community mental health centers available today persist in admitting younger populations more frequently than older ones. Only 4 percent of all patients at these centers are 65 and over (Dagon, 1982). Considering estimated need, few communities have developed special geriatric out-patient mental health programs. In fact, two-thirds of the total 1974 mental health care budget of 14.5 billion dollars went towards institutional care. Recent budget analysis indicates that as little as 1.3 percent of these total direct care funds are used for the community elderly (Cohen, 1980).

Although Medicare and Medicaid are landmark health care programs, their limited support for mental health care has been demonstrated. In 1979, only 2 percent of the Medicare dollar went into mental health care for the elderly and disabled. Slightly over one-tenth of 1 percent of those dollars went to Community Mental Health Centers. Similar figures are reported in previous years of Medicare coverage. Thus, since its beginning in 1965, Medicare has not altered its limited support for mental health care services. Psychiatric hospitalization benefits are limited to 180 lifetime days and many Community Mental Health Centers are not given provider status, thus eliminating Medicare reimbursement. Part B Medicare provides an annual ceiling of only $250 for out-patient mental health services (U.S. Department of Health and Human Services (USDH&HS), 1980). Moreover, from 1980 to 1984, the deductible for Medicare Part B was raised from $60 to $75 per year and Part A deductible was raised from $180 to $356. Limited funding and lack of provider status in community mental health centers greatly precludes use of these services.

Three current features of Medicaid diminish its effectiveness. First, while Medicaid provides limited mental health services to low income elderly, only 15–20 percent of the elderly are eligible. Second, funding for Medicaid increasingly is being diminished. The federal share of Medicaid payments was reduced by 4 percent in 1983 and was further reduced by 4.5 percent in 1984. Third, the program is structured to provide institutional care more readily than community care.

Conceptually, the Mental Health Systems Act was a potential boon for the elderly in that it required a comprehensive and coordinated mental health care system. However, within months after its passage, it was consolidated with alcohol and substance-abuse services into a block grant established through the 1981 Omnibus Budget Reconciliation Act. This essentially masked the intended focus on the needy elderly and reduced prior categorical program funding by 25 percent (Estes & Lee, 1981). Moreover, the block grant concept offers wide discretion to individual states and limits the potential for uniform benefits to a target population such as the elderly.

The budgets of other federal programs supporting research, training, and demonstration projects for the elderly are maintaining current funding levels or being cut back. In 1984, the National Institute on Aging, the National Institute of Mental Health (NIMH) Center on Aging, and Health Care Financing Administration are expected to receive budgets close to 1983 levels. The NIMH Center on Aging expenditures in research on "mental disorders of aging," which constitutes approximately 6 percent of its total research budget, will remain essentially the same—from 9.6 million dollars in 1983 to 10.6 million dollars in 1984. Funding for Title IV of the Older Americans Act that provides for several innovative demonstration projects such as the Retired Senior Volunteer Program, was cut in half from 40.5 million dollars in 1981 to 22.2 million dollars in 1983. The projected budget in 1984 is expected to decrease the program by another 77 percent (Krogh, 1983). While these programs are not involved with direct mental health care for the elderly, they do represent important supportive opportunities for many.

LIMITATIONS OF DEINSTITUTIONALIZATION AND COMMUNITY-BASED CARE

The impetus for publically sponsored community-based mental health care arises from two trends. The first is a growing movement toward the provision of preventive services in the community, and the second is the reduction of admissions to state hospitals.

While prevention of mental illness in the community is a crucial responsibility, it has been given little more than lip service (Braceland, 1972). What has, in fact, evolved is a system that has "prevented" the development of a viable continuum of mental health care. Furthermore, this system often serves as a social-control mechanism that favors providing psychiatric services to younger and potentially more disruptive populations over the geriatric population (Williams, Bellis, & Wellington 1980). Additionally, preventive community mental health care for the elderly is hindered by the lack of reliable access and consistent quality clinical care.

Prior to 1960, the public state hospital was the dominant setting for care of the mentally ill, particularly for the elderly (see Table 16-1). However, in order to shift the fiscal responsibility for mental health care to federal and local governments, states began to discharge patients into the community. Thus by 1979, 30 percent of all state hospital patients were 65 and over, compared to well over 50 percent in 1964 (Pardes, 1981). Unfortunately, outpatient care was often not feasible with patients who required ongoing care to maintain function, and, consequently, over the past twenty years many of these patients have been "transinstitutionalized" into nursing homes (Borus, 1981).

Despite the intent to deinstitutionalize the mentally ill, consequences for the elderly have been relatively unimpressive. Nursing homes and state hospitals still have a disproportionate number of geriatric patients. Previous political statements regarding the elimination of "harmful" public institutional placement have now been reconstituted on the nursing home, which has become the second most frequently used place of referral for discharges from all types of psychiatric institutions (Federal Council on Aging, (FCOA)1981). Considerable debate has emerged regarding the relative quality of mental health care in these settings. However, most nursing homes do not have either the commitment, the professional staff, nor the funding to provide for the chronically disabled mentally ill geriatric patient.

Court decisions have established legal credibility to the goals of appropriate access and quality care in institutional settings. In 1966, the case of Lake versus Cameron affirmed the legal right of access to appropriate alternative community facilities regardless of financial circumstances. In 1975 the case of O'Connor versus Donaldson reinforced the policy of "right-to-treatment" in mental health care institutions. Yet, if given scrupulous support in practice, this would severely tax the capabilities and available resources of the current public mental health care system.

SYSTEMIC FACTORS AFFECTING GERIATRIC MENTAL HEALTH

The Client

The older person who needs mental health care is not only stymied by the aforementioned policy limitations, but also by his or her own individual personal and social context. The relative heterogeneity of personality and adjustment among elderly persons compared to other groups makes the need for individualization of treatment paramount. Critical factors, such as number and quality of family and community supports, lower socioeconomic status, heightened physical disabilities, immobility, poor proximity, and transportation services all serve to modify and often circumvent access to appropriate mental health care.

The attitudes of the current old age cohort add to the complexity of access problems. Few elderly patients voluntarily seek out mental health services (Gurian, 1982). Some feel reluctance for cultural reasons, others fear that they will be institutionalized (Thompson, 1978). Some studies have demonstrated that many elderly do not believe that mental health assistance is appropriate for their needs. In one NIMH study of eight community mental health centers, normal elders expressed opinions that associated mental health care with "crazy people" and long hospitalization. Such problems as depression and anxiety were not viewed as appropriate to present to mental health professionals (Patterson, 1976). Frequently, such complaints are directed to general medical practitioners and often subsumed in a list of organic complaints (Hilkevitch, 1965).

Professionals

Three major obstacles to services for the elderly are imposed by mental health professionals. Ageism, the first obstacle, is difficult to disentangle from mental health professionals' values and biases. The prevailing notion that the conditions of the elderly are irreversible and untreatable is demonstrated by the therapeutic nihilism persistent among many professionals (Cohen, 1976; Gaitz, 1974; Kling, 1981; Patterson, 1976). Those providing institutional care for the geriatric mentally ill often have illustrated negative and inappropriate attitudes toward their patients (Kling, 1981; Teeter, Garetz, Miller et al., 1976).

Interprofessional rivalry in public programs is the second major barrier to quality treatment for the geriatric patient. Professional infighting, the blurring of role-related tasks, and use of paraprofessionals and nonmedical professionals have caused some clinicians to leave publicly funded centers in favor of private practice. Moreover, this interdisciplinary rivalry often results in a lack of clinical service integration for the patient (Gaitz & Hacker, 1970; Mollica, 1983). While effective interdisciplinary evaluation is essential, particularly to the elderly mentally ill patient, often it is sacrificed because of professional rigidity and mutual disrespect.

Overcoming the third professional obstacle, inappropriate and underdeveloped diagnostic and treatment technologies, is especially critical to effective mental health care of the elderly. In one study of two nursing homes in Minneapolis, 61 percent of the 74 patients had undiagnosed psychiatric problems (Teeter, Garetz, Miller et al., 1976). In such cases, missed diagnoses can result in inappropriate treatments. While it is true that psychiatric consultation in nursing homes is sparse, such problems can exist in the community as well. As mentioned earlier, general practitioners are most likely to see psychiatrically distrubed patients and yet often do not refer these patients to psychiatric clinics (Hilkevitch, 1965; Peterson, 1978; Stotsky, 1972). The underdeveloped psychiatric skills of the general practitioner can increase the number of missed diagnoses and treatments. Additionally, ignorance of unique symptom presentations and lack of age-specific assessment instruments among psychiatrists, psychologists, and social workers can result in misapplied therapeutic approaches (Blazer, 1980; Dagon, 1982).

Agencies

Community provision of mental health care to the elderly necessitates an array of programs that offer different types of health and social services. The requirement of a comprehensive and coordinated resource network has been supported by gerontologists and emphasized in a variety of surveys (Cohen, 1976; Jurkiewicz, 1980; Rathbone-McCuan & Claymon, 1979). Where relatively comprehensive services are present, however, turf barriers and competition for funds exist between health and social agencies. In communities with less comprehensive services, interagency coordination and integration of client services are even more sharply curtailed. Such conditions add to the frustrations of the older person with reduced cognitive function and mental disorders.

A mental health agency with internal problems also can restrict availability for the elderly client. Even though an elderly person may be ready to request services, he or she may be faced with an agency that lacks appropriate or sufficient staff and resources or has restrictive eligibility or acceptability requirements (Rathbone-McCuan & Claymon, 1979). Many elderly clients do not fit the service or professional orientation offered at an agency, so clients are assessed and treated in a way that fits the agency services. Treatment and service delivery can also be delayed intentionally or unintentionally to fit the agency's schedule rather than the client's needs.

POSITIVE TRENDS IN GERIATRIC MENTAL HEALTH

Sifting through the morass of political and systemic factors influencing the mental health of the aged, it is evident that these are not times for stalwart optimism. Yet, some heartening advances are beginning to surface. As new assessment and treatment strategies are being developed, so too are public and private programs and policies emerging that support appropriate and humane mental health care for the aged.

Many of the chapters in this book have reported the potential for and success of various diagnostic and treatment methods for mental health care of the aged. Viable treatments for depression, dementia, and special problems such as memory, sexual adjustment, and alcoholism all have been presented. When adequate personnel and resources are applied to older persons' needs, treatment and program efficacy has been demonstrated. Few knowledgeable clinicians would reject the notion that, at the least, mental health needs of the aged have potential for amelioration (Braceland, 1972).

In a 5½ year study done in Yorkton, Canada, it was found that the vast majority of mental health conditions that require treatment in the elderly are controllable and conducive to home or community placement (Lipscomb, 1971). One large research survey on clinical outcomes in private psychiatric hospitals found that nearly three-quarters of patients over 65 were returned home improved after relatively short hospitalizations (Butler, 1975). Similar encouraging findings were found in a geropsychiatry center in Wisconsin, where only 3 percent of elderly patients required nursing home placement (Dagon, 1982).

A variety of treatment strategies have been implemented throughout the mental health care system with specific emphasis on the aging clients. Table 16-2 lists a number of major approaches employed. These promising efforts are signs of growing interest and commitment to the mental health care of the aged. In addition to these therapeutic techniques, are the expansion and development or roles such as consultants, case managers, volunteer counselors, advocates, and ombudsman.

An impressive array of institutional and community resources are available in many larger metropolitan areas. Table 16-3 illustrates major resources that include special programs to improve access and prevent mental health breakdown among the elderly. In some communities, where these programs are either absent or minimal, there is a growing awareness that these types of services are conducive to healthy community living (Jur-

Table 16-2.

Summary of Major Therapeutic Approaches to Mental Health Problems in the Elderly

Individual	Group	Special
Individual psychotherapy	Psychotherapy groups	Drug therapy
Supportive therapy	Family groups	Milieu therapy
Behavior modification	Reminiscence groups	Reality orientation therapy
Crisis intervention	Resocialization groups	Multidisciplinary team treatment
Life review therapy	Remotivation groups	Network analysis and intervention
Cognitive therapy	Activity therapy	Exercise therapy
Peer counseling	Self-help/Social	
Leisure counseling	Self-advocacy groups	

Table 16-3.

Summary of Mental Health and Related Programs for the Aged

Institutional-Based Programs	Community-Based Mental Health related	Community-Based Social & Health Related Programs
State & government hospital	Geriatric day hospital	Senior centers
Private psychiatric hospital	Geriatric day care	Transportation
General hospital	Aftercare	Nutrition
Special unit	Adult foster care	Meals on wheels
Geropsychiatric unit	Community mental health center	Congregate dining
Nursing home	Screening centers/programs	Recreation
Home for the aged	Outreach	Senior volunteer groups
Domiciliary	Friendly visitors	Information & referral
Board & care	Advocacy-ombudsman	Health care centers
		Visiting nurse services
		Home health aides
		Homemaker services
		Respite services
		Legal services
		Pre-retirement training

kiewicz, 1980). Geriatric day hospitals have served to expedite in-patient discharges, reduce readmissions, and maximize rehabilitation efforts in the community (Matlack, 1975). Preliminary studies of screening centers for long-term care applicants have demonstrated that such an approach can actually reduce by as much as 85 precent the use of institutional care for geriatric mental illness (Brody, 1974; Epstein & Simon, 1968).

The Older Americans Act enacted by Congress in 1965 has served to assist persons over 60 to live independently by providing such community services as home health, homemaker, chore, and friendly visitors. These auxiliary services often reduce isolation and circumvent unnecessary institutionalization. Moreover, along with a network of 640 community mental health centers and 5000 senior centers, nearly 700 Area Agencies on Aging are available to work collaboratively with agencies providing services to the elderly. These Area Agencies on Aging can serve as an effective integrating mechanism for all aging programs. Ongoing interagency collaboration and effective linkages with both public and private sectors help to establish a more comprehensive and available social and health resources network. Successful collaboration has resulted in preventive and restorative benefit for the elderly in many communities (Jurkiewicz, 1980; Santore & Diamond, 1974).

Professional mental health-care specialists also appear to be gaining broader public acceptance. Similar national surveys from 1956 and 1976 showed a marked increase in the use of services provided by mental health professionals (Gurin, Veroff, & Feld, 1960; Veroff, Kulka, & Donvan, 1981). As general acceptance increases and better assessment and treatments are developed, this rise should be reflected in the elderly population as well.

The need for special treatments and programs for mental health care of the elderly has stimulated the development of geropsychiatric clinical training programs, research, and political and professional commissions. Since 1979, seven specialty training programs in geropsychiatry were developed at major universities in North Carolina, Pennsylvania, Texas, Illinois, Michigan, California, and Washington. Research in the mental health needs of the elderly has been increasing, particularly through the support of the National Institute of Mental Health (NIMH), which has created the Center for the Study of the Mental Health of the Aging. NIMH support has tripled in this area from $2.5 million in 1975 to $7.5 million in 1980 (Pardes, 1981). Over the past 15 years there has been special professional and political attention focused on mental health of the elderly. This includes the Committee on Mental Health and Mental Illness of the Elderly, the President's Commission on Mental Health, the Congressional Forum on Mental Health and Mental Illness of the Elderly, and special inquiries and program recommendations by the Group for the Advancement of Psychiatry, the American Psychological Association, and the Mental Health Association.

Private sector support and advocacy for the aged can be seen in such groups as the American Association for Retired Persons, the National Retired Teachers Association, the National Association of Retired Federal Employees, the National Council of Senior Citizens, the National Council on Aging, the National Caucus on Black Aged, and the Gray Panthers. Collectively these groups represent a substantial number of senior citizens.

Other private sector developments include the organization of the American Association of Geriatric Psychiatry and the Alzheimer's Disease and Related Disorders Association (ADRDA). The ADRDA, formed in 1979 to support families and advance understanding of dementia, has evolved from 12 to 60 national chapters with an additional network of social and professional support groups to facilitate its efforts.

In his analysis of mental health services, Cohen (1980) cited other global positive signs: (1) an improved perception of mental health problems; (2) new interest in personal, family, and cultural roots; (3) a changing emphasis from producing to experiencing, involving more interpersonal exploration and development emphasis; and (4) an emerging spirit of intergenerationalism.

PLANNING GERIATRIC MENTAL HEALTH SERVICES

Critical Issues in Planning Effectively

As indicated previously, a number of policy, program, and treatment strategies can affect care of the elderly. It is therefore, clear, that effective planning of services must be greatly influenced by the extent of mental illness in the elderly and by the structures and types of treatments available to address the problem.

The data on prevalence of mental illness in the elderly is highly variable. Since most cases are reported through institutional and community-based agencies only, the actual incidence of mental health problems is difficult to determine with certainty. Relatively little definitive data is available on geriatric patients with emotional stress who are seen in physician's offices, clinics, and in isolated rural and some urban neighborhoods. While better epidemiologic studies are needed, each neighborhood or community that is planning to provide mental health services should invest in an appropriately designed survey to measure the extent of local need. These studies would be greatly enhanced by psychiatric consultation aimed at clearly defining the nature and types of maladjustment in the target population and at developing appropriate instruments to adequately gauge depression and dementia.

The organized structures already available to provide mental health care for the aged require close examination by planners. Deciding on the appropriate structure within which to treat a given mental health problem is not achieved easily. Planners need to be aware of what in- and out-patient services are available in their community and what each of these settings can offer the aged patient. Some communities will have state hospitals and nursing homes available; others may have only general hospitals available for in-patient care. Review of utilization patterns can provide important data on the type of care to which patients are most frequently referred in a given community. Additionally, an evaluation of the services and professionals available in the setting will help planners measure relative appropriateness and limitations of the treatment contexts available to meet mental health care needs.

General hospitals, not generally equipped for geropsychiatric patients, may be used to provide care. Given proper preparation, training, and consulting staff, this context can serve as a temporary care facility, and more importantly, a screening center for impending mental health problems of elderly patients. State psychiatric hospitals and nursing homes are usually the structure for care of the long-term mentally ill elderly. Mechanisms and funding must be developed to improve the quality of care, enliven the treatment milieu, and educate staff. Investigation of the comparative efficacy of these and community-based settings has been limited. Alternatives outside institutions that should be considered also include halfway homes, foster care, sheltered care, and group homes. Planners require further data on which of these contexts of care provides the most effective management in terms of financial and psychosocial costs to the patient, family, and community.

Out-patient care provided in mental health clinics and by private clinicians may be the most appropriate treatment context for many patients. A number of studies have demonstrated equal or superior results to in-patient care with older persons (Braun, 1981). Yet, budgetary and eligibility constraints limit the opportunity to utilize these services in many communities. Planners need to consider political and fiscal realities on both the national and community level before the community mental health care concept can be applied in a local area. In some communities, mental health centers are unavailable and the context of care may be a senior center, hotel, apartment building, church, or a patient's home. The locus of care is variable from community-to-community, and planners must design a budget and policy that maximize the effectiveness of the extant, albeit incomplete, settings.

Beyond the officially designated mental health care settings exists a larger community network with programs and policies that may support or hinder mental health of the elderly. A complete inventory of private and public health and social welfare resources in a community is the critical first step in rational planning. Public policy imposes a series of limitations on the structure and nature of programs that can be developed. In a national survey and site visit study done in middle-sized communities in 1979, a number of policy problems were cited that prevented appropriate service development and interorganizational and interagency collaboration for the care of the aged. Categorical funding and inconsistent or contradictory eligibility requirements for services were frequent obstacles. In many communities, resources such as foster care, day care, nursing home grievance/ombudsman, and adult protective services were either missing or severely inadequate (Jurkiewicz, 1980).

The availability of these programs in a community can serve, in many cases, as an excellent alternative to (sometimes inappropriate) institutionally-based mental health care. On the other hand, difficulties emanating from a lack of domain consensus between agencies can disrupt the most well-intentioned mental health programs. Despite these problems, some positive community experiences with interorganizational and case coordination models that help access services for the elderly have emerged and should be analyzed for exportability and relevance to other communities (Jurkiewicz, 1980).

In addition to direct and indirect structures for delivering mental health care to the elderly, are treatments that clinicians provide. These individual, group, and special therapies cited throughout this book and partially summarized in Table 16-2 have frequently been shown to be effective with different elderly groups. In order to plan effectively within a given context of care, it is important that types of treatments available are known to providers, can generate support, and can be proven efficacious for the elderly target population.

Another factor to be considered in effective planning is the type of professionals selected to provide care. Mental health professionals include psychiatrists, psychologists, social workers, and nurses. These professionals often share common goals and use similar therapeutic techniques. In fact, with the exception of private mental health care settings, an increasing "blurring of professional roles" has been found particularly in public in-patient and out-patient facilities providing mental health care. With the obvious exception of physical exams and prescribing drugs, task differences between psychiatrists and other professional groups in many public settings appear minimal (Redlich & Kellert, 1978).

Greater differences between mental health professionals occur in setting location and therapeutic techniques used. In a study done by Redlich and Kellert in a northeastern region of the United States, the following breakdown of professionals occurred: nurses were concentrated in state in-patient facilities, social workers in out-patient facilities, psychologists in out-patient and private practice, and psychiatrists in administrative positions in in-patient facilities and in private practice. Other findings indicated that psychiatrists were involved principally in individual psychotherapy, group therapy was practiced mostly by nurses, and family therapy was practiced mostly by social workers (Redlich & Kellert, 1978). Thus, the type of professional may influence where and what types of services will be provided.

Beyond traditional roles are a growing number of expanded roles for the professional and non-professional. Such roles as a personal representative, case manager, consultant/resource person, advocate, and outreach worker are emerging as especially relevant and effective roles in providing mental health care for the elderly (Davis, 1983; Gaitz & Hacker, 1970; Rathbone-McCuan & Claymon, 1979; Santore & Diamond, 1974; Stotsky, 1972). These roles aid the elderly person in bridging the social network and reducing frustration. Developing self-help organizations and the training and use of skilled volunteers is another mechanism that can facilitate independence of the elderly and maximize resources available in many communities. Planners need to know about and utilize available professionals, non-professionals, and other groups.

Values in Planning and Policy

When the history of mental health care in the United States is examined, two prevailing values emerge. The first is based on the concept of need and the value that the best services should go to the most needy. The second involves the concept of gain and the value that results attained should be equal to the investment (Mechanic, 1969). In providing care to the elderly person with mental health problems, these two values may compromise each other. Mechanic points to this dilemma when he suggests that treatment that cares for the illness when it happens, and also slows the potential for recurrence, is an efficient approach that meets these two values. "Thus, when all other factors are constant . . . we would expect curing the condition of a child or a young adult to result in continuing gains throughout the person's life. [Yet] the same cure in the case of an older person would not produce an equal yield" (Mechanic, 1969). The values of preventive mental health care and early treatment have been the desired aim of many planners, policy-makers, and practitioners. It is little wonder then that mental health care for the elderly has been seen as unattractive and inherently futile to many professionals and planners. However, recent research in dementia and depression, and treatment successes with the elderly have potentiated outcomes more in keeping with the investment of resources. The values of need and gain now appear relevant to the elderly and underline the importance of prevention and early treatment for a group that is becoming increasingly long-lived.

The value of prevention in mental health services to the aged has been expressed in the development of a number of programs, roles, and therapeutic techniques. Social action programs that involve senior clients and address larger social issues, and that provide crisis-oriented centers and milieu treatment in in-patient facilities, case managers, advocates, outreach workers, and educational and community support projects, can all serve to prevent or reduce mental health problems among the elderly. Professionals who provide education and develop support systems that involve families, friends, and neighborhoods offer efficient and creditable prevention. Planners and policy-makers who support these efforts are endorsing the validity of prevention for the elderly population.

The value of traditional or curative mental health services is also well recognized. Such services are critical to slowing and eliminating disabilities of chronically mentally ill elderly. In times of scarce resources, money and care are focused generally on this type of care. Elderly patients with chronic dementias and severe depression must be provided with the best therapeutic opportunities for maximum self-care and independence.

Pitting the relative value of social (preventive) solutions against medical and psychiatric (curative) solutions to the mental health needs of the elderly is not only unproductive but actually harmful. Fortunately, among many professionals and community planners, an integrated system of mental health care for the elderly is an emerging value. The efforts borne of the Older Americans Act and the Area Agencies on Aging confirm the value of preventive programs and interagency coordination. Additionally, the need for a multidisciplinary approach to providing care for mental health problems of the elderly has been demonstrated (Gaitz & Hacker, 1970). An effective integration of the tasks and roles of various professionals and programs can enhance recognition and treatment of elderly clients on a community level. As an example, mental impairment accompanying physical illness is a frequent occurrence in the elderly and early involvement by mental health professionals may decrease the seriousness of such an impairment and aid in an earlier and longer return to the community. When effective medical care is backed with consistent supportive treatments, a community can go a long way toward promoting the mental health care of the elderly. Mutual communication and education between medical, psychiatric, and social disciplines should be supported and sustained.

Although there are a number of differences in professional values and skills that circumvent a wholly integrated system, the basic need and value of such an approach in many communities cannot be denied. Planners and policy-makers that fiscally support and reward interagency and interprofessional collaborations will have contributed to a system that provides both prevention and cure and integrates the biopsychosocial needs of the elderly population.

RECOMMENDATIONS TO PLANNERS AND POLICY-MAKERS

Over 25 years ago, Kolb suggested a broad-based geriatric mental health program on a state and community level that would provide opportunities for the aged to live at home. His recommendations included: "assisted housing prospects for the aged, mental health clinics, home treatment plans, . . . day centers, pensions, discriminating employment practices and fixed age versus flexible retirement policies need attention and study so that agencies, services, and practices may develop along lines designed to give maximum efficiency in preventing premature mental decay" (Kolb, 1956). In some communities, most of these recommendations have been given considerable attention in recent years and successful policies and programs have been initiated. Yet, overall, many of these still valid suggestions have not been applied to the current mental health scene for the elderly. At best, some communities require expansion or maintenance of these efforts; at worst, such efforts are virtually non-existent. These unfulfilled recommendations from the past highlight the need for greater commitment and concentration on special requirements and programs that can enhance the quality of life for elderly persons.

This chapter has given testimony to the fact that social policies significantly influence the planning and implementation of programs. Similarly, professionals and community planners can create and develop new programs that support the mental health care of the elderly. What follows is a summary of feasible recommendations that can be applied in many communities.

Recommendations that involve legislative policy and funding include:

1. Expansion and support for Adult Protective Services and home care.
2. Improvement of existing institutional and community settings providing mental health care by increasing professional personnel and renovating substandard facilities.
3. A shift in emphasis on institutional to appropriate community care by expansion of coverage for out-patient care, extending Medicare provider status to community mental health care centers, elimination of separate health and mental health care deductibles, and tripling the reimbursement rate under Medicare.
4. Utilization of the Area Agency on Aging as an external mechanism to enforce coordination and integration of physical, mental, and social services on an interorganizational level.
5. Maintenance and augmentation of community health and social support networks such as Visiting Nurse Services and Senior Centers.
6. Provision of education, training, and personnel development in geriatric mental health.
7. Continuation and extension of research on dementia and other mental health problems of the elderly.
8. Broadening of Medicaid coverage for out-patient mental health services for the elderly.
9. Development of reliable standards of mental health care in all treatment settings with particular focus on chronic-care facilities and nursing homes.

Recommendations that involve program design and enhancement include:

1. Implementation of high quality innovative programs such as outreach, advocacy, respite, case management, screening health centers, day care, and day hospitals.
2. Application of systematic and well-designed evaluations of programs.
3. Coordination and integration of physical and mental health services on an intra-agency level.
4. Provision of indirect supportive programs such as legal aid, telephone reassurance, Meals on Wheels, volunteer services, and friendly visitors.
5. Development of highly visible, accessible programs that are appealing and demonstrate a readiness to deliver care to the mentally disabled aged.
6. Incorporation of aged and their families in the planning and development of community mental health programs.
7. Facilitation of public education about dementia and other mental health care problems of the aged.

In general, legislative recommendations emphasize the need for mental health services to become defined more clearly, available, and reimbursible. Suggested program innovations emphasize the enhancement of community supports, improvement of physical and mental health collaboration, and the provision of viable alternatives to institutional care. Other programs that support social networks, train and use older volunteers, provide recreational and educational opportunities, and develop work roles for the aged, are also commendable strategies for improving the quality of geriatric mental health.

GUIDELINES FOR CLINICIANS

The recommendations for policy program development are only partial answers to the complex issues of geriatric mental health care. Mental health professionals must be involved in the resolution of many practice and philosophical dichotomies that reduce effective care.

As pointed out earlier, the physical and mental health care needs of the elderly are frequently divided into discrete categories of care. Except in a few communities, physicians provide medical care, and psychiatrists and other professionals provide mental health care to the elderly. Relatively little is known about the number of elderly seen by physicians who may have unrecognized emotional disease and are not referred to psychiatrists (Hilkevitch, 1965). Likewise, psychiatrists may be unprepared to handle the range of chronic and acute medical problems unique to the elderly. A greater recognition of the importance of integrating these two into a health care continuum for the elderly is necessary.

A second dichotomy involved clinicians and researchers. Despite the need for better mutual collaboration, use of research design is often marginal. Dissemination and interpretation of the relevance of research to practice (see Chapter 1) is essential to challenging values and myths and validating assessment tools and therapeutic techniques. Clinicians can offer useful input to researchers by clearly articulating their goals, treatments, and dilemmas in providing care to the mentally ill elderly.

A third dichotomy is represented in the proponents of traditional models of care versus environmental models. With the blurring of some professional roles, this phenomena may appear to be declining. However, in times of diminishing resources, these divisions may become entrenched more firmly and the relative value of intrapsychic and social network strategies become issues of political and professional debate. The need to design a system of mental health care for the elderly that incorporates both of these strategies in the continuum of care must not be overlooked.

A corollary to this dilemma is the dichotomy of institutional versus community care. While mental health professionals recognize the need for both, the choice of one kind of care over another is determined most often by the availability of certain settings and by biases and skills of providing professionals. Decisions about locus of care should also involve consideration of the therapeutic possibilities of community living with nonprofessional supports. When institutional care is seen as inappropriate, yet is the only available alternative, professionals have a responsibility to document such information in patient records.

Examination of these dichotomies underscores the need for more effective utilization of a variety of professional and nonprofessional groups who serve the needs of the elderly. Physicians need broader education, including information on screening of geropsychiatric problems. Psychiatrists need to utilize their knowledge of internal medicine to effectively treat and refer elderly clients. A multidisciplinary education strategy with these, and other mental health professionals, will strengthen the effectiveness of community geropsychiatric care. Additionally, mental health professionals must be prepared to broaden their traditional roles to include the roles of advocate, consultant, and educator. The need for professional flexibility is paramount in providing mental health care services to the aged.

Mental health professionals should strive for "an understanding of and skill at working with psychosocial cultural variables" (Dagon, 1982). A working knowledge of how the older person interfaces with his or her environment and the nature of available personal and social resource support network is required as well. Each clinician should be capable of effectively communicating with other professionals and being an effective member of an interdisciplinary mental health care team. In addition, mental health professionals should recognize and understand the basic heterogeneity of the elderly, as illustrated by the different adaptational styles of the young-old, the old-old, racial and ethnic groups, and men and women.

Before planning any specific agency program for mental health care of the elderly, a feasibility study is recommended. Assuming that the needs of the community elderly have been established, this process involves the actual providers of care in an inventory of their resources. Essentially, a feasibility study "considers what staff are involved in geriatrics, how much time they can work, and what specific skills and interests they have" (Dagon, 1982). The critical proviso is to begin a feasible program that can systematically demonstrate success and can deliver all that is promised. Evaluation and re-evaluation over time should be planned and designed to provide necessary data on program and professional efficacy.

Principal challenges remaining to mental health professionals include the need to:

1. Define effective clinical assessment and treatment strategies.
2. Support appropriate medical, social, and rehabilitation technologies.
3. Set decent minimal standards for all publicly supported clinical services that would assist the courts in evaluating "right to treatment" cases and would provide a standardized mechanism for determining adequacy of treatment provided.
4. Increase interprofessional and interagency understanding, coordination and integration.
5. Know the limitations of and support expansion of policy and agency supports for the elderly.
6. Teach social skills and organize community resources to sustain elderly clients.
7. Advocate for the elderly by calling attention to policies and practices that negatively affect care of the mentally ill aged.

Formulation of guidelines for the mental health care of the elderly is essential in order for professionals, planners, and policy makers to design appropriate treatments, programs, and policies. Despite the current trend of political incrementalism and retrenchment, public awareness and professional commitment to the mental health needs of the aged is significant. Planning and developing innovative integrated programs that include training, education, research, and political advocacy should be the hallmarks of the field. It is important to remember today that short-sighted policies and programs have unavoidable ramifications for geriatric mental health care in the future.

REFERENCES

Birren, J.E., & Renner, V.J. A brief history of mental health and aging. In *Issues in mental health and aging,* (Vol. 1, *Research*). Rockville, Maryland: National Institute of Mental Health, Nov. 1975, 1–26.

Blazer, D. The epidemiology of mental illness in late life. In E. Busse, & D. Blazer (Eds.), *Handbook of geriatric psychiatry*. New York: Van Nostrand and Reinhold Company, 1980, 249–271.

Borus, J.F. Deinstitutionalization of the chronically mentally ill. *New England Journal of Medicine*, 1981, *305*, 339–342.

Braceland, F.J. The mental hygiene of aging: Present-day view. *Journal of American Geriatrics Society*, 1972, *20*, 467–472.

Braun, P. Overview: Deinstitutionalization of psychiatric patients; A critical review of outcome studies. *American Journal of Psychiatry*, 1981, *138 (6)*, 736–749.

Brody, S.J. Evolving health delivery systems and older people. *American Journal of Public Health*, 1974, *64*, 245–248.

Butler, R.N. Psychiatry and the elderly: An overview. *American Journal of Psychiatry*, 1975, *132*, 893–900.

Cohen, G.D. Mental health services and the elderly: Needs and options. *American Journal of Psychiatry*, 1976, *133*, 65–68.

Cohen, G.D. Prospects for mental health and aging. In J.E. Birren and R.B. Sloan (Eds.), *Handbook of mental health and aging*. Englewood Cliffs, New Jersey: Prentice-Hall, Inc., 1980, 971–993.

Dagon, E.M. Planning and development issues in implementing community-based mental health services for the elderly. *Hospital and Community Psychiatry*, 1982, *33*, 137–141.

Davis, J. Mental well being of elders: Seeking positive solutions. *Generations*, 1983, *7*, 30–35.

Epstein, L.J., & Simon, A. Alternatives to state hospitalization for the geriatric mentally ill. *American Journal of Psychiatry*, 1968, *124*, 955–961.

Estes, C.L., & Lee, P.R. Policy shifts and their impact on health care for elderly persons. *The Western Journal of Medicine*, 1981, *135*, 511–517.

Federal Council on Aging, Department of Health and Human Services. The need for long term care information and issues: A chartbook of the Federal Council on Aging. DHHS Publication No. (OHDS) 81-20704. Washington, D.C.: U.S. Government Printing Office, 1981.

Gaitz, C.M. Barriers to the delivery of psychiatric services to the elderly. *The Gerontologist*, 1974, *14*, 210–214.

Gaitz, C.M., & Hacker, S. Obstacles in coordinating services for the care of the psychiatrically ill aged. *Journal of the American Geriatrics Society*, 1970, *18*, 172–182.

Gurian, B. Mental health outreach and consultation services for the elderly. *Hospital and Community Psychiatry*, 1982, *33*, 142–147.

Gurin, G., Veroff, J., & Feld, S. *Americans view their mental health: A nationwide survey*. New York: Basic Books, 1960.

Hilkevitch, A. Psychiatric disturbances in out-patients of a general medical outpatient clinic. *International Journal of Neuropsychiatry*, 1965, *1*, 371–375.

Jurkiewicz, V.C. An exploratory descriptive study of interorganizational and case coordination programs for the multi-problem, frail and minority elderly. *Dissertation,* Los Angeles: University of California, 1980.

Kling, A. Mental illness in the elderly. In A.R. Somers & D.R. Fabian (Eds.), *The geriatric imperative: An introduction to gerontology and clinical geriatrics.* New York: Appleton-Century-Crofts, 1981, 221–235.

Kolb, L. The mental hospitalization of the aged: Is it being overdone? *American Journal of Psychiatry, 1956, 112,* 627–636.

Krogh, L. President's proposed budget fiscal year 1984. *Gerontology News.* Washington, D.C.: The Gerontological Society of America, March 1983, 5.

Lipscomb, C.F. The care of the psychiatrically disturbed elderly patient in the community. *American Journal of Psychiatry,* 1971, *127,* 1067–1070.

Matlack, D.R. The case for geriatric day hospitals. *Gerontologist,* 1975, *15,* 109–113.

Mechanic, D. *Mental health and social policy.* Englewood Cliffs, New Jersey: Prentice-Hall, Inc., 1969.

Mollica, R.F. From asylum to community: The threatened disintegration of public psychiatry. *New England Journal of Medicine,* 1983, *308,* 367–373.

National Retired Teachers Association, and American Association of Retired Persons. The 1982 federal legislative policy and 1982–1983 joint state legislative committee policy guidelines. Washington, D.C.: 1902 K Street, N.W., 20049.

Pardes, H. The aging: Mental health problems. *New York State Journal of Medicine,* 1981, *81(5),* 798–801.

Patterson, R.D. Services for the aged in community mental health centers. *American Journal of Psychiatry,* 1976, *133,* 271.

Peterson, O.L. Geriatrics: The need for science and policy. *Annals of Internal Medicine,* 1978, *89,* 279–280.

Rathbone-McCuan, E., & Claymon, C. Counseling the isolated elderly. *Journal of the American Geriatrics Society,* 1979, *27,* 355–358.

Redick, R.W., & Taube, C.A. Demography and mental health care of the aged. In J.E. Birren & R.B. Sloan (Eds.), *Handbook of mental health and the aged.* Englewood Cliffs, New Jersey: Prentice-Hall, Inc., 1980.

Redlich, F., & Kellert, S.R. Trends in American mental health. *American Journal of Psychiatry,* 1978, *135,* 22–28.

Rosen, B.M., Anderson, T.E., & Bahn, A.K. Psychiatric patterns for the aged: A nationwide survey of patterns of utilization. *American Journal of Orthopsychiatry,* 1967, *35,* 223–224.

Santore, A.F., & Diamond, H. The role of community mental health centers in developing services to the aging. *Gerontologist,* 1974, *14,* 201–206.

Sherwood, S., & Mor, V. Mental health institutions and the elderly. In J.E. Birren & R.B. Sloan (Eds.), *Handbook of mental health and aging.* Englewood Cliffs, New Jersey: Prentice-Hall, Inc., 1980, 854–884.

Stotsky, B.A. Social and clinical issues in geriatric psychiatry. *American Journal of Psychiatry,* 1972, *129,* 117–126.

Teeter, R.B., Garetz, F.K., Miller, W.R., & Heiland, W.F. Psychiatric disturbances of aged patients in skilled nursing homes. *American Journal of Psychiatry,* 1976, *133,* 1430–1433.

Thompson, P.W. The aged, out-patient services and community mental health programs. *Journal of National Association of Private Psychiatric Hospitals,* 1978 *10*, 62.

U.S. Department of Health and Human Services, Social Security Administration. *Your Medicare handbook.* Washington, D.C.: SSA Publication No. 05-10050, July 1980.

U.S. Senate Special Committee on Aging. *Mental health care and the elderly: Shortcomings in public policy.* U.S. Senate Report No. 92-433. Washington, D.C.: U.S. Government Printing Office, 1971.

Veroff, J., Kulka, R.A., & Donvan, E., *Mental health in America.* New York: Basic Books, 1981.

Williams, D.H., Bellis, E.C., & Wellington, S.W. Reinstitutionalization and social policy: historical perspectives and present dilemmas. *American Journal of Orthopsychiatry,* 1980, *50,* 54–64.

INDEX

A

B

C

I

J

L

M

N

O

P

R

S